PRINCIPLES OF PHARMACOLOGY
FOR RESPIRATORY CARE

PRINCIPLES OF PHARMACOLOGY FOR RESPIRATORY CARE

Georgine W. Bills, MBA, RRT
Program Director
Respiratory Therapy Program
College of Health Professions
Weber State University
Odgen, Utah

Robert C. Soderberg, DDS, MS (Pharmacology)
Program Director
Health Sciences Program
College of Health Professions
Weber State University
Odgen, Utah

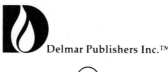
Delmar Publishers Inc.™

I(T)P

NOTICE TO THE READER

Publisher does not warrant or guarantee any of the products described herein or perform any independent analysis in connection with any of the product information contained herein. Publisher does not assume, and expressly disclaims, any obligation to obtain and include information other than that provided to it by the manufacturer.

The reader is expressly warned to consider and adopt all safety precautions that might be indicated by the activities described herein and to avoid all potential hazards. By following the instructions contained herein, the reader willingly assumes all risks in connection with such instructions.

The publisher makes no representations or warranties of any kind, including but not limited to, the warranties of fitness for particular purpose or merchantability, nor are any such representations implied with respect to the material set forth herein, and the publisher takes no responsibility with respect to such material. The publisher shall not be liable for any special, consequential or exemplary damages resulting, in whole or in part, from the readers' use of, or reliance upon, this material.

Delmar Staff
Team Leader: David Gordon
Associate Editor: Adrianne Williams
Project Manager: Carol Micheli
Production Coordinator: Mary Ellen Black
Design Coordinator: Mary Siener

For information, address Delmar Publishers Inc.
3 Columbia Circle, Box 15-015
Albany, New York 12212-5015

Copyright © 1994
by Delmar Publishers Inc.
The trademark ITP is used under license

printed in the United States of America
published simultaneously in Canada
by Nelson Canada,
a division of The Thomson Corporation

1 2 3 4 5 6 7 8 9 10 XXX 00 99 98 97 96 95 94

Library of Congress Cataloging-in-Publication Data

Bills, Georgine W.
    Principles of pharmacology for respiratory care / Georgine W.
Bills, Robert C. Soderberg.
        p.   cm.
    Includes bibliographical references and index.
    ISBN 0-8273-5274-3
    1. Respiratory agents.   2. Pharmacology.   3. Respiratory
therapists.   I. Soderberg, Robert C.   II. Title.
    [DNLM: 1. Respiratory Therapy.   2. Bronchodilator Agents—
—administration & dosage.   3. Bronchodilator Agents—pharmacology.
WB 342 B599p 1994]
RM388.B55   1994
615'.72—dc20
DNLM/DLC
for Library of Congress   93-48582
                                                                      CIP

CONTENTS

Preface   xi
List of Figures   xiii

PART I: GENERAL PHARMACOLOGICAL PRINCIPLES

CHAPTER 1   GENERAL PHARMACOLOGICAL CONCEPTS   2

Introduction   2
Pharmacology   3
Sources of Drug Information   3
Terminology   4
Essential General Principles of Pharmacology   7
Factors That Alter Drug Effects   13
Abuse of Prescription Drugs   15

CHAPTER 2   PHARMACOLOGY OF THE AUTONOMIC NERVOUS SYSTEM   18

Introduction   19
Function and Anatomy of the ANS   19
Neurotransmitters   20
Sites of Action, Neurotransmitters and Receptors of Somatic and
     Autonomic Nervous Systems   22
General Physiological Functions Controlled by ANS   22
Overall Effect of Sympathetic Division and Definition of Adrenergic   23
The Sympathetic Nerve Ending   24
Sites of Action of Adrenergic Drugs   25
Definitions of the Adrenergic Drugs   26
α-Adrenergic Drugs   26
β-Adrenergic Drugs   27
α-Blocking Drugs   29
β-Blocking Drugs   30
Adrenergic Neuronal Activators and Blockers   31
Overall Effects of Parasympathetic Division and Definition of Cholinergic 32
The Parasympathetic Nerve Ending   33
Mechanism of Action of Cholinergic Drugs   34
Definitions of Cholinergic Drugs   35

Choline Esters   35
Anticholinesterase Drugs   36
Anticholinergic Drugs   37

CHAPTER 3   PHARMACOLOGY OF THE CENTRAL
                     NERVOUS SYSTEM   42

Introduction   44
General Anatomy of the CNS   44
Effects of Drugs in the CNS   46
General Characteristics of CNS Drugs   46
Sedative Hypnotics and Antianxiety Drugs   48
Barbiturates   49
Alcohol (Ethanol)   51
Psychopharmacology and Treatment of Mental Disorders   52
Epilepsy   58
Parkinsonism   61
General Anesthetics   62
Narcotic Analgesics   66
Nonnarcotic Analgesics   69

CHAPTER 4   SKELETAL MUSCLE RELAXANTS   76

Introduction   76
Peripheral-Acting Muscle Relaxants   77
CNS Muscle Relaxants   79

CHAPTER 5   CARDIOVASCULAR AND RENAL PHARMACOLOGY   82

Introduction   83
Conduction System of the Heart   83
Heart Disease   85
Cardiac Glycosides and CHF   86
Definitions and Types of Arrhythmias   88
Overall Effect of Antianginal Drugs and Effects of Nitrates and Nitrites   91
Hypertension   93
Coagulation Process   100
Effects of High Lipids in Blood   104

CHAPTER 6   PHARMACOLOGY OF THE GASTROINTESTINAL TRACT 108

Introduction	108
Role of Hydrochloric Acid and Pepsin in Digestion	109
Ulcer Disease	109
Drugs Used in Treatment of Ulcers	110
Overall Bowel Function	113
Causes and Treatment of Diarrhea	113
Constipation and Its Treatment	116
Laxatives and Cathartics	116

CHAPTER 7   PHARMACOLOGY OF THE ENDOCRINE SYSTEM 120

Introduction	121
Pituitary Gland and Hypothalamus	122
Control of Hormone Release	123
Corticosteroids and Overall Effects	124
Overall Function of Thyroid Gland	127
Structure and Function of Parathyroid Gland	129
Overall Function of the Pancreas	131
Diabetes Mellitus	132
Antigen–Antibody Reactions	135

CHAPTER 8   ANTIMICROBIAL PHARMACOLOGY 140

Introduction	140
Antimicrobial Agents and Definitions	141
Principles in the Wise Use of Antibiotics	142
Causes of Failure in Antibacterial Therapy	143
Categories of Antibiotic Drugs	144
Beta-Lactam Antibiotics	144
Miscellaneous Antibiotics	148
Broad-Spectrum Antibiotics	151
Sulfonamides and Related Drugs	152
Antifungal Drugs	153
Antiviral Agents	154

CHAPTER 9   PHARMACOLOGY OF CHEMOTHERAPY 158

Introduction	158
Cancer Cells and Definitions	159

Treatment of Cancer   159
Chemotherapy   160

PART II: RESPIRATORY CARE PHARMACOLOGY

CHAPTER 10   PRINCIPLES OF AEROSOLIZED AND INSTILLED
MEDICATION ADMINISTRATION   166

Introduction   166
Aerosolized Medications   167
Instilled Medications   171

CHAPTER 11   BRONCHODILATOR THERAPY   178

Introduction   178
Bronchoconstriction   179
Methods of Bronchodilation   179
Sympathomimetic Bronchodilators   183
Sympathomimetic and Anticholinergic Bronchodilator Drugs   184
Xanthines   190

CHAPTER 12   WETTING AGENTS AND MUCOLYTICS   196

Introduction   196
Bland Aerosols   197
Mucolytics   199
Expectorants and Bronchorrheic Agents   203

CHAPTER 13   AEROSOL ANTIMICROBIAL THERAPY   208

Introduction   208
Indications for Aerosolized Antimicrobial Drugs   209
Disadvantages and Limitations of Aerosolized Antimicrobials   209
Pulmonary Infectious Processes   211
Categories of Antimicrobial Drugs Administered by Aerosol   211
Antibacterial (Antibiotic) Drugs   211
Antifungal Drugs   215
Antiviral Drugs   216
Antiprotozoal Drugs   217
General Conclusions and Considerations Regarding
Aerosolized Antimicrobials   218

CHAPTER 14   ANTI-INFLAMMATORY AND ANTIASTHMATIC DRUGS — 222

Introduction — 222
Bronchoconstriction and Mucosal Edema — 223
α-Adrenergic Sympathomimetic Drugs — 224
Corticosteroid Anti-Inflammatory Drugs — 226
Anti-Asthmatic (Mast Cell Stabilizer) Drugs — 230

CHAPTER 15   SURFACE ACTIVE AGENTS — 240

Introduction — 240
Surface Tension — 241
Surfactant — 242
Infant (or Idiopathic) Respiratory Distress Syndrome — 243
Fulminant Alveolar Pulmonary Edema — 245

CHAPTER 16   SPECIAL APPLICATIONS — 252

Introduction — 253
Dosage Guidelines for Infants and Children — 253
Asthma Management in Children — 254
Advanced Cardiac Life Support — 255
Special Procedures: Bronchoscopy and Bronchial Challenge — 257

APPENDIX A   ANSWERS TO POSTTEST — 265

APPENDIX B   CASE STUDIES — 269

APPENDIX C   PROBLEM SOLVING/DRUG CALCULATIONS — 301

APPENDIX D LIST OF DRUGS BY GENERIC AND TRADE NAMES — 304

GLOSSARY — 311

INDEX — 321

PREFACE

A thorough understanding of general pharmacological principles of action, as well as specific bronchoactive agents, is essential for respiratory care practitioners (RCPs). RCPs are in the unique health-care provider position of not only administering medications but also acting as a consultant to the physician with respect to the most appropriate drug and dosage in a given patient care situation. Development of the necessary level of understanding regarding drugs, and specific medications administered by aerosol or instillation, can be enhanced by information that is readable, applicable, timely, and accurate.

This text is a competency-based approach to pharmacology, comprehensive yet introductory in nature. The text is intended to bridge the gap between a general text and one that is very specific. Each author has been involved in health care and education for over 20 years; Robert Soderberg, MS (Pharmacology), DDS authors Part I (General Pharmacological Principles) and Georgine Bills, MBA, RRT, authors Part II (Respiratory Care Pharmacology). Activities such as self-tests and patient care scenarios, along with decision-making exercises, are provided to enhance the learning and retention of the text's content. Line drawings and clearly organized reference tables are used to illustrate concepts and focus the student's attention on key points of information.

The text comprises two major content areas:

- General pharmacological principles, including medications and their effects relating to the autonomic and central nervous systems, skeletal muscle relaxants, cardiovascular and renal pharmacology, pharmacology of the gastrointestinal tract and endocrine system, antimicrobial agents, and chemotherapy.
- Respiratory care pharmacology, including principles of aerosolized medication, bronchodilators, wetting agents, mucolytics, antimicrobials, anti-inflammatory agents, antiasthmatic agents, and surface-active agents and special applications.
- The introduction of each chapter will establish the rationale for the chapter content (*why* does the student *need* this information?). A list of objectives is provided to help the student focus on the key information to be learned from the chapter and also serve as a framework for the content. Topic headings are related to the stated objectives.

Learning activities help the student integrate and apply the principles presented in the content of the chapter. Clinical application and practice in decision making and patient assessment are very difficult to accomplish with this body of knowledge; this text provides the student with numerous activities that should enhance the learning process and improve retention.

A posttest for each chapter allows the student to assess his or her understanding of concepts presented in the chapter. Use of exam items that are similar in format to the N.B.R.C. exams (multiple-multiple choice) can further improve the students' test-taking skills.

The appendices provide the student with self-test exam keys, a drug dosage calculation review, patient case studies (relating to Part II), a glossary, and reference list of drugs discussed in the text. The "drug cards" are intended as a quick reference for the student who is attempting to master the complexity of drug categories, trade names, and drug actions.

The authors are grateful for the contributions of Betheme Gregg, MS, RRT, Barbara Ludwig, MA, RRT, and Judy Mathewson, MS, RRT, in the development of the patient case studies (Appendix C).

LIST OF FIGURES

Chapter 1

Figure 1–1	Dose–Response Curve
Figure 1–2	Fluid Mosaic Model
Figure 1–3	Drug–Receptor Relationship
Figure 1–4	Absorption, Distribution, Metabolism, and Excretion

Chapter 2

Figure 2–1	Somatic Nervous System
Figure 2–2	Synapses and Ganglia of the ANS
Figure 2–3	Origin and Distribution of the ANS
Figure 2–4	Sympathetic Nerve Ending
Figure 2–5	Parasympathetic Nerve Ending

Chapter 3

Figure 3–1	General Anatomy of the CNS
Figure 3–2	Levels of Excitability and Depression of the CNS
Figure 3–3	Limited Potency and Efficacy of CNS Drugs
Figure 3–4	Additive Effects of CNS Drugs
Figure 3–5	Antagonism between CNS Drugs
Figure 3–6	Chronic Depression followed by Excitation

Chapter 5

Figure 5–1	Conduction System of the Heart
Figure 5–2	Normal Electrocardiogram
Figure 5–3	The Nephron of the Kidney
Figure 5–4	Mechanism of Action of ACE Inhibitors
Figure 5–5	Simplified Version of Clotting Mechanism

Chapter 7

Figure 7–1	Relationship of Pituitary Gland and Hypothalamus
Figure 7–2	Hormones of the Pituitary Gland
Figure 7–3	Negative Feedback Control of Thyroxin
Figure 7–4	The Adrenal Gland

Chapter 8

Figure 8–1	The Beta-Lactam Ring
Figure 8–2	The Beta-Lactam Antibiotics
Figure 8–3	Structure of Cephalosporins

Chapter 10

Figure 10–1   MDI With Spacer/Chamber
Figure 10–2   Method to Determine MDI Contents
Figure 10–3   Description of Spinhaler^R Turbo-Inhaler
Figure 10–4   Description of Rotahaler^R

Chapter 11

Figure 11–1   Effect of Sympathetic Stimulation in Bronchial Cells
Figure 11–2   Effect of Parasympathetic Stimulation in Bronchial Cells
Figure 11–3   Sympathomimetic Drugs: Stimulate cAMP
Figure 11–4   Anticholinergic Drugs: Block Parasympathetic Stimulation
Figure 11–5   Xanthines: Inhibit Phosphodiesterase

Chapter 12

Figure 12–1   Structure of Mucus Molecule
Figure 12–2   Mucolytic Action of N-Acetylcysteine
Figure 12–3   Mucolytic Action of Sodium Bicarbonate

Chapter 13

Figure 13–1   Aerosol Deposition of Antimicrobials

Chapter 14

Figure 14–1   Bronchoconstriction by Mucosal Edema
Figure 14–2   Allergic Response: Ruptured Mast Cell Releases Histamine
Figure 14–3   Cromolyn Sodium: Stabilizes Mast Cell to Prevent Histamine Release
Figure 14–4   Procedure for Using Spinhaler^R Turbo-Inhaler

Chapter 15

Figure 15–1   Normal Surfactant: Normal Work of Breathing
Figure 15–2   Lack of Surfactant: Increased Work of Breathing
Figure 15–3   Interstitial Pulmonary Edema
Figure 15–4   Alveolar Pulmonary Edema
Figure 15–5   Use of Alcohol (ETOH) in Alveolar Pulmonary Edema

PART I
GENERAL PHARMACOLOGICAL PRINCIPLES

CHAPTER 1

GENERAL PHARMACOLOGICAL CONCEPTS

LEARNING OBJECTIVES

After completion of this chapter and its learning activities, the student will be able to:

1. Define pharmacology and list and describe several disciplines within the area of pharmacological study.
2. Describe where detailed and up-to-date information about drugs can be obtained.
3. Define 19 terms essential to the study of pharmacology.
4. Describe and discuss essential general principles of pharmacology and include in the discussion: routes of administration, absorption, cellular and chemical factors, distribution, metabolism, and excretion.
5. Describe factors that alter drug response.
6. Describe some aspects of governmental control of abuse of prescription drugs and generally know the significance of the five schedules of drugs as defined by the federal Comprehensive Drug Abuse Prevention and Control Act of 1970.

INTRODUCTION

As one looks at the broad subject areas covered by pharmacology, one might ask why a respiratory care practitioner needs to be informed about drugs other than those that are used specifically in respiratory care. By studying principles that affect all drugs and having specific knowledge of various drugs that patients are taking, it is possible to make rational assessments and predict possible drug incompatibility and interactions that might be encountered with patients who are being treated for various respiratory diseases.

This chapter discusses the purpose and value of studying pharmacology and indicates where information about drugs can be found. Terminology that is essential to the study of pharmacology is defined. The concepts of what happens to a drug when it is introduced into the body and some biological factors that affect the action of drugs are explained.

PHARMACOLOGY

Pharmacology is the study of drugs, their origin, nature, properties, and effects on living organisms. As a discipline, it is one of the important basic sciences of medicine and other health professions.

Pharmacology as a science can be subdivided into several divisions/categories. Table 1–1 lists some of these areas with a brief definition of each.

SOURCES OF DRUG INFORMATION

There are many sources, reference texts, and the like where pertinent drug information can be found. Some of the main sources other than textbooks are:

- *United States Pharmacopeia* (USP)—published every 5 years; includes single-entity drugs of established manufacturers and sets official, chemical, and physical standards that relate to purity and strength.

TABLE 1–1 Areas of Pharmacology

AREAS OF PHARMACOLOGY	DEFINITION
Pharmacotherapy	Uses a specific medicine to treat a specific disease
Pharmacodynamics	Studies the actions of drugs on living organisms
Pharmacokinetics	Quantifies the time required for absorption, duration of action, distribution in the body, metabolism, and method of excretion of drugs
Pharmacy	Involves the practice of compounding, preparing, and dispensing drugs
Toxicology	Studies the harmful effects of drugs on tissues

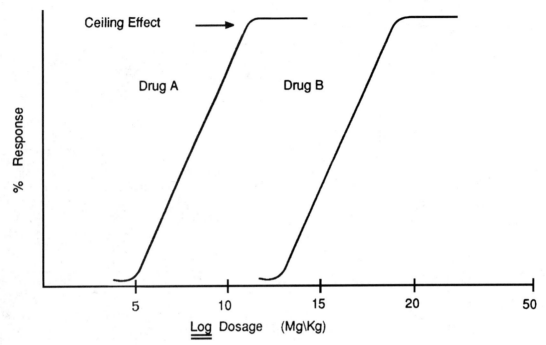

FIGURE 1–1 Dose–Response Curve.

- *National Formulary* (NF)—published every 5 years and establishes formulations not in the USP.
- *Physicians' Desk Reference* (PDR)—published every year and includes a brief description of drugs, including indications, dosage, side effects, and so forth; indexed by manufacturer, product name, generic name, product category, and product information.

TERMINOLOGY

The following terms are important in the study of pharmacology and, in order to understand the concepts discussed throughout this text, they will need to be mastered.

Dose–Response Curve

Whenever a drug is tested for a particular response, a dose–response curve is obtained. This dose–response curve is a graphic representation of the relationship between dose in milligrams and the response to or effect of the drug. Figure 1–1 illustrates the appearance of a typical response.

As indicated by the figure, the dose and response increase in a corresponding fashion. The response increases until additional dosage causes no increase in the effect. This point is called the *ceiling effect*. It should be noted that, if the ceiling effect is reached, increasing the dose has no additional therapeutic advantage and in fact may cause toxic effects. The dose–response curve also can be used to evaluate and compare similar drugs. Regarding potency, as seen in Figure 1–1, drug A and drug B are both effective but drug A is more potent than drug B because a smaller dose of drug A is needed to cause the same effect.

Potency

When comparing one drug to another, the drug that reaches an effective level with a smaller dose is the more potent of the two drugs. It should also be remembered that a more potent drug can reach toxic levels at smaller dosage.

Therapeutic Dose

The therapeutic dose is the recommended amount of a drug that should be used to obtain the desired clinical effect.

Median Lethal Dose (LD$_{50}$)

In order to determine the safety of a drug, the Food and Drug Administration (FDA) requires extensive testing on animals before the drug is allowed for human testing. One of the first tests that is conducted, using several different species of animals, is the median lethal dose. This is the dose at which 50 percent of the test animals die.

Median Effective Dose (ED$_{50}$)

The median effective dose is the dose at which 50 percent of the test animals show the desired effect.

Therapeutic Index (TI)

The therapeutic index is a ratio of the LD$_{50}$ to the ED$_{50}$ and gives a relative indication as to the safety of a drug. The formula for calculation of the therapeutic index is:

$$TI = \frac{LD_{50}}{ED_{50}}$$

If a particular drug has an LD$_{50}$ of 1000 mg and an ED$_{50}$ of 100 mg, the therapeutic index would be 10.

$$TI = \frac{1000}{100} = 10$$

The greater the TI, or the greater the difference between the LD$_{50}$ and the ED$_{50}$, the greater the safety of the drug. Drugs that have low therapeutic indexes must be carefully monitored during clinical use in order to avoid toxic and perhaps lethal results. Another way of expressing this concept is that the closer the TI is to zero the more toxic the drug.

Idiosyncrasy

Idiosyncrasy is an unexplained or unpredictable susceptibility to a drug's action. It can be manifested as an accelerated, toxic, or inappropriate response to the usual therapeutic dose or action.

Allergy

Allergy is an antigen (invader)–antibody (defender) reaction to a foreign substance that causes a release of histamine and other chemical mediators, with resulting manifestations of bronchoconstriction, rash, urticaria, hives, drop in blood pressure, and the like.

Drug

A drug is a biologically active substance that modifies cellular function.

Placebo

A placebo is a substance, chemical or otherwise, that contains no active ingredient but can cause modification of effects either in a positive or negative manner purely on the basis of suggestion.

Tolerance

Tolerance is a phenomenon, occurring after a period of use of some drugs, that necessitates an increase in dosage to maintain an effect.

Therapeutic Effect

The therapeutic effect is the intended effect of a drug (e.g., pain relief or sedation).

Tachyphylaxis

Tachyphylaxis is a rapidly developing tolerance to a drug.

Side Effect

Side effects are drug effects other than those intended. Every drug causes some side effects; they may be very harmful or just a nuisance.

Drug Nomenclature

Every drug has three different names, which often makes the study of pharmacology confusing. The barbiturate phenobarbital is an example. The *chemical name* is 5-ethyl-5-phenyl barbituric acid and the *generic name* (nonproprietary) is phenobarbital, while the *trade* (proprietary) names include Luminal[R] and Eskabarb[R].

Toxic Effect

A toxic effect usually is due to an overdose and occurs when the therapeutic or side effect is harmful.

Teratogens

Teratogens are drugs that are known to cause birth defects.

Carcinogens

Carcinogens are drugs that cause malignant neoplasms (cancers).

Drug Dependence

There are two types of dependence: 1) addiction, an altered physiological state than can cause withdrawal symptoms, and 2) psychological, which is due to reinforcing properties of the drug.

ESSENTIAL GENERAL PRINCIPLES OF PHARMACOLOGY

This section discusses routes of administration, absorption, cellular and chemical factors, distribution, metabolism (*biotransformation*), and excretion. Absorption, distribution, metabolism, and excretion are collectively known as the pharmacokinetics of a drug.

Routes of Administration

In order for a drug to exhibit therapeutic action on the body, it must first enter by one of the routes indicated in Table 1–2. The most common and usually the safest route is orally (PO). This route is the most convenient and is acceptable to most patients. It is also the safest because, in the case of overdose or toxic reaction, the drug can be partially removed by inducing vomiting or by gastric lavage (stomach pumping). The disadvantage of the oral route is that the onset of action is usually 30–60 minutes and the absorption also can be greatly retarded or altered by the presence of food. In some cases the drug may be irritating to the stomach lining and cause nausea, vomiting, or heartburn.

The *parenteral* route denotes any route other than the alimentary canal, however, parenteral usually refers to injection. The most common parenteral route is intramuscular (IM) injection. This route has a rapid onset of action (15–30 minutes) but the injection must be administered with skill and by trained personnel. The parenteral route that has the fastest onset of action is intravenous (IV), which usually is restricted to use in the hospital setting. There is some degree of risk encountered with this route, as well as the IM route, because once the drug is administered, it cannot be withdrawn. Miscalculating dosage can produce serious or even fatal results.

TABLE 1–2 Common Routes of Administration

ROUTE	TIME OF ONSET	WHEN APPROPRIATE	EXAMPLE
Oral (PO)	30–60 min	Outpatient and for convenience	Most drugs and particularly over-the-counter drugs
Rectal	30 min	When patient is unable to take by mouth	Antinausea medications
Sublingual	Minutes	When rapid absorption is needed	Nitroglycerin tablets
Transdermal	Minutes	Continuous low dosage, usually outpatient	Nitroglycerin patches
Inhalation	Within 1 min	Local, effects in respiratory tract	Bronchodilators
Intramuscular (IM)	15–30 min	Drugs that have poor oral absorption and when higher levels are needed rapidly	Narcotics
Intravenous	Within 1 min	Emergency situations and long-term infusions	General anesthetics, nutrient solutions
Subcutaneous (SC)	30–45 min	Drugs that have poor oral absorption and when higher levels are needed rapidly, but slower than IM	Insulin
Intraarterial drugs	Less than 1 min	Deliver drug to a specific organ	Anticancer drugs

Drug Absorption

Absorption means to "pass through." With the exception of IV or intraarterial routes, drug absorption includes passing through the membrane of the gastrointestinal (GI) tract or the membrane of the blood vessels in order to gain access to the bloodstream.

In order for drugs to be absorbed through the complex structure of cell and tissue membranes, there are several factors to consider, such as transport mechanisms, lipid solubility, and drug ionization.

Transport Mechanisms. There are several different mechanisms whereby drugs and other substances pass through membranes. These include passive diffusion, filtration, and active transport. The most common is passive diffusion, which is governed by concentration gradient. For example, when a drug enters the GI tract, it has a high concentration relative to the surrounding blood supply. By moving from high to low concentration, the drug passes from the GI tract into the bloodstream. Other mechanisms, such as filtration and active transport, will be presented as they apply to specific drug groups.

Lipid Solubility.   Because the cell membrane is composed of significant amounts of lipid (fat) material, drugs that are lipid soluble will pass through the cellular membrane rapidly. There are a number of drugs that are very lipid soluble, such as general anesthetics. Because of their lipid solubility, general anesthetics are readily absorbed into the lipid-rich central nervous system (CNS), where they alter neurological activity.

Drug Ionization.   If a drug is primarily water soluble and only partially lipid soluble, it must be either a weak acid or a weak base in order for it to be absorbed rapidly. Weak acids and weak bases, when in solution, are mostly in the un-ionized form and thus have fewer electrical charges that interfere with absorption. If drugs are in an ionized state, absorption of the charged or ionized form of the drug is very difficult because of two factors: 1) the ionized molecules are poorly soluble in the lipid material of the cellular membrane, and 2) the small ionized molecules are highly charged and have difficulty moving through the channels in the membrane because of repulsion by fixed charges in both the channels and the membrane surface.

Because of the above phenomenon, the pH of tissue fluids into which a drug is administered is very important to absorption rate. The more neutral (*un-ionized*) the drug is (weak acid or weak base) the better it will be absorbed. The pH of the tissue fluids in which the drug is present will determine the ratio of un-ionized to ionized forms of the drug. The chemical and mathematical description of this relationship can be explained by the Henderson-Hasselbalch equation:

$$pH \quad pK_a + \log \frac{\text{ionized drug}}{\text{un-ionized drug}}$$

We will not actually use this equation in this text but, in general, the relationship between the pK_a of a drug and the pH of tissue fluids will determine whether or not a drug will be readily absorbed. This equation generally means that weak acids are more readily absorbed in fluids with an acid pH and weak bases are more readily absorbed in fluids with an alkaline pH. For example, when an acid drug such as aspirin is in an acid environment like the stomach, it is mostly in the un-ionized state, which favors absorption.

Cellular and Chemical Factors

In order for a drug to have an effect on the body, there must be some interaction between the drug, cells, and tissues. In order to understand these relationships, we will examine several physical and chemical factors.

Passage of Drugs across Biological Membranes.   The body is well protected from the outside world by skin and mucous membranes. In order for a drug to interact with the basic structure and functional entity of an organism (the cell) a drug must pass through some type of membrane. The membrane can include the multiple cell membranes of the gut and of capillaries, and the plasma membrane of the cell.

The currently accepted molecular structure of the plasma cell membrane is often referred to as a *fluid mosaic model*. The principle structure of the cell membrane is two layers of lipid material (*bilipid*). Situated within the bilipid layer are integral proteins.

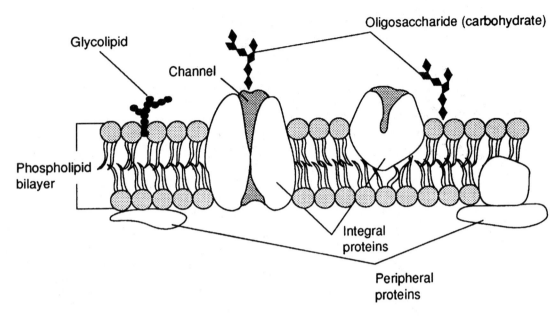

FIGURE 1–2   Fluid Mosaic Model.

Because the integral proteins constantly change their location, a "mosaic-like" distribution is created (i.e., the cell membrane is not a static entity). In addition to this pattern of proteins in a bilipid background, there are also some openings or "channels" that allow water and very small water-soluble molecules to pass through (see Figure 1–2).

Other membranes, such as the capillary endothelium, have intercellular channels that allow the movement of water and water-soluble materials. These channels are much larger than those present in the plasma membrane. Because of their larger size, the channels in the capillary endothelium will allow small and medium-size molecules not only to pass through into blood but also to pass through the intestinal epithelial villi. The major process by which substances pass through this type of channel, either by osmosis or hydrostatic pressure, is termed filtration. It should be noted that capillary membranes in the CNS have very small intercellular channel between cells (*tight junction*) that allow only lipid-soluble and very small substances to pass through. This specialized structural phenomenon is probably responsible for the so-called blood–brain barrier.

Receptor Site.   Most drugs exhibit their effects by specific interaction with molecular configurations on cellular membrane surfaces called *receptors*. A receptor can be defined as a location or reactive chemical configuration on the surface of a cell that combines with a specific substance or drug. When the receptor and a drug combine, a series of events occur in the cell that constitute the *drug action*. Receptors have been shown to consist mainly of large molecules (*macromolecules*) or groups of molecules that are protein in structure. Receptors usually are located on cell membranes but also can be located in the cellular cytoplasm and in the nucleus. Various tissues may contain more than one receptor type, and identical receptors may be located in more than one tissue. Generally, a specific drug will combine with a specific receptor. Some authors compare the binding to a *key-and-lock* arrangement. Such a receptor–drug relationship is illustrated in Figure 1–3.

Drugs that combine with specific receptors to cause a drug action are called *agonists* and drugs that combine with receptors and cause no action are called *antagonists*. Another term for an antagonist is a blocking agent. An example of a blocking agent is the drug naloxone, which blocks the effects of narcotics. Because of its narcotic antagonist properties, naloxone is given to reverse the effects of narcotic overdose. Antagonists and agonists often compete for the same receptor site; an example of this type of competitive antagonism is found in a group of drugs called antihistamines. The antihistamine competes with histamine for the same receptor site and reduces the binding of histamine to that site, therefore reducing the effects of histamine.

Site of Action.   Once a drug passes through a biological membrane, it must be carried to a location in the body where it exhibits its therapeutic effect in order to be effective. The specific site of action is not completely identified or understood for all drugs, but there are many drugs for which the general site has been determined. For example, the hypothalamus controls body temperature, and it has been shown that aspirin alters the activity of the hypothalamus so that the temperature of the body is decreased whenever a fever is present.

Mechanism of Action.   The mechanism of action explains how a drug produces its effect. There are several drugs for which the specific mechanism of action is known. For example, it has been shown that the mechanism of the anticoagulant effect of aspirin is the prevention of the aggregation of platelets, thus interfering with the clotting mechanism of the blood. Obviously, knowledge of the specific mechanism of action for a particular drug, is extremely helpful for the proper clinical application of the drug.

Drug Distribution

Once a drug has gained access to the blood plasma, it is carried by the blood to various tissues and compartments throughout the body, where it can combine with receptor sites. There are several factors that determine how much drug actually reaches the receptor site, such as plasma protein binding, tissue affinity, and blood flow.

Plasma Protein Binding.   In the plasma, there are hundreds of circulating proteins (albumins, globulins, and others). These molecules, because of their large molecular size, do not pass through membranes readily. However, these plasma proteins chemically attract certain drugs and, because of this attraction, many drugs become bound and are not available for pharmacological action. Only the free drug is available for drug action. For those drugs that do have an affinity for plasma proteins, an equilibrium is established between free drug and bound drug, and changes in the fraction of the bound drug can alter the amount of drug effect. For example, there are many drugs that compete for the same plasma binding site, and this can result in a sudden release of drugs that are normally bound. This could cause exaggerated drug effects or in some cases toxic drug reactions.

Tissue Affinity.   Some drugs have a strong affinity for certain tissues of the body, and this tends to create a potential reserve of drugs that may later be released into the blood-

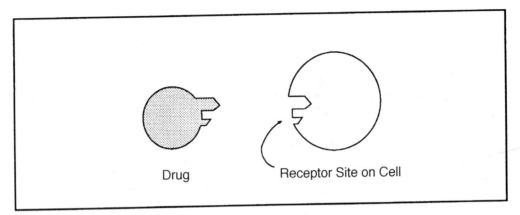

FIGURE 1–3   Drug–Receptor Relationship.

stream. One example of the phenomenon is the barbiturates, which are bound in fatty tissue of the body and have a slow release into the plasma over a long period of time. This partially explains the long duration of action of phenobarbital or the "hangover" feeling that patients sometimes experience when using this drug.

Blood Flow.   Obviously, different tissues and organs receive varying amounts of blood. Organs such as the liver, kidney, and brain receive the largest amount of blood, and therefore these organs ultimately are exposed to the largest amount of drug.

Drug Metabolism

Drug metabolism is the process by which drugs and other foreign chemicals that enter the body are altered, changed, inactivated, and prepared for elimination. This process also is referred to as *biotransformation*. Some drugs that enter the body are not metabolized but are excreted unchanged; however, most drugs are altered by the process of biotransformation. Most biotransformations occurs in the liver, but they can occur in other organs as well. Located within the parenchymal (functional) cells of the liver are a group of enzymes that specifically alter the structure of drugs. This enzyme system is called the *microsomal enzyme* system.

. An interesting phenomenon that occurs in the liver is that some drugs have the ability to stimulate the rate of action of this enzyme system and thus increase the metabolic rate of other drugs. This phenomenon is called *enzyme induction* and means that more enzymes are produced, which in turn increases the rate of reaction with drugs. A group of drugs that are enzyme inducers are the sedative/hypnotic drugs such as the barbiturates.

Drug Excretion

There are several different sites where drugs are excreted from the body; these include the kidney, respiratory system, and GI tract. The great majority of drugs are excreted by the

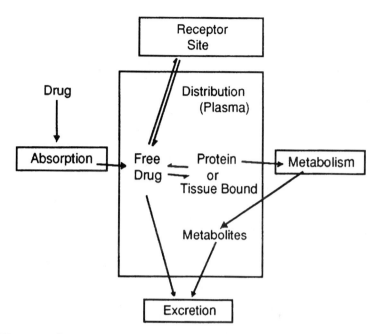

FIGURE 1–4 Absorption, Distribution, Metabolism, and Excretion.

kidney. Most substances in the blood are filtered in the glomerulus of the nephron, followed by reabsorption of essential substance/electrolytes back into the blood by the renal tubule. The substances that are not reabsorbed are urinary waste products and drugs that are metabolized in a water-soluble form. In other words, many of the metabolized drugs have been converted to an ionized form so that they will not be readily reabsorbed into the bloodstream. It is possible, and sometimes desirable, to alter the pH of the urine in order to enhance excretion of some drugs or increase their absorption. The relationships between absorption, distribution, metabolism, and excretion are presented in Figure 1–4.

FACTORS THAT ALTER DRUG EFFECTS

In addition to physical–chemical and physiological factors that alter drug responses, there are several other factors that can have a profound modifying effect on a drug.

Patient Compliance

In order for a drug to be maximally effective, it must be used according to specific directions given by the prescribing practitioner. This is particularly true when patients are taking medication on an outpatient basis.

Placebo Effect

As mentioned before, this can have a positive as well as a negative effect, and the magnitude of the effect depends on the patient's own perception of what a drug should or should not do. In addition, the power of suggestion by the health practitioner can have profound results.

Pathological State

Patients in various disease states will respond very differently to a given drug. For example, a patient who has hyperthyroid disease would metabolize a drug very rapidly. Also, impaired metabolism or elimination in a patient who has chronic liver or kidney disease could cause toxicity with a normal or regular dose of a drug.

Time of Administration

The time of day (morning, noon, nighttime, mealtime, etc.) that a drug is administered can have dramatic effects. Some drugs are less toxic and have fewer side effects when taken with meals, whereas other drugs are not absorbed well at mealtimes and have to be taken on an empty stomach. Sedative drugs would be more appropriate when taken at bedtime or when alertness and certain skills are not necessary.

Sex of Individual

It is a common misconception that females are "more sensitive" to medication than males. There is very little scientific information to substantiate this concept on the basis of sex. There are, however, important differences in sensitivity based on total body weight, physical size, muscle mass, and metabolic rate.

Age

Generally, the very young and the elderly are most sensitive to drug dosage. This is partially a result of total body weight and size but is also a result of immature liver and kidney function in the young and decreased liver and kidney function in the elderly.

Genetic Variations

There are many differences in a patient's response to drug therapy, and some of these differences are due to genetic variation. In most individuals, this probably occurs at the level of the liver microsomal enzymes system. That is, some individuals have different genetically determined enzymes that are capable of metabolizing different drugs, at different rates, resulting in differences in drug inactivation and/or elimination.

Drug Interaction

We are truly a medicated society and often take several different drugs simultaneously, either during a stay in a hospital or as an outpatient. There are many different mechanisms by which drugs affect each other. One of the most common is the stimulation of the liver microsomal enzyme system by one group of drugs, which in turn speeds up the metabolism of other drugs that are also metabolized by the same system. Such an interaction would reduce drug effects.

ABUSE OF PRESCRIPTION DRUGS

Many drugs are abused today in our society, and those that are most often abused are those controlled by prescription. In order for the FDA to maintain control over the dispensing of drugs with significant abuse potential, the Comprehensive Drug Abuse Prevention and Control Act was passed in 1970. This act is summarized in Table 1–3.

It should be noted that Schedule II drugs cannot be prescribed over the phone and must be filled with a hand-carried written prescription. Additionally, refills must be hand-

TABLE 1–3   Drug Schedules Defined in Federal Comprehensive Drug Abuse Prevention and Control Act of 1970

SCHEDULE	CONTROLLED DRUGS
Schedule I, drugs with high abuse potential and no accepted medical use	Heroin, hallucinogens; these drugs are not to be prescribed
Schedule II, drugs with high abuse potential and accepted medical use	Narcotics (morphine and pure codeine), cocaine, amphetamines, short-acting barbiturates; no refills without a new written prescription from the physician, dentist, etc.
Schedule III, drugs with moderate abuse potential and accepted medical use	Moderate and intermediate-acting anabolic steroids and accepted medical use barbiturates, glutethimide, preparations containing codeine plus another drug; because therapist's prescription is required, may be refilled 5 times in 6 months when authorized by the physician
Schedule IV, drugs with low abuse potential and accepted medical use	Phenobarbital, chloral hydrate, and antianxiety drugs (Librium, Valium); prescription required, may be refilled 5 times in 6 months when authorized by the physician
Schedule V, drugs with low abuse potential and accepted medical use	Narcotic drugs used in limited quantities for antitussive and antidiarrheal purposes; drugs can be sold only by registered pharmacist and buyer must be 18 years old and show identification

written in the same manner, and certain Schedule II drugs can be refilled only within a set period of time.

POSTTEST: GENERAL PHARMACOLOGICAL CONCEPTS

For each of the following questions, try to select the *one* best answer from those choices given.

1. It is important for a respiratory therapist to have a general knowledge of drugs:
   a. in order to administer the proper dose
   b. in order to treat a specific disease
   c. in order to avoid potential drug incompatibility
   d. in order to prevent side effects

2. All of following are categories of pharmacology except:
   a. pharmacodynamics
   b. pharmacy
   c. therapeutics
   d. pharmacokinetics
   e. pathology

3. The dose–response curve represents all of the following except:
   a. the ceiling effect
   b. relationship between the drug effect and dose
   c. the relative potency of one drug compared to another drug
   d. therapeutic effect
   e. the dose at which maximum effect occurs

4. An unexplained drug effect is called:
   a. potency
   b. allergic reaction
   c. hypersensitivity
   d. idiosyncrasy
   e. exaggerated response

5. An agonist is a drug that combines with a receptor causing a drug action to occur. True or False.

6. If the LD_{50} of a drug is 50 mg and the ED_{50} is 10 mg, the following are all true except:
   a. the therapeutic index is 0.2.
   b. the therapeutic index is 5.
   c. the drug is relatively nontoxic.
   d. the drug does not have to be monitored too closely.

7. A cell membrane can be termed a fluid mosaic because of:
   a. a bilipid membrane
   b. proteins that change position within the membrane
   c. pores
   d. lipid solubility

8. The location in the body at which a drug interacts with its receptor site is called the:
   a. receptor site
   b. site of action
   c. interface
   d. mechanism of action

9. Drugs in the following forms are more readily absorbed except:
   a. lipid soluble
   b. ionized
   c. un-ionized
   d. small molecules

10. All of the following factors are important in distribution of a drug except:
    a. plasma protein binding
    b. blood flow
    c. tissue affinity
    d. molecular structure

REFERENCES/RECOMMENDED READING

Dipalma JR, Digregorio JG: *Basic Pharmacology in Medicine*, 3rd ed. McGraw-Hill, New York, 1990.

Hitner H, Nagle BT: *Basic Pharmacology for Health Occupations*, 2nd ed. Glencoe Publishing Co, San Jose, CA, 1987.

Kenakin TP: *Pharmacologic Analysis of Drug Receptor Interaction*. Raven Press, New York, 1987.

Partidge WM: Recent advances in blood-brain barrier transport. *Annu Rev Pharmacol Toxicol* 28:25–39, 1988.

Waterman MR, Estabrook RW: The induction of microsomal electron transport enzymes. *Molec Cell Biochem* 53/54:267–278, 1983.

CHAPTER 2

PHARMACOLOGY OF THE AUTONOMIC NERVOUS SYSTEM

LEARNING OBJECTIVES

After completion of this chapter and its learning activities, the student will be able to:

1. Describe the overall function and describe the anatomical differences between the somatic nervous system, the sympathetic divisions, and the parasympathetic divisions of the autonomic nervous system (ANS).
2. Describe the concept of neurotransmitters.
3. In the somatic, the sympathetic, and the parasympathetic nervous systems, indicate the site of action, neurotransmitter, and receptor type.
4. Describe some of the characteristic physiological functions that are controlled by the sympathetic and parasympathetic divisions.
5. Describe the overall effect of the sympathetic division and describe the term *adrenergic*.
6. Describe the sympathetic nerve ending at the neuroeffector site, list the neurotransmitter involved and the names of the sympathetic receptors, and in general know the location of these receptors.
7. Describe the basic mechanism by which adrenergic drugs work at the neuroeffector site.
8. Define the terms *α-adrenergic*, *β-adrenergic*, *α blockers*, *β blockers*, and *neuronal blockers*.
9. List and describe the main effects of α-adrenergic drugs; also list possible adverse effects.
10. List and describe the main effects of β-adrenergic drugs; also indicate possible adverse effects. (*Note*: Some drugs have both α and β effects.)
11. List and describe the main effects of α-blocking drugs; also indicate possible adverse effects.
12. List and describe the main effects of β-blocking drugs; also indicate possible adverse effects.

13. List and describe the main effects and describe the mechanism of action of adrenergic neuronal activators and blocking drugs; also indicate possible adverse effects.
14. Describe the overall function of the parasympathetic division and define the term *cholinergic*.
15. Describe the parasympathetic nerve ending at the neuroeffector site, list the neurotransmitters and the name of the parasympathetic receptors, and in general know the location of these receptors.
16. Describe the basic mechanism by which the cholinergic drugs work at the neuroeffector site.
17. Define the following terms: choline esters, anticholinesterase, anticholinergic, and antimuscarinic.
18. List and describe the main effects of choline esters or cholinergic drugs; also indicate possible adverse effects.
19. List and describe the main effects of anticholinesterase drugs; also indicate possible adverse effects.
20. List and describe the main effects of anticholinergic drugs; also indicate possible adverse effects.

INTRODUCTION

The pharmacology of the ANS is a useful model for understanding how a drug interacts with its receptor site. Much of the early theory of mechanism of action, identification of neurotransmitters, and identification and location of receptor sites was established on the basis of research on the ANS. Therefore, we will go into some detail in this section so that the student not only will understand the pharmacological principles in other drug groups, but will better understand some of the commonly used respiratory care drugs.

FUNCTION AND ANATOMY OF THE ANS

The ANS is the division of the body's nervous system controlling physiological functions that generally are involuntary. These involuntary functions, such as control of heart rate, blood pressure, glandular secretions, and digestion, also are sometimes called automatic or vegetative. In order to understand how the ANS functions, the student needs to understand the basic anatomical makeup of the ANS and compare this to the structural arrangement of the somatic nervous system.

Figure 2–1 shows that, in the somatic nervous system, the nerve cell body originates in the central nervous system (CNS) and then an axon travels to the site of innervation

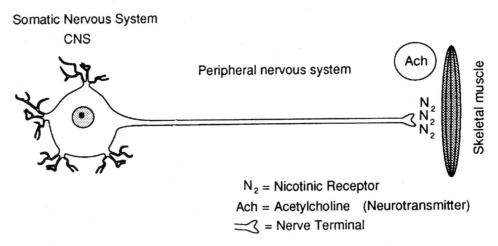

FIGURE 2–1   Somatic Nervous System.

at the skeletal muscle without any interruption or synapse. In the ANS, in both the sympathetic and parasympathetic divisions, there is an interruption between the CNS and the site of innervation. This interruption or break in the nerve pathway is called a *synapse* and it is located in a ganglion (Figure 2–2).

In both the parasympathetic and the sympathetic divisions, the interruptions (synapses) between the CNS and the receptor sites occur in autonomic *ganglia*. In the sympathetic division most of these ganglia are located close to the spinal cord; in the parasympathetic division most are located close to the effector site. With few exceptions, this is the typical anatomical arrangement of the autonomic ganglia. Because of the existence of these ganglia, there must be a *preganglionic* neuron and a *postganglionic* neuron. In the sympathetic division, the preganglionic neurons are short and the postganglionic neurons are longer, whereas in the parasympathetic division, the preganglionic neurons are very long and the postganglionic neurons are short. One other important anatomical feature is that the parasympathetic division branches off of the CNS through the cranial and sacral segments of the spinal cord and the sympathetic division branches off of the CNS through the thoracic and lumbar segments of the spinal cord (Figure 2–3). It should be noted that multiple synapses occur in the ganglia and that, because neurotransmitters are released at the ganglion site, drugs also can have an effect here.

NEUROTRANSMITTERS

An important concept in the function of the ANS is that of the neurotransmitter (Figure 2–2). In the nervous system, when nerves communicate with other nerves or neuroeffector sites, there is a gap between nerves or between the nerve and the organ that is innervated.

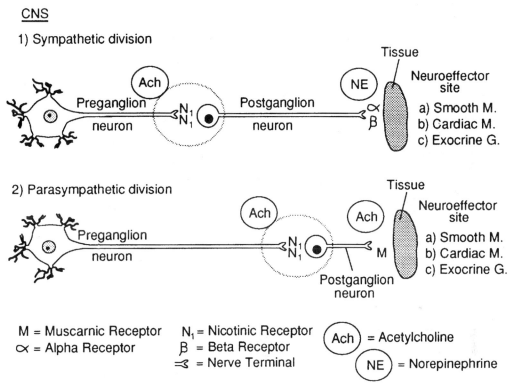

FIGURE 2–2   Synapses and Ganglia of the ANS.

This gap is called a *synaptic cleft*, or *neuroeffector junction*, and is generally 100–200 angstroms in width (an angstrom is equal to 10^{-8} cm). Because of this gap, the obvious question that arises is how a nerve transmits an electrical signal to postsynaptic nerves or a neuroeffector junction. This question is answered by the existence of *neurotransmitters*. A neurotransmitter is a chemical substance that "transmits messages" across synaptic clefts and neuroeffector junctions. The end of a nerve fiber is called the nerve terminal and contains neurotransmitters that are stored in small membrane-bound vesicles. When an impulse is transmitted along the axon to the nerve terminal, these vesicles fuse with the nerve terminal membrane and the contents are released into the synaptic cleft or the neuroeffector junction. The neurotransmitter then diffuses across the cleft to the *postsynaptic* or *postjunctional* site, where it interacts with receptors. The interaction between neurotransmitter and receptor initiates a chain of events leading to the production of electrical signals in the postsynaptic neuron or physiological changes in the neuroeffector organ.

In summary, most drugs that affect the ANS do so by affecting the synapses or neuroeffector sites in a manner similar to that of neurotransmitters. In other words, drugs are biologically active chemicals that combine with receptor sites in a manner similar to neurotransmitters.

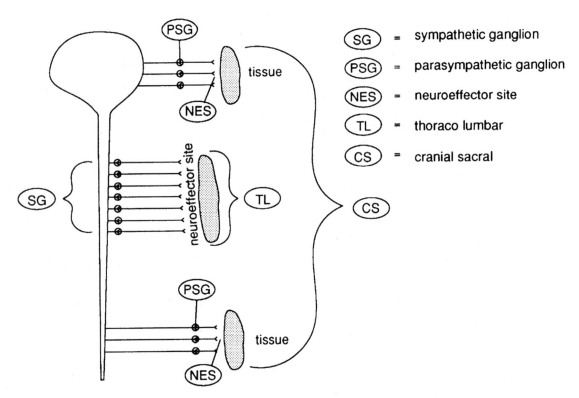

FIGURE 2–3 Origin and Distribution of the ANS.

SITES OF ACTION, NEUROTRANSMITTERS, AND RECEPTORS OF SOMATIC AND AUTONOMIC NERVOUS SYSTEMS

As seen in Figures 2–1 and 2–2, there are different sites of action, neurotransmitters, and receptors for the various divisions of the nervous system. These are summarized in Table 2–1.

GENERAL PHYSIOLOGICAL FUNCTIONS CONTROLLED BY ANS

In general, both parasympathetic and sympathetic divisions innervate most organs of the body, and usually the two systems have opposite effects. In other words, one system will enhance a certain function and the other will decrease that same function; for example, the sympathetic innervation to the heart causes an increase in heart rate, whereas the parasympathetic innervation causes a decrease in heart rate. The innervation by both systems to a particular organ is also known as *dual innervation*. Table 2–2 illustrates the dual innervation and opposite effects in selected areas of the body.

TABLE 2–1   Sites of Action, Neurotransmitters (NT), and Receptors of Somatic Nervous System and ANS

NERVOUS SYSTEM	NEUROEFFECTOR SITE	NT AT GANGLION SITE	NT AT NEURO-EFFECTOR SITE	RECEPTOR
Somatic	Skeletal muscle	None	ACh*	Nicotinic-2
Autonomic	Smooth muscle,	ACh	NE*	α_1, α_2, β_1, β_2
Sympathetic	cardiac muscle,		ACh (to sweat	
division	glands		glands)	
Parasympathetic	Smooth muscle,	ACh	ACh	Nicotinic-1,
division	cardiac muscle,			muscarinic
	glands			

*ACh = acetylcholine, NE = norepinephrine.

OVERALL EFFECT OF SYMPATHETIC DIVISION AND DEFINITION OF ADRENERGIC

Generally the sympathetic division is the dominant system when the body is under stress or in a state of increased activity. Sympathetic activity also is prominent when the body is in a dangerous or life-threatening situation. This condition is called the *fight or flight*

TABLE 2–2   Effects of Parasympathetic and Sympathetic Divisions

NEUROEFFECTOR SITE	SYMPATHETIC EFFECT (NE)*	PARASYMPATHETIC EFFECT (ACh)*
Arteries	Vasoconstriction (*Exception*: coronary and skeletal arteries are dilated)	Most are not affected
Heart	Increased rate and force of contraction	Decreased rate and force of contraction
Intestines and gastrointestinal activity	Decreased	Increased
Pupil of eye	Dilation (mydriasis)	Constriction (miosis)
Respiratory tract	Bronchodilation	Bronchoconstriction
Urinary bladder	Relaxation	Contraction
Urinary sphincter	Constriction	Relaxation

*NE = norepinephrine, ACh = acetylcholine.

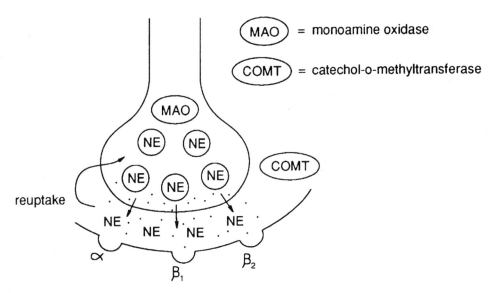

FIGURE 2–4 Sympathetic Nerve Ending.

response, and, if the homeostatic balance is kept in this state for a prolonged period of time, complete exhaustion can occur and may lead to death.

The term *adrenergic* often is used to describe drugs that mimic the action of the sympathetic nervous system, and the term literally means "adrenalin-like." Another term that often is used and has the same meaning is *sympathomimetic* ("sympathetic-like").

THE SYMPATHETIC NERVE ENDING

The basic anatomy of the sympathetic nerve ending at the neuroeffector site is presented in Figure 2–4. The neurotransmitter at the neuroeffector site is norepinephrine (NE), which is synthesized in the nerve ending and packaged in vesicles. When an impulse reaches the nerve ending, NE is released into the synaptic cleft and combines with the type of receptor present. In the parasympathetic system there is an enzyme located wherever acetylcholine (ACh) is released, and any excess ACh that does not combine with the receptor site is metabolized by this enzyme. However, in the sympathetic system there is no enzyme that immediately breaks down NE; thus it takes time for the effects of NE to dissipate. The physiological effects of NE are terminated by two means: 1) NE is actively transported back into the nerve terminal and repackaged into the vesicles (*reuptake*), or 2) NE diffuses away from the site where enzymes—monoamine oxidase (MAO) and catechol-0-methyltransferase (COMT)—ultimately metabolize NE. Although these enzymes do metabolize NE, they usually do not interfere with the neurotransmitter's synaptic action.

TABLE 2–3   Location and Action of Adrenergic Receptors

RECEPTOR	ORGAN	NE	EPI*
α	Most arteries and veins	Vasoconstriction	Vasoconstriction
β_1	Heart	Moderate increase in rate, force of contraction	Greater increase in rate, force of contraction
β_2	Lungs, bronchiolar smooth muscle	None	Bronchodilation
	Uterus	None	Relaxation
	Skeletal muscles (blood vessels)	None	Vasodilation

*Epinephrine (EPI) is not a neurotransmitter but is released by the adrenal gland. When the sympathetic nervous system is active, the adrenal gland is innervated by presynaptic sympathetic nerves, which cause the adrenal gland to release epinephrine.

Drugs administered to a patient move to different organs (neuroeffector sites) throughout the body. The adrenergic receptors have been classified according to the response of various organs when their receptors interact with adrenergic drugs or NE, and are identified as α_1, α_2, β_1, and β_2 receptors. (*Note*: There are a number of α_2 receptors that have been identified but do not play a major role in the autonomic drugs. Therefore, in this text we will consider all α receptors to be the same.) Table 2–3 indicates the general locations and actions of α, β_1, and β_2 receptors; the general responses of these receptors to NE and epinephrine also are listed.

SITES OF ACTION OF ADRENERGIC DRUGS

Referring back to Figure 2–4, it can be seen that there are many possibilities for drug–receptor interactions at the various sites with which NE combines. First, there are several drugs that affect the adrenergic transmission presynaptically in the nerve ending. Some of the mechanisms by which these drugs work are altering NE transmission by creating false transmitters, blocking the reuptake of NE, depleting NE from storage vesicles, increasing release of NE from nerve endings, and blocking release of NE from nerve terminals. The various drugs that work by these mechanisms are collectively called "neuronal activators" or "neuronal blockers."

Second, at the postjunctional site where the receptors are located, there are also many possibilities for drug–receptor interaction. Some drugs stimulate α receptors, β receptors, or both, and some drugs block α receptors or β receptors. (*Note*: It has recently been shown that chronic medication can alter the number of receptors and thus increase or decrease tolerance to drugs; i.e., the number of receptors can vary according to pharmacological, physiological, and pathological factors. It is not within the scope of this text to discuss these phenomena.)

DEFINITIONS OF THE ADRENERGIC DRUGS

As discussed previously, there are many possible mechanisms by which adrenergic drugs can work. The following list defines the mechanisms of action of the adrenergic drugs:

- *α-adrenergic*—drugs that stimulate the α receptor sites.
- *β-adrenergic*—drugs that stimulate the β receptor sites.
- *α-blockers*—drugs that block the α receptors.
- *α-blockers*—drugs that block the β receptors.
- *Neuronal activators or blockers*—drugs that either increase or inhibit the levels of NE in the nerve ending.

α-ADRENERGIC DRUGS

These drugs stimulate the α receptor sites; a few stimulate both α and β receptors but have a stronger affinity for the α receptor sites (Table 2–4).

Norepinephrine (Levophed^R)

The most dominant clinical effect of NE is vasoconstriction. It has a slight effect on the $β_1$ receptors in the heart but no effect on $β_2$ receptors in the lungs. **Therapeutic uses:** to elevate blood pressure in cases of acute hypotension or shock rarely used for this purpose because of adverse effects. **Adverse effects:** as a result of extreme vasoconstriction, can cause hypertension, renal shutdown, skin pallor, and possible tissue necrosis.

TABLE 2–4 α-Adrenergic Drugs

DRUG	CLINICAL USE
Norepinephrine (Levophed^R)	Increase blood pressure, helpful in hypovolemic shock
Epinephrine	See Table 2–5
Ephedrine	Shock, bronchodilation
Phenylephrine	Increase blood pressure, nasal decongestant
Metaraminol (Aramine^R)	Increase blood pressure
Phenylpropanolamine	Anorexiant (mild)

Epinephrine

This is also an endogenous substance that is released by the adrenal gland. It has a profound effect on both α and β receptors, with a stronger affinity for the $β_1$ and $β_2$ receptors. We will discuss the clinical uses and adverse effects of this drug in the section on β-adrenergic drugs and also in the chapter on bronchodilators.

Ephedrine

This drug affects both α and β receptors, with a moderate effect on the α receptors and relatively strong effect on the $β_1$ and $β_2$ receptors. **Therapeutic uses:** to elevate blood pressure in cases of hypotension or shock, and improve blood flow to vital organs; also used as a mild bronchodilator in order to reduce airway resistance. **Adverse effects:** because of both α- and β-stimulatory effects, can cause tachycardia, arrhythmias, and CNS stimulation leading to insomnia, anxiety, and tremor.

Phenylephrine

This substance is primarily an α stimulator, and its overall effect is vasoconstriction. **Therapeutic uses:** to increase blood pressure; main use is as a topical nasal decongestant and also a pupil dilator. **Adverse effects:** can cause rebound congestion when overused as a nasal decongestant and can cause mild discomfort in the eye when used as a pupil dilator.

Metaraminol (Aramine^R)

This substance works on both α and $β_1$ receptors but is used primarily for its α effects. **Therapeutic uses:** to increase blood pressure and arterial pulmonary pressure. **Adverse effects:** arrhythmia, hypotension, and tissue necrosis.

Phenylpropanolamine

This substance has both α and β effects and is basically similar to ephedrine in its actions. **Therapeutic use:** common over-the-counter agent used as an anorexiant because it has slight CNS properties similar to those of amphetamines. **Adverse effects:** minor if used according to directions.

β-ADRENERGIC DRUGS

These drugs stimulate mainly the $β_1$ and $β_2$ receptors but some also stimulate α receptors. A brief discussion of some of the more common β-adrenergic drugs follows, along with some clinical uses and pertinent adverse effects (Table 2–5).

TABLE 2–5   β-Adrenergic Drugs

DRUG	CLINICAL USE
Epinephrine	Cardiac stimulation, increase blood pressure, bronchodilator
Ephedrine	Bronchodilator and cardiac stimulant, treatment of asthma
Isoproterenol (Isuprel[R])	Bronchodilator, cardiac stimulant
Dopamine (Intropin[R])	Decongestant, cardiac stimulant
Albuterol (Proventil[R])	Bronchodilator
Isoetharine (Bronkometer[R])	Bronchodilator
Metaproterenol (Alupent[R])	Bronchodilator
Terbutaline (Brethine[R])	Bronchodilator

Epinephrine

This substance is released by the adrenal medulla and thus is an endogenous substance. Epinephrine also can be used as a drug and has a prominent effect on β_1 and β_2 receptors as well as α receptors. Because it has such a widespread effect on all sympathetic receptors, it has a number of clinical uses. **Therapeutic uses:** for elevated blood pressure; as a vasoconstrictor to reduce bleeding, as a heart stimulant to increase heart rate and cardiac output, as a bronchodilator, particularly in emergency treatment of bronchial spasm and bronchial constriction during anaphylactic shock. **Adverse effects:** arrhythmia, palpitations, hypertension.

Ephedrine

This drug is discussed here as well as with the α-adrenergic drugs, because of its β_1 and β_2 effects. **Therapeutic uses:** as a mild bronchodilator; also reduces airway resistance. **Adverse effects:** same as those of epinephrine.

Isoproterenol (Isuprel[R])

This drug is closely related to NE and epinephrine in chemical structure but has pure β effects. **Therapeutic use:** one of the original bronchodilator drugs; occasionally used today but, because it has strong β_1 effects causing undesirable cardiac stimulation, it has been replaced by more effective β_2 stimulators. **Adverse effects:** cardiac arrhythmia, tachycardia, and hypotension.

Dopamine (Intropin[R])

This is an α and β_1 stimulator. **Therapeutic uses:** primarily to increase heart rate and cardiac contraction in open heart surgery, and for correction of hemodynamic imbalances. **Adverse effects:** arrhythmia, vasoconstriction, and hypertension.

Albuterol (Proventil^R), Isoetharine (Bronkometer^R), Metaproterenol (Alupent^R), and Terbutaline (Brethine^R)

These drugs are β_2 stimulators and currently are used as bronchodilators. They will be discussed in detail in Chapter 11 of this text.

α-BLOCKING DRUGS

This group of drugs block the α receptor sites and have an overall effect of vasodilation. Because they produce a competitive blockade of the α receptor sites, NE cannot cause vasoconstriction. The drugs create such a generalized, nonselective vasodilation that they have only limited clinical use (Table 2–6).

Phenoxybenzamine (Dibenzyline^R)

This drug causes a profound blockade of α receptors that lasts 3–4 days. **Therapeutic uses:** initially used to treat peripheral vascular disease (Raynaud's disease, which causes profound vasoconstriction of the extremities when exposed to cold and can lead to tissue necrosis). Because of the development of less potent drugs, it is not used for this purpose today. This drug is used, however, to treat a rare kind of adrenal gland tumor called a pheochromocytoma, and causes a massive release of epinephrine and NE in the body. **Adverse effects:** orthostatic hypotension, reflex tachycardia, profound drop in blood pressure, and miosis (blocks α receptors in the radial muscle of the eye).

Tolazoline (Priscoline^R) and Phentolamine (Regitine^R)

These drugs produce moderately effective competitive blockades of the α receptors and have a short duration of action. **Therapeutic use:** peripheral vascular disease (Raynaud's disease). **Adverse effects:** can produce hypertension and cardiac stimulation; also can cause an increase in gastric secretion. There are few rational uses for these drugs, and their administration should be left to the experts.

TABLE 2–6 α-Blockers

DRUG	CLINICAL USE
Phenoxybenzamine (Dibenzyline^R)	Peripheral vascular disease
Tolazoline (Priscoline^R)	Peripheral vascular disease, pulmonary hypertension in newborns
Prazosin (Minipress^R)	Hypertension

Prazosin (Minipress[R])

This drug selectively blocks the α receptors in the vasculature without producing tachycardia. **Therapeutic uses:** very effective when given orally and clinically useful when treating hypertension; also can be used in peripheral vascular disease, and has a short duration of action. **Adverse effects:** similar to those of tolazoline.

β-BLOCKING DRUGS

These drugs include a group of agents that are extremely useful and heavily prescribed in medical practice. There are many different β blockers available, with some affecting both β_1 and β_2 receptors and some that are relatively selective for β_1 receptors (Table 2–7). Propranolol was one of the earliest β blockers used and today is one of the top 10 most prescribed drugs in the United States.

Propranolol (Inderal[R])

This is the prototype drug of the β blockers. It is a nonselective drug that affects both β_1 and β_2 receptors, but has become one of the most popular and useful drugs available today. **Therapeutic uses:** in treating hypertension, angina, cardiac arrhythmias, myocardial infarction, open-angle glaucoma, and tremors; also used prophylactically in the prevention of migraine headache. (*Note:* We will mention various mechanisms of action of propranolol as we discuss several clinical uses in later sections of this text.) **Adverse effects:** should not be used in asthmatics, or patients with chronic obstructive pulmonary disease, congestive heart failure, hypotension, and bradycardia; can also cause CNS problems such as weakness, fatigue, and depression.

TABLE 2–7 β-Blockers

DRUG	CLINICAL USE
Propranolol (Inderal[R])	Hypertension, angina, cardiac arrhythmia, migraine headache
Timolol (Blocadren[R])	Same as propranolol but also used in treating open-angle glaucoma (very potent)
Metoprolol (Lopressor[R])	Hypertension
Nadolol (Corgard[R])	Hypertension
Atenolol (Tenormin[R])	Hypertension, cardiac arrhythmia

Timolol (Blocadren[R])

This is a nonselective β_1 and β_2 blocker that is 10 times more potent than propranolol. **Therapeutic uses:** same as those of propranolol; should be used with caution because of its potency. Because it is short acting, it also is used after myocardial infarction because it prevents subsequent reinfarction. Also used in treating open-angle glaucoma. **Adverse effects:** same as with propranolol.

Metoprolol (Lopressor[R])

This is a selective β_1 blocker with short duration of action. **Therapeutic uses:** same as those of propranolol but, because of its specific β_1 effects, it is used in cardiac disorders. **Adverse effects:** same as with propranolol.

Nadolol (Corgard[R])

This is a nonselective β_1 and β_2 blocker that is longer acting than propranolol. **Therapeutic uses:** same as those of metoprolol but longer acting. **Adverse effects:** same as with propranolol.

Atenolol (Tenormin[R])

This is a selective β_1 blocker that has a long duration of action. **Therapeutic uses:** same as those of propranolol, with primarily β_1 cardiac indications. **Adverse effects:** same as with propranolol.

ADRENERGIC NEURONAL ACTIVATORS AND BLOCKERS

In general, these agents decrease adrenergic nerve function by affecting the release of NE from the presynaptic nerve terminal. In addition, these drugs affect all sites where NE is released and thus tend to influence both α and β receptors. (In addition, some of these drugs activate the effects of NE.) The actions of the various drugs are quite complex, and only the clinically useful mechanisms of action are discussed (Table 2–8).

TABLE 2–8 Neuronal Blocking Drugs

DRUG	CLINICAL USES
Reserpine (Serpasil[R])	Antihypertensive
Guanethidine (Ismelin[R])	Severe hypertension
α-Methyldopa (Aldomet[R])	Moderate hypertension
Clonidine (Catapres[R])	Moderate hypertension

Reserpine (Serpasil[R])

This drug depletes NE from nerve terminals by preventing storage of NE in the vesicles. This results in less NE being available for combination with receptors. Although this drug seldom is used today, it is presented here as a classic antihypertensive. **Therapeutic uses:** treatment of mild hypertension, and used in conjunction with diuretics; also occasionally used to treat Raynaud's disease. **Adverse effects:** CNS sedation, gastrointestinal (GI) distress, exacerbation of peptic ulcer, and nasal congestion.

Guanethidine (Ismelin[R])

This drug is used in treating severe hypertension and blocks the release of NE from nerve terminals. This drug also takes several weeks to reach therapeutic levels and has a long duration of action. **Therapeutic use:** to treat moderate to severe hypertension. Because of potency, hospitalization and adjustment of dose by experts is essential. **Adverse effects:** *postural hypotension*, bradycardia, may aggravate asthma, impotence, *orthostatic hypotension*, and diarrhea. (*Note:* Because of severe and unpleasant side effects, and the development of newer effective antihypertensive drugs, this drug is becoming obsolete.)

α-Methyldopa (Aldomet[R])

This drug works with either presynaptic or postsynaptic nerve endings and causes activation of the receptor site by a metabolite (α-methylnorepinephrine), and probably stimulates α_2 receptors. **Therapeutic use:** antihypertensive. **Adverse effects:** similar to those of reserpine.

Clonidine (Catapres[R])

This drug reduces sympathetic tone and acts directly on the cardiovascular center in the brain. **Therapeutic use:** antihypertensive. **Adverse effects:** similar to those of α-methyldopa.

OVERALL EFFECTS OF PARASYMPATHETIC DIVISION AND DEFINITION OF CHOLINERGIC

Generally the parasympathetic division is dominant when the body is at rest. When the body is in a quiet state, this division controls and stimulates digestion, waste elimination, and the genitourinary systems. Also, the activity level of the cardiovascular system generally is decreased. The term *cholinergic* often is used to describe drugs that mimic the parasympathetic system and literally means "acetylcholine-like." Another similar term is *parasympathomimetic*, which means "parasympathetic-like."

THE PARASYMPATHETIC NERVE ENDING

The basic anatomy of the parasympathetic nerve ending at the neuroeffector site is represented in Figure 2–5. As stated previously, the neurotransmitter at the neuroeffector site in the parasympathetic division is acetylcholine. This substance is synthesized in the nerve ending and packaged in vesicles. When a nerve impulse reaches the nerve ending, ACh is released into the synaptic cleft and combines with the type of receptor present. In the sympathetic division, there is no enzyme available to metabolize excess NE; however, in the parasympathetic division, or wherever ACh is released, there is *acetylcholinesterase* (AChE), which metabolizes any excess ACh that does not combine with the receptor. The significance of this fact is that the effect of ACh throughout the body is rather short lived. Thus, the parasympathetic division is more discrete in its action and, in contrast to the sympathetic division, does not have a generalized effect.

The cholinergic receptors have been classified and named based on two experimental drugs, *muscarine* and *nicotine*, that initially were used to identify the action of the receptor sites when these drugs were administered. The names of the receptors are *muscarine* (M), *nicotinic*-1 (N_1), and *nicotinic*-2 (N_2). The neuroeffector sites of the parasympathetic division contain M receptors, the N_1 receptors are located at all ganglion sites in the ANS, and the N_2 receptors are located at the neuromuscular junctions in the somatic nervous system. With knowledge of the responses when these receptors are stimulated and knowledge as to their location, one can predict the action of various cholinergic drugs when they combine with their respective receptors. (*Note:* Although the neuromuscular junctions in the somatic nervous system have N_2 receptors, they are stimulated by ACh. The effects of

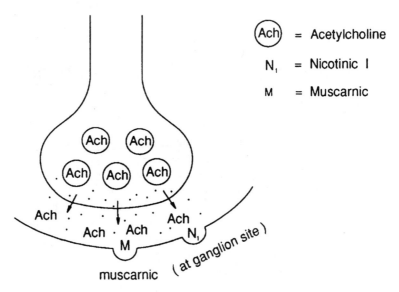

FIGURE 2–5   Parasympathetic Nerve Ending.

TABLE 2–9   Location and Action of Cholinergic Receptors

RECEPTOR*	ORGAN	ACh
Muscarinic (M)	Not located in most arteries and veins	None
	Pupils of eye (miosis)	Constricting
	Heart	Decrease in heart rate
	Bronchial smooth muscle	Bronchoconstriction
	Uterus	Contraction of smooth muscle
	Urinary bladder	Contraction of muscle
	GI tract	Increased mobility and peristalsis
Nicotinic-1 (N_1)	All autonomic ganglia	Stimulation of postganglia neuron
Nicotinic-2 (N_2)	Neuromuscular junction of skeletal muscle	Contraction of skeletal muscle

*The muscarinic receptors recently have been subdivided into M_1, M_2, and M_3 types. However, there are few drugs that have yet been identified as specific for these types. Also, the N_1 and N_2 (nicotinic receptors) have been changed in some texts to N_n and N_m. In this text we will use M, N_1, and N_2.

drug action at this site will be discussed in Chapter 4.) Table 2–9 indicates the general location of the cholinergic receptors and their response to ACh.

MECHANISM OF ACTION OF CHOLINERGIC DRUGS

Referring back to Figure 2–2, one can observe that, because of the many locations wherein ACh acts as a transmitter, there are more possibilities for drugs to interact with cholinergic receptors. Thus, cholinergic drugs produce a much broader spectrum of unwanted side effects because the parasympathetic system, unlike the sympathetic system, does not function as a unit. Therefore, most clinically useful cholinergic drugs are quite specific and affect the postsynaptic receptor site.

At the postsynaptic site, there are three possible drug–receptor interactions. First, drugs can stimulate the muscarinic receptor, producing a cholinergic effect (i.e., these drugs mimic the activity of the parasympathetic nerves). Second, there are drugs that block the cholinergic receptors and prevent ACh from interacting. Thirdly, there are drugs that block acetylcholinesterase. These drugs are called *anticholinesterase* drugs, which increase the accumulation of ACh and enhance the duration of parasympathetic impulses or cholinergic drugs.

DEFINITIONS OF CHOLINERGIC DRUGS

There are various mechanisms by which cholinergic drugs can work. The definitions and categories of these drugs are as follows:

- *Choline esters*—stimulate the muscarinic receptors and in general mimic the effects of ACh.
- *Anticholinesterases*—block the enzyme AChE.
- *Anticholinergics*—block the receptor sites where ACh interacts.
- *Antimuscarinic*—specifically block the muscarinic receptor sites.

CHOLINE ESTERS

This group of drugs stimulate the muscarinic receptors. Some of the commonly used drugs are discussed, along with their therapeutic uses and adverse effects (Table 2–10).

Acetylcholine

This substance is an endogenous neurotransmitter. It has no clinical use, primarily because of its short duration of action brought about by its rapid destruction by AChE. Also, because of acetylcholine's wide distribution throughout the body at both ganglionic and neuroeffector sites, the clinical effects are too widely spread. **Therapeutic use:** not used clinically. **Adverse effects:** not applicable.

Methacholine (Provocholine[R])

This is a synthetic choline ester with a longer duration of action because it is slowly metabolized by AChE. It has only a slight effect on nicotinic receptors. **Therapeutic use:** has a strong affinity for the cardiovascular system but is used mainly to stimulate muscarinic receptors in the sphincter muscle of the iris, causing miosis. **Adverse effects:** severe bronchial constriction.

TABLE 2–10 Choline Esters	
DRUG	**CLINICAL USES**
Acetylcholine	None
Methacholine (Provocholine[R])	Miosis, bronchial provocation testing
Bethanechol (Urecholine[R])	Urinary retention
Pilocarpine (Adsorbocarpine[R])	Miotic, treatment of glaucoma

Bethanechol (Urecholine[R])

This is a synthetic choline ester that has a longer duration of action than methacholine. It primarily stimulates muscarinic receptors. **Therapeutic use:** to treat urinary retention following general anesthesia; rarely used today. **Adverse effects:** abdominal cramps, bronchial constriction, and miosis.

Pilocarpine (Adsorbocarpine[R])

This is a naturally occurring alkaloid that stimulates muscarinic receptors. **Therapeutic use:** topical administration in treating glaucoma by causing miosis. **Adverse effect:** myopia, blurred vision, hypertension, and bradycardia.

ANTICHOLINESTERASE DRUGS

As the name implies, this group of drugs inhibits the effects of AChE at receptor sites throughout the CNS as well as the peripheral nervous system. Because these drugs are not very selective, their therapeutic use is limited (Table 2–11), and they are generally used by medical specialists such as anesthesiologists or ophthalmologists. The major therapeutic uses of these drugs are for treating myasthenia gravis, certain types of glaucoma, and urinary retention, antagonizing the effects of neuromuscular blocking agents, and treating toxic overdose of anticholinergic drugs.

Edrophonium (Tensilon[R])

This agent combines directly with the enzyme AChE and produces a short-acting, reversible blockade. Also, it does not penetrate the blood–brain barrier and thus has few CNS effects (this is also true of neostigmine and pyridostigmine). **Therapeutic uses:** in diagnosing myasthenia gravis, in treating certain kinds of tachycardia, and as an antidote for curare. **Adverse effects:** causes excessive parasympathetic response, hypotension, bradycardia, and miosis.

TABLE 2–11 Anticholinesterases

DRUG	CLINICAL USE
Edrophonium (Tensilon[R])	Diagnosis and treatment of myasthenia gravis
Neostigmine (Prostigmin[R])	Myasthenia gravis
Pyridostigmine (Mestinon[R])	Myasthenia gravis
Physostigmine (Eserine[R])	Overdose reactions to anticholinergics and tricyclic antidepressants

Neostigmine (Prostigmin[R])

This drug has a strong affinity for the nicotinic receptors and thus is used in treating myasthenia gravis. Also, this drug is considered the prototype of the anticholinesterase drugs. **Therapeutic uses:** treatment of myasthenia gravis and urinary retention; also, to reverse the effects of curare-type muscle relaxants. **Adverse effects:** similar to those of edrophonium.

Pyridostigmine (Mestinon[R])

This drug is similar to neostigmine and is more currently used today. **Therapeutic uses:** same as those of neostigmine. **Adverse effects:** same as with neostigmine.

Physostigmine (Eserine[R])

This drug is similar to neostigmine but is more lipid soluble and more readily crosses the blood–brain barrier. **Therapeutic use:** treatment of overdose of anticholinergic and tricyclic antidepressant drugs. **Adverse effects:** similar to those of the other anticholinesterases, plus it causes CNS depression.

ANTICHOLINERGIC DRUGS

These drugs block the muscarinic receptors throughout the body but also can affect the nicotinic receptors if given in high enough doses. As a group, these drugs are used in management of peptic ulcers, as a pupil dilator in ophthalmology, as a preanesthetic medication, and in treating motion sickness. In addition to the many clinical uses, there are five different terms that can be used to describe these drugs: antimuscarinic, anticholinergic, atrophic, antiparasympathetic, and parasympatholytic. The following drugs are those that are clinically significant (Table 2–12).

Atropine (Atripison[R])

This is the prototype drug of the anticholinergics and can be used for a number of clinical situations. In low doses it mainly affects the muscarinic receptors, but in higher doses it can block nicotinic receptors. **Therapeutic uses:** as a preanesthetic agent to decrease salivary and respiratory secretions, as an agent to increase heart rate, and for pupillary dilation. **Adverse effects:** dry mouth, constipation, mental confusion, palpitations, tachycardia, urinary retention, and decrease in sweating.

Scopolamine

This drug is similar to atropine but is more readily absorbed by the CNS. This fact makes it useful as an anti–motion sickness drug. **Therapeutic use:** mainly as a preventive for motion sickness (available as a *transdermal* patch). **Adverse effects:** same as with atropine.

TABLE 2–12   Anticholinergic Drugs

DRUG	CLINICAL USE
Atropine (Atripison^R)	Stimulant and before anesthesia to decrease secretions
Scopolamine	Treatment and prevention of motion sickness
Tropicamide (Mydrasil^R)	Short-acting pupil dilator used in routine eye examinations
Dicyclomine (Bentyl^R)	Decreases GI motility, treatment of ulcers
Propantheline (Pro-Banthīne^R)	Decreases GI motility, treatment of ulcers

Tropicamide (Mydrasil^R)

This is a short-acting pupil dilator. **Therapeutic use:** routine eye examination. **Adverse effects:** similar to those of atropine.

Dicyclomine (Bentyl^R)

This agent has a strong affinity for the muscarinic receptors in the GI tract. **Therapeutic uses:** to reduce GI motility and increase healing of ulcers. **Adverse effects:** same as with atropine.

Propantheline (Pro-Banthīne^R)

Therapeutic uses and adverse effects: same as with dicyclomine.

POSTTEST: PHARMACOLOGY OF THE AUTONOMIC NERVOUS SYSTEM

For each of the following questions, try to select the *one* best answer from those choices given.

1. The overall function of the ANS includes all of the following except:
   a. controls involuntary functions
   b. controls heart rate
   c. controls skeletal muscle
   d. controls digestion

2. The structural arrangment of the sympathetic nervous system includes all of the following except:
   a. the preganglionic fibers emerge from the CNS through thoracolumbar outflow.
   b. the sympathetic ganglia are located close to the spinal cord.
   c. in the sympathetic nervous system the preganglionic fibers are short and the postganglionic fibers are long.
   d. the preganglionic fibers emerge from the CNS through the cranial–sacral outflow.

3. The structural arrangement of the parasympathetic nervous system includes all of the following except:
   a. the parasympathetic preganglionic fibers are long and the postganglionic fibers are short.
   b. the parasympathetic ganglia are located close to the organ that is innervated.
   c. the parasympathetic preganglionic fibers emerge from the cranial–sacral outflow.
   d. the parasympathetic preganglionic fibers emerge from the thoracolumbar outflow.

4. All of the following statements about neurotransmitters are true except:
   a. neurotransmitters are chemical substances.
   b. neurotransmitters are produced in the presynaptic nerve terminal.
   c. neurotransmitters are produced in the postsynaptic terminal and combined with receptors in the synapse.
   d. communication between a nerve and a nerve cell body or organ occur in areas called synapses.

5. The neurotransmitter at the ganglion site of the sympathetic nervous system and the parasympathetic nervous system is acetylcholine. True or False?

6. The parasympathetic nervous system causes all of the following except:
   a. increase in heart rate
   b. increased function in GI tract
   c. contraction of urinary bladder
   d. pupillary constriction

7. Stimulation of the β_2 receptors by epinephrine causes:
   a. constriction of the uterus
   b. bronchoconstriction
   c. bronchodilation
   d. vasoconstriction of the blood vessels of the skeletal muscle

8. All of the following statements about propranolol (Inderal^R) are true except:
   a. affects both β_1 and β_2 receptors
   b. used in treating cardiac arrhythmias
   c. used in treating high blood pressure
   d. used in treating anaphylactic shock

9. Which one of the following effects is not a function of the parasympathetic nervous system?
   a. increase in cardiovascular activity
   b. increase in digestive system

    c. waste elimination

    d. increase in activity of genitourinary system

10. The mechanism of action of cholinergic drugs may include all of the following except:

    a. stimulates nicotinic-1 receptors

    b. stimulates nicotinic-2 receptors

    c. stimulates acetylcholinesterase

    d. blocks acetylcholinesterase

REFERENCES/RECOMMENDED READING

Aflaro-LeFevre R, Blicharz ME, Flynn NM, Boyer MJ: *Drug Handbook: A Nursing Process Approach.* Addison-Wesley Nursing, a division of the Benjamin/Cummings Publishing Co, Inc, Redwood City, CA, 1992.

Dipalma JR, Digregorio JG: *Basic Pharmacology in Medicine*, 3rd ed. McGraw-Hill, New York, 1990.

Handbook of Nonprescription Drugs, 9th ed. American Pharmaceutical Association, Washington, DC, 1990.

Hitner, H, Nagle BT: *Basic Pharmacology for Health Occupations*, 2nd ed. Glenco Publishing Co, Mission Hills, CA, 1987.

Physicians' Desk Reference for Nonprescription Drugs, 12th ed. Medical Economics Company, Montvale, NJ, 1991.

Tortora GJ, Anagnostakus NP: *Principles of Anatomy and Physiology.* Harper & Row, New York, 1990.

CHAPTER 3

PHARMACOLOGY OF THE CENTRAL NERVOUS SYSTEM

LEARNING OBJECTIVES

1. Review the general anatomy of the central nervous system (CNS) and list the functions of each area.
2. Describe the overall effect of CNS drugs regarding complex circuitry, types of neurotransmitters, and possible general mechanisms of action.
3. Describe the general characteristics of CNS drugs.
4. Describe as a group the sedative hypnotic/antianxiety drugs and define the terms *sedative, hypnosis,* and *antianxiety.*
5. Describe the barbiturates as a historical prototype of the sedative hypnotics, along with their therapeutic effects and their effect on rapid eye movement sleep.
6. Name and classify the barbiturates as to their duration of action and clinical uses.
7. Discuss the nonbarbiturate sedative hypnotics, along with duration of action and clinical use.
8. Discuss the benzodiazepines as sedative hypnotics and antianxiety agents and indicate their main clinical uses, mechanism of action, and adverse effects.
9. Describe alcohol as a pharmacological agent, along with its adverse effects and addiction liability.
10. Describe what is meant by psychopharmacology and briefly describe the therapeutic approach to mental and behavioral disorders.
11. List the categories of psychopharmacological agents along with the prototype drugs that are used to treat various disorders.
12. Define the term *antipsychotic* and describe the prototype drug, chlorpromazine, along with its therapeutic uses and adverse effects.
13. Define the types of depression that are treated by pharmacological agents and list the categories of antidepressant drugs used to treat these disorders.
14. Describe the mechanism of action of tricyclic antidepressant and monoamine oxidase inhibitor antidepressant drugs used in treating depression; also, indicate therapeutic uses and adverse effects of each group.

15. Describe the mechanism of action of the new generation of antidepressant drugs, giving examples of these agents, their therapeutic uses, and their adverse effects.

16. Describe the conditions that are treated by the mood stabilizer drugs, along with their mechanism of action, therapeutic uses, and adverse effects.

17. Describe the conditions that are treated by psychostimulant drugs, along with their mechanism of action, therapeutic uses, and adverse effects.

18. Describe the drugs currently used to treat anxiety, along with their therapeutic uses and adverse effects.

19. List some of the miscellaneous clinical conditions that are treated by psychopharmacological agents and be familiar with some of the drugs used for these purposes.

20. Define epilepsy and give a brief description of the classification, diagnosis, and overall management of the disease.

21. Describe the five main antiepileptic drugs currently used, along with a general description of mechanism of action, their therapeutic uses, and adverse effects.

22. Describe the overall cause of parkinsonism, along with the symptoms and the relationship of symptoms to dopamine levels.

23. Describe and list the current drugs used to treat parkinsonism, along with their mechanism of action, therapeutic uses, and adverse effects.

24. Define the term *general anesthesia* and describe the current theory as to the mechanism of action of general anesthetics; list and describe the stages of anesthesia.

25. List the properties of an ideal general anesthetic and relate these properties to the need for administering a combination of drugs.

26. List the classifications of general anesthetics.

27. List the inhalation general anesthetic agents currently used and classify them as volatile liquids or gases.

28. List four injectable general anesthetics currently used and discuss the advantages of the injectable general anesthetic agents.

29. List the reasons for using preanesthetic agents prior to administration of a general anesthetic, along with examples of each.

30. Define narcotic analgesics, describe the mechanism of action, and indicate the type of pain narcotic analgesics are used for.

31. Describe the physiological effects of narcotics, using morphine as a prototype, on various systems of the body.

32. Describe the classification of narcotic analgesics and list the commonly used agents in each category.

33. List some commonly used narcotic analgesics and describe them according to addiction potential, analgesic potency, respiratory depression, and other adverse effects.

34. Describe how narcotic antagonist drugs are used to treat overdose reactions to narcotics.

35. Define nonnarcotic analgesics and compare the major differences between narcotics and nonnarcotic drugs.

36. Describe the salicylates as the prototype drugs of nonnarcotics in terms of examples, mechanism of actions, and therapeutic effects.
37. Describe the various adverse effects of the salicylates.
38. List and describe various nonnarcotic drugs that are not salicylates and indicate their mechanism of action and adverse effects.
39. Define nonsteroidal anti-inflammatory drugs and indicate their main clinical use.
40. List some of the more common nonsteroidal anti-inflammatory drugs, along with their mechanism of action, therapeutic uses, and adverse effects.

INTRODUCTION

The drugs discussed in this chapter are the most widely used and abused group of drugs in patient care. They have a broad range of effects and a great deal of overlap regarding their therapeutic use. Also, because of the wide range of effects, there is ample opportunity for self-medication and abuse. The therapeutic CNS drugs include sedative hypnotics, psychopharmacologic drugs, antiepileptics, antiparkinson drugs, general anesthetics, and analgesics. This chapter reviews the anatomy of the CNS, discusses some general characteristics of CNS drugs, and discusses the more important groups of drugs that are therapeutically useful in the various categories of CNS pharmacology.

GENERAL ANATOMY OF THE CNS

The general anatomy of the CNS is extremely complex, with many different nuclear centers and locations that interact with each other. In order to simplify the study of the CNS function, the brain is divided into four parts: the cerebrum, the diencephalon, the brain stem, and the cerebellum (Figure 3–1). These parts are described below, with a brief discussion of the functions of each area.

Cerebrum

The cerebrum is the largest area of brain tissue and occupies the superior part of the CNS. It is composed of a left and a right cerebral hemisphere. The cortex of each hemisphere contains billions of nerve cell bodies that directly or indirectly control most functions of the body. This area of the brain is where interpretation, judgment, feelings, and the like are registered. The cerebral cortex is divided into lobes, and these lobes control both sensory and motor functions that involve involuntary and voluntary actions, the special senses, and intellectual abilities.

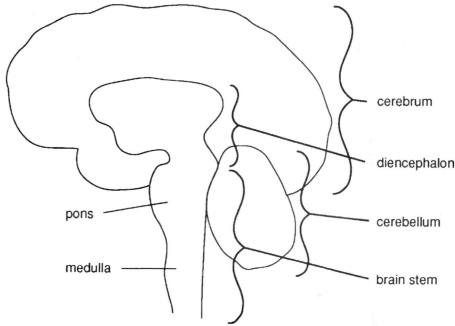

FIGURE 3–1   General Anatomy of the CNS.

Diencephalon

This area is located immediately above the brain stem and is composed mainly of the thalamus and hypothalamus. The main function of the *thalamus* is to serve as a relay station for most sensory input into the CNS. It functions as a center for interpretation of pain, touch, and control of body temperature. The functions of the *hypothalamus* are to control temperature, water balance, sleep cycles, the autonomic nervous system, and certain emotions.

Brain Stem

The brain stem extends from the foramen magnum to the base of the diencephalon and consists of the *medulla* and the *pons*. The functions of the pons are to act as a sensory relay center and respiratory rhythmicity center. The functions of the medulla are to control respiration, vascular tone, heart rate, and gastrointestinal (GI) function.

Cerebellum

This area is located inferior to the cerebrum and posterior to the brain stem. The main function of the cerebellum is coordination of motor skills and *proprioception*.

EFFECTS OF DRUGS IN THE CNS

In general, drugs manifest their effects in the CNS in a fashion similar to their effects in the peripheral nervous system, but because of the complexity of the organization of the CNS, drug action there is much harder to predict and understand. For example, drugs in the CNS work at synapses just as they do in the peripheral nervous system, but in the CNS there are multiple neurotransmitters and multiple receptor sites. A few CNS drugs are quite selective but most are nonspecific regarding their site of action, and many side effects can result from this lack of specificity. A major problem in studying CNS pharmacology is that there are 50–100 billion neurons interconnected by complex circuitry. Unlike the autonomic and somatic nervous systems, where there are few neurotransmitters, the CNS contains multiple neurotransmitters, neuromodulators, and neurohumoral substances such as acetylcholine, norepinephrine, epinephrine, dopamine, serotonin (5-hydroxytryptamine; 5-HT), amino acids, and various neuropeptides. These multiple neurotransmitters, along with multiple excitatory and inhibitory inputs, cause a variety of effects. As a result, it is often difficult to predict the effect of a particular drug in the CNS.

Finally, some of the mechanisms of action of drugs in the CNS are similar to those in the peripheral nervous system but, because of the complexity of organization of the CNS, the possibilities of drug action at the synaptic site are greatly increased. CNS drugs can alter the effect of transmitters by enhancement, prolongation, antagonism, or various other mechanisms. Also, CNS drugs can alter the amount of neurotransmitters released by increasing or reducing the synthesis of these substances.

Therefore, because of the great complexity in the CNS, many mechanisms of action are not completely understood and, for some CNS drugs, the specific mechanism of action, the receptor site, and the site of action are still unknown.

GENERAL CHARACTERISTICS OF CNS DRUGS

The following characteristics are common to most CNS drugs and, although they are not applicable to all, they do apply to most. In order to understand these characteristics, we will use a balance diagram as shown in Figure 3–2. (*Note:* The terms used in the scale in Figure 3–2 only approximate the levels of excitability and depression in the CNS.)

1. **The potency or efficacy of CNS drugs is limited.** If a stimulant drug is administered, the level of excitation of one excitatory drug is not necessarily the same as that of another. The same characteristic applies to depressant drugs (see Figure 3–3).
2. **Many CNS drugs are additive when administered together.** This is particularly true of depressant drugs. For example, when alcohol is taken with barbiturates, the depressant effect is intensified as a result of the *synergistic* effect of both drugs (see Figure 3–4).

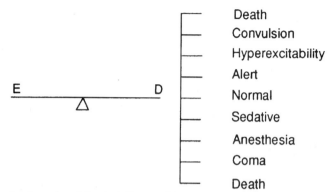

FIGURE 3–2   Levels of Excitability and Depression of the CNS.

3. **Antagonism between stimulants and depressants is variable.** Clinically, if one wants to offset the depressant effect of a drug by administering a stimulant or vice versa, the effect often is unpredictable and extremely variable (see Figure 3–5).
4. **Low doses of some depressant drugs often cause some excitation.** When some depressant drugs are administered, there is often a brief period of excitation that occurs. For example, when a general anesthetic is administered, there is an excitement phase that occurs before the patient reaches a deeper state of anesthesia.
5. **Acute or chronic excitation that is drug induced often is followed by a period of depression.** When the CNS has been functioning at a high level of excitation over a period of time, either drug induced (e.g., following the long-term use of amphetamines) or in a convulsive state, a period of depression usually follows.
6. **Chronic depression that is drug induced is followed by a period of excitation.** This often is manifest when an individual has been taking depressant drugs such as narcotics or barbiturates for a period of time and then terminates the medication (see

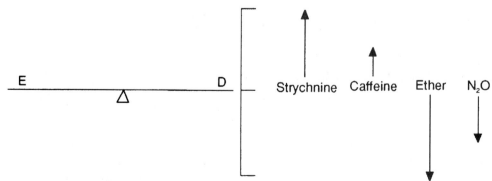

FIGURE 3–3   Limited Potency and Efficacy of CNS Drugs.

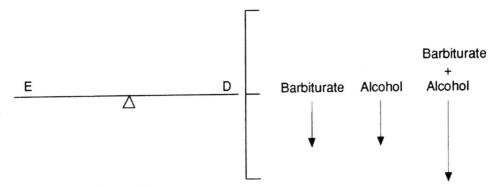

FIGURE 3–4   Additive Effects of CNS Drugs.

Figure 3–6). For example, this type of mechanism probably occurs when withdrawal symptoms are seen after the patient stops taking a depressant-type drug.

SEDATIVE HYPNOTICS AND ANTIANXIETY DRUGS

These drugs represent a diverse group of therapeutic agents that are widely used and also often abused by the patient. The original sedative hypnotic drugs were the barbiturates and nonbarbiturate-type agents, but these drugs have been replaced by the benzodiazepines (antianxiety agents) because of their greater selectivity, improved safety, fewer drug interactions, and a lower dependency and abuse potential. In order to better understand the sedative hypnotic and antianxiety drugs, the appropriate terminology used for clinical classifications follows:

- *Sedative*—produces a calming effect, decrease in CNS activity, and drowsiness.

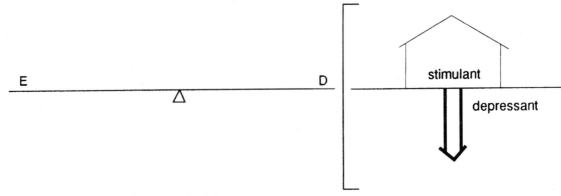

FIGURE 3–5   Antagonism between CNS Drugs.

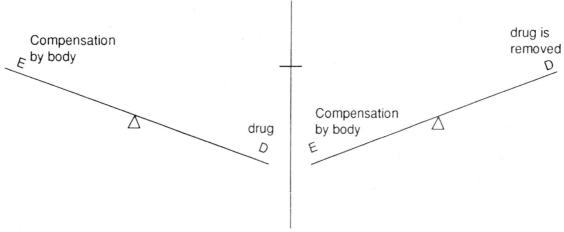

FIGURE 3–6 Chronic Depression followed by Excitation.

- *Hypnotic*—produces drowsiness and facilitates the onset of sleep.
- *Antianxiety agent* (anxiolytic) reduces anxiousness, particularly an incapacitating or inappropriate anxiety.

It should be noted that sedation and hypnosis are related to dose; that is, if the dose of a sedative drug is increased, it will lead to either hypnosis or sleep. Also, if a hypnotic drug is given at a less than a therapeutic dose, it will create sedation.

BARBITURATES

Historically the barbiturates have been the prototype agents used as sedative hypnotics, but with the introduction of the benzodiazepines and some recently developed newer drugs, they are considered obsolete as sedative hypnotics. They do, however, have a number of valid uses in other areas of medicine, and therefore a brief description of their pharmacology is presented.

As a group, the barbiturates are powerful CNS depressants, and the amount of CNS depression is dose related. This means they have the potential to depress the CNS to the level of coma or even death. Because these agents have no anagelsic property, any type of surgical procedure that is performed using these agents should be done in combination with an analgesic. They are metabolized in the liver and produce a clinically significant induction of the hepatic microsomal enzyme system that affects the metabolism of other drugs. They have little effect on the cardiovascular system in terms of altering heart rate or blood pressure, unless given in excessive amounts. They exhibit the phenomenon of *redistribution*, which means that, following absorption, barbiturates often are redistributed or stored in fatty tissue throughout the body. This tends to create a secondary site for

TABLE 3–1 Classification of Barbiturates

DRUG	DURATION OF ACTION	CLINICAL USE
Thiopental (Pentothal[R])	Ultra short (less than 1 hr)	Induction of surgical anesthesia
Pentobarbital (Nembutal[R])	Intermediate (30 min–3 hr)	Sedative/hypnotic
Phenobarbital (Luminal[R])	Long-acting (6 hr)	Anticonvulsant

release of drug later on, and thus many barbiturates tend to have a long-acting or *hangover* effect. Also, the barbiturates have a strong addiction liability, which can cause a life-threatening withdrawal scenario. Finally, they can be used as sedatives or hypnotic drugs but, when used as sleeping agents, they do not produce a normal physiological rapid eye movement (REM) sleep pattern.

In summary, the main therapeutic uses of the barbiturates today include induction agents in general anesthesia, anticonvulsants in treating epilepsy, and backup sedative hypnotic agents. Table 3–1 shows a brief summary of a few of the more common barbiturates, with an approximate range of their duration of action and some main clinical uses.

Nonbarbiturate Sedative Hypnotics

This group of drugs has some historical significance, because they were developed with the intent to reduce the tolerance and addiction liability prevalent with the barbiturates. However, many of these drugs have become obsolete because of the successful long-term use of the benzodiazepines. For the sake of completeness in their role as sedative hypnotics, a few of the more common drugs, along with their duration of action and clinical uses, are listed in Table 3–2.

Benzodiazepines

These drugs are the most widely used sedative hypnotic and antianxiety agents today and have replaced the older barbiturates and related drugs. The shift in usage toward these

TABLE 3–2 Nonbarbiturate Sedative Hypnotics

DRUG	DURATION OF ACTION	CLINICAL USE
Chloral hydrate (Noctec[R])	Short	Hypnotic
Glutethimide (Doriden[R])	Intermediate	Hypnotic
Meprobamate (Miltown[R])	Short	Hypnotic
Ethylchlorvynol (Placidyl[R])	Short	Hypnotic

drugs has occurred because of their greater selectivity, fewer side effects, fewer drug interactions, and lower addiction potential. The benzodiazepines were first introduced in the 1950s with the development of the drug **chlordiazepoxide (Librium[R])**. Since that time numerous other drugs have been introduced, and basically all the agents have similar properties, with some being used for specific conditions.

On a worldwide scale, these drugs represent the most widely prescribed class of drugs. The main clinical use of these drugs is as antianxiety agents, and all of the benzodiazepine drugs produce selective antianxiety effects, with some patients experiencing mild sedation. In some cases the sedative effect may be desirable, but most patients become tolerant to the sedation without losing any therapeutic result. All of these agents can produce dose-related sedation and hypnosis, and most can decrease sleep latency (onset time). When used as sleep agents, discontinuation may lead to rebound effects, especially regarding REM sleep. Many of the drugs have additional CNS effects, and various agents are used for clinical indications such as anticonvulsants, antiepileptics, CNS muscle relaxation, induction of anesthesia, and alcohol and sedative hypnotic withdrawal, and as antidepressants and antipanic agents (see Table 3–3 for specific agents and their therapeutic uses). The overall mechanism of action of the benzodiazepines is that they enhance the effects of the inhibitory γ-aminobutyric acid (GABA) neurotransmitters in the brain.

Benzodiazepines have relatively few adverse effects, and, in contrast to the barbiturates and related agents, overdosage is rarely fatal. In therapeutic doses, these agents do not significantly depress respiration and cardiovascular function; however, when combined with other CNS depressants, especially alcohol, additive effects can cause severe depression. These agents do not have a serious abuse potential; however, tolerance does develop to the sedative and hypnotic effects and occasionally some patients may seem like *zombies* when these drugs have been taken in high doses. Finally, the main side effects are extensions of the therapeutic effects and may include sedation, *ataxia*, dizziness, and hangover.

ALCOHOL (ETHANOL)

Although alcohol (ethyl alcohol) rarely is used as a therapeutic agent, it does have a number of pharmacological actions that affect the whole body. Also, because of its wide social use, it is appropriate that mention be made about its major actions on the body, adverse affects, and addiction liability.

The most prominent effect of alcohol is its ability to depress the CNS, and, like many of the sedative hypnotic drugs, the amount of depression is dose related. Many individuals have the misconception that drinking alcohol provides a stimulatory effect. This apparent stimulation is actually caused by the fact that, in small doses, the inhibitory areas of the brain are depressed first and the "stimulation" is manifested by lack of inhibition, lack of self-consciousness, and, in some cases, violent or obnoxious behavior. As the dose is increased, both the excitatory and inhibitory areas of the brain are depressed, and this gradually leads to sedation, hypnosis, and eventually coma. The exact mechanism of this depression is not fully understood, but it is extremely important that patients are

TABLE 3–3   Benzodiazepines

DRUG	DURATION OF ACTION	CLINICAL USE
Diazepam (Valium[R])	Long	Antianxiety
Chlordiazepoxide (Librium[R])	Long	Antianxiety
Alprazolam (Xanax[R])	Short	Antipanic
Triazolam (Halcion[R])	Short	Sleep aid
Flurazepam (Dalmane[R])	Short	Sleep aid
Buspirone (BuSpar[R])*	Short	Antianxiety/antipanic

*Buspirone is a member of a new group of antianxiety agents that are chemically unrelated to the benzodiazepines. It is included here because of its effectiveness as an antianxiety agent with minimal sedation and no hypnotic effects. It also has few side effects but has shown no potential for tolerance, physical dependency, or abuse.

aware that alcohol has an additive effect when taken with other CNS depressants. Also, it is well documented that chronic use of alcohol leads to neurological and mental disorders, memory loss, sleep disorders, and psychosis.

Other areas that are affected by alcohol include the cardiovascular system, GI tract, and fetal development. In the cardiovascular system, alcohol causes peripheral vasodilation that may create the feeling of warmth, but actually an increase in heat loss and potential hypothermia can occur. In moderate doses, alcohol does not appear to have any affect on coronary blood flow, but, with chronic use, cardiomyopathy may occur. In the GI tract, alcohol can stimulate saliva flow and increase hydrochloric acid secretion in the stomach. With chronic use, this can lead to gastric and duodenal ulcer formation, which is similar to the irritation caused by heavy aspirin use. In regard to fetal development, alcohol consumption can lead to fetal alcohol syndrome (FAS), with the possibility of causing mental dysfunction in the child.

Ethanol has application in respiratory care as a surface active agent (this is discussed in greater detail in Chapter 13). Finally, alcohol has an antiseptic/disinfection action on bacteria and will inhibit bacterial growth when used at 70–90 percent concentration. The major adverse effects of alcohol are well known and include persistent thirst, nausea, vomiting, gastritis, acidosis, fatigue, and headache. Also, it is well established that alcohol is highly addictive; the withdrawal symptoms associated with alcohol addiction can lead to anxiety, tremor, nervousness, delirium, hallucinations, and seizure.

PSYCHOPHARMACOLOGY AND TREATMENT OF MENTAL DISORDERS

Psychopharmacology involves the use of drugs to control or correct the chemical imbalances that may be associated with various mental disorders. Some of the psychological disorders that are treated pharmacologically include schizophrenia, bipolar affective disorder (manic depression), and other major depressions. Research regarding some of these conditions has shown that many have a genetic basis that may lead to an underlying biochemical imbalance; thus many of the clinical conditions can be treated by attempting to correct chemical imbalances with the appropriate use of drugs.

The modern era of psychopharmacology began in the early 1950s with the introduction of the drug chlorpromazine. This drug literally revolutionized the treatment of various mental disorders such as *schizophrenia*. Since the 1950s there has been continual pharmacological progress in the treatment of a variety of psychiatric conditions and behavioral disorders. Presently, the treatment approach to these disorders is pharmacological rather than by incarceration or institutionalization. Psychiatrists today have at their disposal a number of medications that have greatly expanded their ability to treat mental illness. The knowledge of the biology of behavior is growing at a rapid rate and with reasonable diagnostic skill and knowledge of appropriate drugs, many physicians can treat cases of psychiatric disorders that are encountered in general medical practice.

Categories of Psychopharmacological Drugs

The major categories of the psychopharmacological drugs are listed in Table 3–4. Each of these categories is discussed in the following sections.

Antipsychotics

The antipsychotics are a group of agents that are used to treat various types of psychosis, and the prototype drugs are the phenothiazines. There are at least 15 different phenothiazine drugs currently used today. All of these agents have similar properties; therefore, we will discuss only **chlorpromazine (Thorazine^R)** as a representative. In general, chlorpromazine, as well as the other phenothiazines, are used to treat psychiatric disorders by decreasing anxiety, anger, psychomotor excitement, social withdrawal, aggression, and hallucinations. These drugs also improve an individuals coherency and organization of thought and improve speaking ability. The beneficial effects are particularly evident in the treatment of schizophrenia. Chlorpromazine produces a greater sedative effect than many of the other phenothiazines, and this property is useful in treating acutely psychotic patients who have sleep disorders and severe emotional turmoil. In addition, chlorpromazine has a narcotic potentiating effect and sometimes is administered with narcotics to amplify the pain relief in terminally ill patients. Although phenothiazine drugs are effective adjuncts to psychiatric therapy, when the drugs are administered for long periods of time, they result in a variety of side effects.

A number of adverse effects associated with phenothiazine drugs include agranulocytosis, photosensitivity (sensitivity of the cornea of the eye), hypotension, and, most commonly, the development of *extrapyramidal* movements. Extrapyramidal movements, or Parkinson-like movements, are more common with high doses of the more potent phenothiazine drugs. The most serious chronic condition that occurs with long-term use of chlorpromazine is *tardive dyskinesia*, which consists of a variety of involuntary movements

TABLE 3–4 Psychopharmacological Drugs

CATEGORY	MAIN DRUGS	RELATED PSYCHIATRIC DISORDER
Antipsychotics	Chlorpromazine (Thorazine[R])	Psychosis
Antidepressants	Tricyclic antidepressant (TCA) Imipramine (Tofranil[R])	Various types of depression
	MAO inhibitors Isocarboxazid (Marplan[R])	Various types of depression
	New-generation antidepressants	
	Fluoxetine (Prozac[R])	Various types of depression
	Trazodone (Desyrel[R])	Various types of depression
	Bupropion (Wellbutrin[R])	Various types of depression
Mood stabilizers	Lithium carbonate, carbamazepine (Tegretol[R])	Manic depression
Psychostimulants	Methylphenidate (Ritalin[R]) various amphetamines	Hyperactivity
Antianxiety/sedative agents	Chlordiazepoxide (Librium[R]), diazepam (Valium[R])	Anxiety
Miscellaneous		
Nocturnal enuresis	Imipramine (Tofranil[R])	Nocturnal enuresis
Panic attack	TCAs and MAOs*	Panic attacks
Anxiety	Propranolol (Inderal[R])	Public speaking, stage fright, and examination problems
Opiate addiction	Clonidine (Catapres[R])	Opiate withdrawal
Gilles de la Tourette syndrome	Haloperidol (Haldol[R])	Tourette syndrome

*TCA = tricyclic antidepressant, MAO = monoamine oxidase.

in the face, mouth, and tongue. Tardive dyskinesia, along with other extrapyramidal movements tends to disappear during sleep and is suppressed by voluntary movements.

Table 3–5 lists some of the more commonly used phenothiazine drugs.

Treatment of Depression

The main treatment modality of major depressive disorders in todays medical practice is the use of pharmacological agents. Some of the conditions that respond to drug therapy include the depressive phase of manic depression, unipolar depression, and chronic organic brain syndromes with severe depression. The conditions that respond most favorably to drugs are those with biological factors resulting from a decrease of or imbalance in brain

TABLE 3–5 Phenothiazine Drugs

DRUGS	POTENCY (LOW TO HIGH)	CLINICAL USE
Thioridazine (Mellaril[R])	Least	Antipsychotic
Chlorpromazine (Thorazine[R])	Low	Antipsychotic
Perphenazine (Trilafon[R])	Higher	Antipsychotic
Fluphenazine (Prolixin[R])	Most	Antipsychotic

neurotransmitters. There are various other types of short-term depressions that occur throughout life, such as a death in the family, divorce, or financial loss. These short-term depressions can be treated with medications, but their response to drug therapy is unpredictable and not well documented. However, these mood changes should not be ignored; probably these patients should be referred to a psychiatrist or psychologist for evaluation.

Table 3–6 lists the categories of drugs used in treating various types of depressive disorders.

Tricyclic Antidepressants and Monoamine Oxidase Inhibitors. The principal drugs that are used in treating various depressive disorders are the tricyclic antidepressants (TCAs) and the monamine oxidase inhibitors (MAOIs). The TCAs are used more often because the MAOIs have a greater potential for toxicity and interaction with certain foods and drugs. The current theories of mechanisms of actions are that both the TCAs and the MAOIs increase the levels of norepinephrine and/or serotonin in brain tissue. It is thought

TABLE 3–6 Drugs Used to Treat Depressive Disorders

DRUG CATEGORY	EXAMPLES	CLINICAL USE
Tricyclic antidepressants (TCAs)	Imipramine (Tofranil[R])	Depression
	Amitriptyline (Elavil[R])	Depression
Monoamine oxidase inhibitors (MAOIs)	Isocarboxazid (Marplan[R])	Depression
	Phenelzine (Nardil[R])	Depression
	Tranylcypromine (Parnate[R])	Depression
New-generation antidepressants*	Trazodone (Desyrel[R])	Depression, sleep disorders
	Doxepin (Sinequan[R])	Depression
	Fluoxetine (Prozac[R])	Depression
	Bupropion (Wellbutrin[R])	Depression
	Amoxapine (Asendin[R])	Depression

*Both Wellbutrin[R] and Asendin[R] have the potential to induce seizures, and Asendin[R] also can cause an increase in extrapyramidal effects.

that low levels of these neurotransmitters, or a functional imbalance of these substances, are responsible for various forms of depression. The TCAs increase the levels of norepinephrine and serotonin by blocking the reuptake of each of these neurotransmitters into the nerve ending. The MAOIs inactivate the enzyme monoamine oxidase in the nerve ending, and thus increase the levels of norepinephrine and serotonin being secreted by the nerve ending. Regardless of what mechanism is operative, the TCAs and MAOIs increase levels of these excitatory neurotransmitters that somehow counteract the effect of depression. For reasons that are not understood, both of these drug groups have a latency of onset of about 2–3 weeks, which often can be frustrating for a patient suffering from severe depression.

The side effects of the TCAs are very similar to those of the phenothiazine drugs, except that there are fewer extrapyramidal movements. Both categories exhibit an anticholinergic property that produces blurred vision, dry mouth, constipation, impotence, and urinary retention. In therapeutic doses, some of the TCAs can cause tachycardia and arrhythmias, and this can also occur with use of MAOIs. Cardiovascular side effects can be very serious with the use of MAOIs, primarily as a result of interactions with other drugs and foods containing the amino acid tyrosine, which is metabolized to tyramine. Tyramine precedes the release of norepinephrine and epinephrine, and patients who are taking chronic doses of MAOIs should be carefully monitored and instructed to avoid foods containing tyrosine. In a patient taking MAOIs, the levels of norepinephrine are already elevated, and with the addition of tyramine in the diet, more norepinephrine is released. Thus the norepinephrine levels increase to a point at which increased vasoconstriction can occur, causing a severe hypertensive crisis.

New-Generation Antidepressants. In the past few years there have been a number of new-generation antidepressant drugs introduced. In general, these drugs are more selective regarding their effects on various neurotransmitters in the CNS. Several drugs of this group block the reuptake of norepinephrine, whereas others specifically block the reuptake of serotonin (5-HT). Regardless of which neurotransmitter is affected, current technologies are unavailable to link a specific biochemical abnormality to a given clinical disease. Because the newer drugs have fewer side effects and have a more rapid onset of action, prescriptions for these agents have been rapidly growing over the last few years.

Although the new drugs do have their own set of adverse effects, they are less dangerous, but some can be annoying. The adverse effects of the new-generation antidepressants include anorexia, dizziness, increased seizure activity, and extrapyramidal effects. Table 3–7 lists some of the "new generation" antidepressants.

Mood Stabilizers

These drugs are used in two clinical conditions: to treat acute manic attacks and as preventative agents against recurrence of manic–depressive episodes. For years **lithium carbonate** has been the main drug used to control these two conditions. Mania is a condition wherein the patient is in an extremely high level of excitation, and in manic–depression the patient alternates between high activity and a depressed state. Lithium reduces the frequency of manic–depression cycles, and in higher doses can control the

TABLE 3–7 "New Generation" Antidepressants		
GENERIC NAME	BRAND NAME	CLINICAL USE
Trazodone	Desyrel[R]	Sleep disorders
Doxepin	Sinequan[R]	Antidepressant
Fluoxetine	Prozac[R]	Antidepressant
Bupropion	Wellbutrin[R]	Antidepressant
Amoxapine	Asendin[R]	Antidepressant

*Both Wellbutrin[R] and Asendin[R] have potential to induce seizures and Asendin[R] can also cause an increase in extrapyramidal effects.

manic phase of the disorder. However, some manics do not respond to lithium, and recently an anticonvulsant drug, **carbamazepine (Tegretol[R])**, has proven to be effective when given in combination with lithium. Carbamazepine is a drug that is related to the TCAs and is used not only as an anticonvulsant but also in treating various neuralgias, such as *trigeminal neuralgia*. Carbamazepine recently has been shown in a number of studies to be an effective antimania drug. However, it is much more toxic than lithium and can cause problems in the hematopoietic system, leading to aplastic anemia.

The mechanism of action of lithium is to exert its effect as a *cation* similar to sodium and potassium. It increases the reuptake of norepinephrine and serotonin and thus decreases the levels of these excitatory neurotransmitters in the synaptic cleft. Adverse effects of lithium are seldom seen when the dosage is maintained at normal therapeutic levels, but individuals who are taking higher levels of these drugs can experience some of the following side effects: in the GI tract, nausea, vomiting, and diarrhea; in the CNS, tremors, confusion, and, in some cases of overdose, coma; and in the cardiovascular system, arrhythmia and hypotension. It also should be noted that, in some individuals, chronic doses of lithium can lead to an enlarged thyroid gland along with altered renal function.

Psychostimulant Drugs

This group of drugs usually includes the amphetamines and methylphenidate (Ritalin[R]). Although these drugs are not classified as antidepressants, they may be used to treat certain types of depression or temporary grief reactions. The main effect of these drugs is to increase the levels of norepinephrine in the brain tissue, and this is brought about by several mechanisms: direct stimulation of adrenergic receptors, release of norepinephrine from storage sites, and prevention of norepinephrine reuptake. In addition, amphetamines stimulate physical activity and are also powerful *anorexic* agents.

Their major clinical use today is in the treatment of the hyperactivity syndrome in children. Because these drugs increase mental and physical activity, it is paradoxical that they are the drug of choice in treating hyperactive individuals. The exact mechanism by which these stimulant drugs cause a calming effect in hyperactivity is not understood.

When the drugs are used therapeutically in treating hyperactive children, they improve attention span and ability to concentrate and cause a decrease in diffuse hyperactivity. The drugs are effective in about 70 percent of hyperactive children with normal intelligence. Response is less predictable in hyperactive patients with mild to borderline retardation, and individuals with moderate to severe retardation become worse when treated with the psychostimulant drugs.

These drugs also are used as temporary appetite suppressants in the treatment of overweight individuals. The adverse effects include stimulation of the sympathetic nervous system, dry mouth, increased heart rate, increased blood pressure, restlessness, and insomnia. A major problem associated with these drugs when used as appetite suppressants is the development of addiction, with rapidly developing tolerance. Abrupt withdrawal of the drug is very dangerous and may lead to extreme agitation and paranoia.

Table 3–8 lists some common psychostimulant drugs used today.

Antianxiety Drugs

The antianxiety drugs are a group of medications that have been discussed earlier under the heading of sedative hypnotic/antianxiety drugs. These drugs were at one time labeled *minor tranquilizers*, but this term is no longer used. As a group, the antianxiety drugs can include barbiturates, nonbarbiturate sedative hypnotics, alcohol, and the benzodiazepines. Recently a new drug, not related chemically to the benzodiazepines or the barbiturates, has been introduced. This drug, **buspirone (Buspar**[R]**)**, has excellent antianxiety effects, no anticonvulsant effects, and little sedation.

The benzodiazepines have become the "mainstay" agents for treating anxiety because they have the highest therapeutic index and safety. All of the drugs in the group have some value in treating short-term severe anxiety or reactive depression, but many can cause behavioral and physical dependence. Some cause withdrawal that is complicated by convulsive seizures. Physical dependence on the benzodiazepines is relatively uncommon, and they are the main antianxiety agents currently used.

Some of the common antianxiety drugs are listed in Table 3–9.

Miscellaneous Disorders Treated by Psychopharmacological Agents

There are a number of miscellaneous clinical conditions in the area of psychopharmacology that respond to drug therapy. This chapter does not discuss any detail regarding etiology and clinical manifestations, but Table 3–10 lists some of the disorders and current medications used.

EPILEPSY

Epilepsy is a fairly common CNS disorder that occurs in both the old and the young. There are many ways of defining epilepsy but, most simply stated, it is a *paroxysmal*

TABLE 3–8 Psyychostimulants		
DRUG	**TRADE NAME**	**USE**
Dextroamphetamine	Dexedrine[R]	Anorexia and hyperactivity
Methamphetamine	Desoxyn[R]	Anorexia and hyperactivity
Methylphenidate	Ritalin[R]	Hyperactivity

(sudden onset) increase of CNS activity that is recurrent, has *stereotypic* clinical characteristics, and is associated with a massive discharge of electrochemical activity that is self-limiting. The frequency and severity of episodes is dependent on the portion of the CNS that is involved. There are many etiological factors that are associated with the various forms of epilepsy; these may include trauma, infection, stroke, alcohol, various drugs, hypoglycemia, anorexia, and genetic predisposition.

The classification of seizure activity is very lengthy, and, because of the introductory level of this text, only the following broad categories are described:

1. Partial seizure
   a. **Simple**—relatively localized discharge in the brain without loss of consciousness.
   b. **Complex**—loss of consciousness with many autonomic nervous system behaviors (this is the most difficult type to diagnose).
2. Primary generalized seizure
   a. **Absence** (petit mal)—characterized by rapid onset, loss of consciousness, and mild rhythmic movements.
   b. **Tonic–clonic** (grand mal)—counts for about 4–10 percent of seizures and can occur during both sleep and wakeful periods; also, some of these can be precipitated by sleep deprivation, alcohol intake, and fatigue.

Diagnosis of epilepsy can be very complicated and difficult and is best done by a neurologist and/or neurosurgeon. First, it requires an accurate and complete family history, a description of a seizure by the patient and a witness, a detailed

TABLE 3–9 Antianxiety Drugs		
DRUG	**TYPE**	**USE**
Phenobarbital (Luminal[R])	Barbiturate	Antianxiety/sedative hypnotic
Meprobamate (Miltown[R])	Nonbarbiturate/sedative hypnotic	Antianxiety agent
Diazepam (Valium[R])	Benzodiazepine	Antianxiety agent
Alprazolam (Xanax[R])	Benzodiazepine	Antianxiety agent
Triazolam (Halcion[R])	Benzodiazepine	Antianxiety agent
Buspirone (BuSpar[R])	New	Antianxiety agent

TABLE 3–10 Miscellaneous Disorders

DISORDERS	DRUG
Nocturnal enuresis	Imipramine (Tofranil[R])
Panic attack	TCAs and MAIOs
Public speaking, stage fright, test anxiety	Propranolol (Inderal[R])
Opiate addiction, withdrawal	Clonidine (Catapres[R])
Tourette syndrome	Haloperidol (Haldol[R]) and clonidine

neurological and physical examination, and an initial electroencephalogram (EEG) to try to identify the seizure type. In addition to the standard techniques, specialized diagnostic procedures such as computerized tomographic (CT) scanning and magnetic resonance imaging (MRI) also can be helpful. Once the diagnosis has been established, overall management of epilepsy is dependent on the selection of an appropriate drug. The long-term goal should be the use of one-drug *monotherapy*, and only when monotherapy medication has failed should a second agent be added to the regimen. Management of the patient with only one medication offers many advantages, such as better control of toxicity, improved patient compliance, avoidance of unpredictable drug interactions, and better control of unusual side effects.

Antiepileptic Drugs

Because of the many types of epilepsy, precise diagnosis is extremely important in order to make an appropriate drug selection. Although there are many alternative drugs and drug combinations that can be used, this chapter discusses only six main antiepileptic drugs.

Phenytoin (Dilantin[R]). Therapeutic use: one of the first-choice drugs in treating a primary generalized grand mal-type seizure. **Mechanism of action:** prevents the spread of seizure in the brain by blocking sodium channels and inhibiting sustained repetitive firing. **Adverse effects:** astigmatism of the eyes, thinking impairment, incoordination, and dyskinesia.

Carbamazepine (Tegretol[R]). Therapeutic use: one of the first-choice drugs to treat primary generalized grand mal-type seizures. **Mechanism of action:** same as that of phenytoin. **Adverse effects:** ocular problems, vertigo, lethargy, and dyskinesia.

Valproic Acid (Depakene[R]). Therapeutic uses: same as that of phenytoin and carbamazepine but also used in certain types of petit mal seizure. **Mechanism of action:** prevents spread of seizure activity by enhancing the inhibitory GABA pathways and blocking repetitive firing. **Adverse effects:** GI problems, tremor, behavioral changes, and, in some individuals, hepatic failure when used in combination with other antiepileptic drugs.

Ethosuximide (Zarontin[R])   **Therapeutic use:** the first-choice drug in the treatment of petit mal seizures. **Mechanism of action:** raises seizure threshold by reducing calcium current. **Adverse effects:** anorexia, nervousness, fatigue, and insomnia.

Phenobarbital (Luminal[R]).   **Therapeutic uses:** as an alternate in treatment of grand mal seizure, particularly in children and in individuals who cannot tolerate phenytoin; also used in treating status epilepticus. **Mechanism of action:** enhances inhibitory GABA pathways and blocks repetitive firing. **Adverse effects:** sedation, changes in sleep patterns, and cognitive impairment.

Diazepam (Valium[R]).   **Therapeutic use:** treating status epilepticus. **Mechanism of action:** same as that of phenytoin. **Adverse effects:** some lethargy and depression.

PARKINSONISM

Parkinsonism is a disease that usually occurs in middle age and becomes progressively worse. It is caused by a lack of dopamine-containing neurons in the CNS. In the substantia nigra area of one of the cerebral nuclei (the area where the dopamine neurons are located), there is normally a balance between excitatory and inhibitory neurons. The excitatory neurons release acetylcholine and the inhibitory neurons release dopamine. Because there is a decrease in the amount of dopamine released in parkinsonism, there is a resultant increase in influence by acetylcholine-containing neurons; this causes an increase in skeletal muscle contraction. The symptoms of parkinsonism occur rather slowly at first, but gradually become chronic and include tremor, rigidity, *akinesia, bradykinesia*, and loss of balance. The exact cause of parkinsonism is considered idiopathic (unknown), but some authorities have linked the onset of the disease with such problems as postencephalitic disease, arteriosclerosis, neuroepileptic disease, and toxin-induced disease.

Treatment of Parkinsonism

The current approach to treating parkinsonism is to increase the levels of dopamine in the CNS. Although dopamine does not pass the blood–brain barrier, it was discovered in the mid-1960s that the immediate precursor to dopamine, levodopa, is readily absorbed into the CNS and is then converted to dopamine by the enzyme dopadecarboxylase. Therefore, the main objective of treatment is to administer levodopa or any other medication that directly or indirectly increases the level of dopamine. The following drugs currently are used in the treatment of parkinsonism.

Levodopa.   **Therapeutic use:** the essential drug in treating Parkinson disease and the cornerstone of all therapy. **Mechanism of action:** passes the blood–brain barrier and is converted to dopamine by dopadecarboxylase. **Adverse effects:** causes postural hypotension, mental confusion, and hallucinations. After long-term use, this drug can have a great deal of variability in its effectiveness and a condition called dyskinesia (abnormal involuntary movements) often occurs.

Levodopa plus Carbidopa (Sinemet[R]).   **Therapeutic use:** increases the absorption of levodopa and provides a longer duration of action. **Mechanism of action:** inhibits the action of the enzyme dopadecarboxylase in the blood so that more levodopa is transported to the brain. **Adverse effects:** same as with levodopa; the combination sometimes makes dosage regulation difficult.

Dopamine Agonists: Bromocriptine Mesylate (Parlodel[R]), and Pergolide (Permax[R]). **Therapeutic use:** used in combination with levodopa to decrease the amount of levodopa needed. **Mechanism of action:** act as substitutes for dopamine by combining with the same dopamine receptors in the CNS. **Adverse effects:** nausea, some hypertension, nervousness, hallucinations, and anemia.

Trihexyphenidyl (Artane[R]). **Therapeutic use:** given in combination with levodopa in the early stages of the disease. **Mechanism of action:** is an anticholinergic thought to restore the balance between dopamine and acetylcholine in the CNS by blocking the action of acetylcholines. **Adverse effects:** anticholinergic effects such as dry mouth, constipation, and urinary retention; also memory loss, speech difficulty, and confusion.

Amantadine (Symmetrel[R]). **Therapeutic use:** used in combination with levodopa in the early stages of the disease. **Mechanism of action:** increases levels of dopamine by inhibiting dopamine reuptake at the nerve terminal. **Adverse effects:** causes edema, decrease of sexual drive, nervousness, and insomnia.

Deprenyl (selegiline; Eldepryl[R]). **Therapeutic use:** used in combination with Sinemet[R] in the early stages of disease and extends the time before levodopa is needed. It has very little effect in the advanced stages. **Mechanism of action:** thought to reduce breakdown of dopamine by inhibiting the enzyme monoamine oxidase. **Adverse effects:** hypertension, nervousness, and insomnia.

GENERAL ANESTHETICS

A general anesthetic can be defined as a drug that induces the absence of all sensation. There are many theories as to the mechanism of action of general anesthetics. They represent a clinically diverse group of drugs that the evidence seems to suggest work less specifically on membrane function rather than working through a specific receptor site. Although there are probably several different types of mechanisms operating, the current theory is that general anesthetics stabilize membranes of excitable tissue by influencing synaptic transmission. When general anesthetic agents are administered, they cause direct depression of the CNS so that various surgical procedures can be performed without regard to patient discomfort. However, there are other effects that occur, such as cardiovascular depression caused by a direct effect on the myocardium and vascular smooth muscle. The effect that general anesthetics exert on neuronal structures mainly occurs on synaptic transmission. They have little effect on neuronal conduction of impulses in the axons of nerves of the CNS.

With the introduction of ether as a general anesthetic agent in the mid-1800s, various clinical stages of anesthesia were observed and documented. These stages of anesthesia were particularly important in the early days of general anesthetic administration in order to determine the approximate level of CNS depression. With the development

TABLE 3-11	Stages of Anesthesia
STAGE	DESCRIPTION
I	*Stage of Analgesia*: affects the midbrain medullary centers and certain spinal cord areas
II	*Stage of Excitation*: affects the subcortical inhibition centers and causes excitation, delirium, and amnesia
III	*Stage of Surgical Anesthesia*: can be subdivided into four planes*: Plane 1: affects midbrain with surgical anesthesia Plane 2: affects midbrain with surgical anesthesia Plane 3: spinal cord/deep surgical anesthesia Plane 4: spinal cord/deep surgical anesthesia
IV	*Stage of Medullary Suppression*: affects the respiratory and cardiovascular center, causing apnea, coma, and death

*The four distinct planes of surgical anesthesia are only seen when using ether.

of sophisticated monitoring devices, the observation of the various stages of anesthesia is not quite as important. However, a well-qualified anesthesiologist must be able to observe the clinical signs of these stages along with the use of monitoring devices. The stages of anesthesia are presented in Table 3–11 in order to acquaint the student with the levels of CNS depression that occur during administration of general anesthesia.

When a general anesthetic is administered, it is important that the patient passes through the "excitement stage" as quickly and smoothly as possible. Most general surgery is performed in stage III anesthesia supplemented by infusion of a muscle relaxant drug. Obviously stage IV is avoided because of the danger of coma and death.

Properties of an Ideal General Anesthetic

There is no single agent available today that combines all of the qualities that are desirable for an ideal general anesthetic. Table 3–12 lists all the properties deemed necessary for safe and effective anesthesia. An anesthesiologist uses a combination of agents in an attempt to achieve as many of the desirable characteristics as possible.

Classification of General Anesthetics

General anesthetics are a diverse group of drugs that include gases, volatile liquids, and intravenous agents. Table 3–13 lists the available agents according to method of administration and form.

Inhalation General Anesthetics

Since the demonstration of anesthesia with the gas nitrous oxide (N_2O) by Wells in 1844 and the volatile liquid ether (C_2H_5O) by Morton in 1846, the inhalation anesthetics have

TABLE 3–12   Characteristics of an Ideal General Anesthetic

1. High margin of safety at all levels
2. Capable of producing surgical anesthesia
3. Rapid and pleasant during induction and recovery
4. Easily controlled and regulated at all levels
5. Few side effects or toxicity
6. Not depressive to the cardiovascular system and respiratory center
7. Nonflammable and nonexplosive
8. Good analgesia
9. Good muscle relaxation
10. Low cost

been the mainstay of general anesthesia. The following discussion describes the various inhalation agents available along with some advantages, disadvantages, and current uses.

Nitrous Oxide.   A gas introduced in 1844, this is the most widely used general anesthetic agent and often is used as an adjunct with general anesthetic agents in order to decrease the need for high concentrations of more potent agents. **Advantages:** rapid induction, good analgesia; not metabolized in the liver, excreted by the lungs, and has little effect on the cardiovascular system. **Disadvantages:** low level of potency; also, if used alone, requires a high concentration and thus endangers adequate levels of O_2. **Current uses:** widely used as an adjunct to other general anesthetics and as an analgesic agent.

Cyclopropane.   A gas introduced in 1934. **Advantages:** potent, rapid induction with little effect on the cardiovascular system, and pleasant induction. **Disadvantages:** causes cardiac arrhythmias, metabolized in the liver, excreted by lungs, and is highly explosive when mixed with oxygen. **Current use:** not used today.

Diethyl Ether.   A volatile liquid introduced in 1846. **Advantages:** slow induction that allows management for safety; stimulates respiration and has very little effect on the cardiovascular system. **Disadvantages:** slow and sometimes stormy induction because of

TABLE 3–13   General Anesthetics

Inhalation
   Gases-nitrous oxide, cyclopropane
   Volatile liquids–ether, halothane, methoxyflurane
Intravenous agents–narcotics, narcotic-N_2O combination, neurolep-anesthesia, high/
   dose-high/potency narcotics

laryngeal irritation, nausea, and vomiting, and slow emergence; highly flammable. **Current use:** very little use today.

Halothane (Fluothane^R).   A volatile liquid introduced in 1956. **Advantages:** smooth, rapid induction, little laryngeal and bronchial spasm, and good muscle relaxation; relatively inexpensive. **Disadvantages:** depression of respiratory and cardiovascular centers, cardiac arrhythmias; can cause smooth muscle relaxation (uterine *atony*), and severe liver failure (rare). **Current use:** widely used, particularly in pediatrics.

Methoxyflurane (Penthrane^R).   A volatile liquid introduced in 1959. **Advantages:** very potent, and thus provides substantial analgesia and muscle relaxation in small doses, minimal effects on the cardiovascular system. **Disadvantages:** slow induction because of high blood solubility, and renal toxicity. **Current use:** limited; mainly used for analgesia.

Isoflurane (Forane^R)   A volatile liquid introduced in 1971. **Advantages:** rapid induction, good potency, good muscle relaxation, and low organ toxicity because of inert quality; causes good cardiac output even at high doses. **Disadvantages:** irritating to the airway and relatively expensive; causes respiratory depression. **Current use:** widely used today.

Enflurane (Ethrane^R).   A volatile liquid introduced in 1966. **Advantages:** relatively inexpensive. **Disadvantages:** low potency; depresses the cardiovascular system and respiratory center, can produce seizure activity and some hypotension, and metabolized to some extent in the kidney with minimal kidney toxicity. **Current use:** rarely used today.

Intravenous General Anesthetics

The intravenous anesthetics are an alternative method of producing general anesthesia and are used primarily in short-term procedures or for outpatient surgeries, such as oral, ophthalmologic, and minor surgery.

Droperidol or Diazepam and (Narcotic).   **Advantages:** control of cardiovascular system, profound analgesia, good postoperative analgesia, minimal toxicity, rapid emergence; generally inexpensive and can be reversed with naloxone (narcotic antagonist). **Disadvantages:** risk of postoperative respiratory depression, no muscle relaxation, does not block auditory input during procedure. **Current use:** frequent.

Fentanyl (High-Dose Narcotic Agent).   **Advantages and disadvantages:** the same as with the narcotic combinations above. **Current use:** Rarely used today.

Ketamine (Phencycline^R) (High-Dose Narcotic Agent).   PCP derivative introduced during the early 1960s. **Advantages:** intravenous route, profound analgesia; cardiovascular stimulant with little effect on the respiratory system, and rapid onset and short duration. **Disadvantages:** direct cardiac depressant; increased muscle tone and prolonged vivid dreams and unpleasant nightmares. **Current use:** rarely used today.

Propofol (Diprivan^R) (High-Dose Narcotic Agent).   A newer hypnotic agent used for anesthetic induction and maintenance. **Advantages:** Very potent, intravenous route, rapid induction, rapid recovery. **Disadvantages:** Respiratory depression; causes brief periods of apnea. **Current use:** occasionally used today.

TABLE 3–14 Preanesthetic Agents

CATEGORY	EXAMPLE	USE
Analgesic	Morphine, fentanyl	To relieve pain and create sedation
Antianxiety agent	Diazepam, triazolam (Halcion)	Decrease apprehension
Sedative hypnotic	Barbiturates	Decrease apprehension
Anticholinergic agent	Atropine, glycopyrrolate	Decrease salivary and bronchial secretions

Preanesthetic Medications

Prior to a surgical procedure, patients usually are very apprehensive, frightened, and extremely anxious. This extreme anxiety can increase the overall level of excitability of the CNS, which in some cases can necessitate administering higher levels of general anesthetics to obtain the proper level of surgical anesthesia. In order to control these levels of excitability and anxiety, various drugs can be administered prior to the procedure that have the following effects: analgesia, antianxiety, sedation, hypnosis, and decrease in secretions. Used in various combinations and administered according to specific need, these agents can relieve preoperative and postoperative pain, decrease the amount of general anesthetic agent needed, and decrease adverse side effects. Table 3–14 lists several categories and examples of drugs that are used as preanesthetic agents.

NARCOTIC ANALGESICS

The narcotic analgesics are a group of drugs that decrease pain sensation without the loss of consciousness. Also, in large doses these drugs can depress the CNS, producing sleep and/or sedation. Today most narcotic agents are termed *opioids*, although morphine and codeine are the only naturally occurring substances that can be obtained from the poppy plant (natural source of opium). In this chapter the term *opioid* will be used to include all naturally occurring and synthetic congeners of opium derivatives (morphine and codeine). Thus the terms *narcotic* and *opioid* will be used interchangeably.

In the 1970s, new light was shed on the mechanism of action of narcotic analgesics with the discovery of endogenous "morphine-like substances" called *beta-endorphins* and, later, a group of substances called *dynorphines*. Since the discovery of these agents, many additional groups of substances have been identified. Also, several different receptor sites have been located in the thalamus and other areas of the CNS where these substances can combine. It is currently believed that the combination of endogenous peptides released at these receptor sites is similar to that seen following administration of morphine and other narcotic analgesics. Thus, these receptor sites often are referred to as "morphine-like receptors." It should be noted that there are many different receptors and subreceptor groups that have been identified, but in this text they will be collectively called "opioid receptors" or "morphine receptors."

The type of pain against which narcotic analgesics are effective obviously depends on the patient and the patients level of tolerance to pain. The analgesic action of the narcotic agents does not interfere with the pain sensation at the nerve ending or the conduction of pain impulses to the brain. Rather, these agents depress the cerebral areas in the brain where the interpretation of pain sensation is registered. Given the variability of pain tolerance among patients, narcotics usually are used in treating moderate to severe pain following trauma, myocardial infarction, and surgery, and during terminal illness. With the exception of trauma (which may be somatic), these types of pain are often referred to as *visceral pain*.

Physiological Effects of Morphine

Morphine is the oldest naturally occurring analgesic. It is the best understood, and therefore the standard against which all other analgesics are compared. We will discuss the effects of morphine on various systems of the body with the realization that most other narcotics or opioids have effects similar to those of the "prototype" morphine.

Central Nervous System.   In the CNS, morphine is a potent analgesic and is effective against all levels of pain. Morphine produces a great deal of sedation in most individuals, but not the kind of sedation that one would see with a barbiturate. Morphine causes, in most patients, a condition called *euphoria* (or a sense of well-being); however, there are a number of individuals who experience a *dysphoria* response. Also morphine has a direct effect on the smooth muscles of the eye and causes *miosis* (pupillary constriction).

Respiratory System.   Morphine is a powerful respiratory depressant and directly affects the medullary center, causing a decrease in respiratory rate and tidal volume that in turn increases CO_2. Respiratory arrest is a common cause of death with overdose of morphine, and, in individuals who are elderly, debilitated, or have chronic lung disease, a normal therapeutic dose of morphine can be lethal. Morphine also should be used with caution in asthmatics because of their broncospastic tendencies.

Cardiovascular System.   Morphine causes orthostatic hypotension in patients who are ambulatory by suppressing the vasomotor center in the medulla. However, if the patient is kept quiet or nonambulatory when taking morphine, there are very few problems involving the cardiovascular system.

Gastrointestinal System.   Morphine stimulates the chemoreceptor trigger zone in the medulla and activates the *emesis* (vomiting) center in the brain, causing severe nausea and vomiting. However, if the patient is kept quiet and if larger doses are given, the nausea and vomiting often are decreased because the *chemoreceptor* trigger zone is suppressed. Morphine also stimulates the smooth muscle of the gut, causing local spasms that break up or delay peristalsis. This can lead to severe constipation, which can become a serious problem with long-term morphine use.

Hepatic System.   Morphine has no major effect on the liver except in high dosage. It can affect the smooth muscle of the bile duct and sphincter muscle, causing biliary *colic*.

Skin.   Morphine occasionally causes *urticaria* and mild dermatitis. This is the result of histamine release, which also causes some vasodilation, leading to redness of the skin and eyes, as well as *puritis* (itching).

Genitourinary System.   Morphine can cause a decrease in urine formation as a result of the stimulation of the posterior pituitary, causing release of antidiuretic hormone. Morphine causes spasm of smooth muscles of the urinary bladder, leading to decrease in urine output (*oliguria*). This can become clinically significant with chronic doses. Morphine also can also decrease sexual activity and causes a decrease in libido.

Tolerance and Dependence.   This occurs with morphine and all related opioids to varying degrees. When narcotic agents are administered over long periods of time, tolerance and physical dependence occur at varying rates depending on the dose and individual variation.

Classification of Narcotics Analgesics

Opioids are classified into three major subgroups according to the activity at the various opioid receptors: 1) agonist (stimulates receptors), 2) agonist–antagonist (stimulates some receptors or blocks some receptors), and 3) antagonist (blocks receptors). The opioid agonists stimulate the opioid receptors and thus mimic the effects of the endorphin substances. The agonists–antagonist are similar to morphine and stimulate some receptors and antagonize others. The antagonists bind to the receptors throughout the body but fail to activate them. Table 3–15 classifies the commonly used narcotic analgesics according to activity, generic name, and trade name.

Comparison of Morphine, Meperidine, and Codeine

Morphine, meperidine, and codeine are commonly used narcotic analgesics. To gain an understanding of the properties of these three commonly used drugs, a comparison of the analgesic potency, addiction potential, respiratory effects, and other side effects is made in Table 3–16. By comparing these three agents, one can predict the effects of other analgesics that are related to them.

Narcotic Antagonists

These agents have a marked antagonist property and pose no agonist or analgesic effect. They are used primarily in the treatment of opioid overdose. Care should be used when giving these drugs to individuals who are physically dependent on opioids because they can precipitate a withdrawal syndrome. The main antagonist is **naloxone (Narcan**[R]**)**. It should be noted that the reversal of the overdose effect may only be temporary, and the patient should be observed closely for possible relapse into withdrawal.

TABLE 3–15   Narcotic Analgesics

CLASSIFICATION (DERIVATIVES)	GENERIC NAME	TRADE NAME
Agonist		
Opium alkaloids	Heroin*	
	Morphine	
	Codeine	
Semisynthetic derivatives	Morphine derivatives	Dilaudid[R]
of morphine and codeine	Hydromorphone	Numorphan[R]
	Oxymorphone	
	Codeine derivatives	
	Hydrocodone	Hycodan[R], Lortab[R], Hy-Phen[R], Hycomine[R], Vicodin[R], Hycodophen[R]
	Dihydrocodeine	Synalgos[R]
	Oxycodone	Percodan[R], Percocet[R], Tylox[R]
Synthetic derivatives	Meperidine	Demerol[R]
	Propoxyphene	Darvon[R]
	Levorphanol	Levo-Dromoran[R]
	Methadone	Dolophine[R]
Agonist–antagonist		
	Buprenorphine	Buprenex[R]
	Butorphanol	Stadol[R]
	Nalbuphine	Nubain[R]
	Pentazocine	Talwin[R]
Antagonist		
	Naloxone	Narcan[R]
	Naltrexone	Trexan[R]

*Currently used in advanced cardiac life support.

NONNARCOTIC ANALGESICS

The nonnarcotic drugs are not related chemically or structurally to the narcotic agents. They relieve mild to moderate pain without the loss of consciousness. In addition, these agents produce analgesia through a peripheral as well as a central mechanism of action and do not produce tolerance or physical dependence with chronic use. Also, most of the nonnarcotic agents produce an antipyretic effect and some produce an anti-inflammatory effect.

TABLE 3–16 Comparison of Narcotic Analgesics

	ANALGESIC POTENCY	ADDICTION POTENTIAL	RESPIRATORY SUPPRESSION	OTHER SIDE EFFECTS
Morphine	Most potent (dose 10 mg)	High	High	Constipation
Meperidine	1/10th to 1/5th as potent as morphine (dose 50–100 mg)	Moderate to High	High	Few
Codeine	1/6th as potent as morphine (dose 60 mg)	Low	Low	Few

Salicylates

The salicylates, which include aspirin, are the most widely used therapeutic agents. Their clinical use dates back to ancient times, with the first pharmacological data appearing in the literature in 1899. Because of the common use of salicylates, they serve as a prototype of all of the nonnarcotic analgesic agents. They include the following drugs:

- *Acetylsalicylic acid* (ASA; aspirin)—the main compound in most salicylate over the counter drugs.
- *Salicylamide*—a compound similar to ASA and also found in many over-the-counter drugs; it is not as potent as ASA but has similar properties.
- *Methylsalicylate*—a common substance found in over-the-counter topically applied liniments, which create a feeling of warmth (Ben-Gay^R, etc.); also sometimes known as "oil of wintergreen."

The main mechanism of action of the salicylates is to decrease the synthesis of prostaglandins in both the periphery and the hypothalamus. This mechanism of action creates the therapeutic effects of analgesia, anti-inflammatory action, and antipyresis.

Therapeutic Effects. Because of their broad range of therapeutic effects, the salicylates have become very popular and are widely used. These therapeutic effects include:

- *Analgesia*—these drugs are effective against mild to moderate pain, including headache, muscle and joint pain, and toothache; they are not as effective for visceral pain as narcotics, but also do not cause physical dependence and tolerance.
- *Antipyresis*—these drugs lower the body temperature when it is elevated as a result of various disease conditions, but do not lower body temperature if the temperature is normal; the mechanism of the antipyresis is probably interference with prostaglandin synthesis in the hypothalamus.
- *Anti-inflammatory action*—these drugs inhibit the synthesis of prostaglandins in the joints and ligaments; therefore, they are effective in treating rheumatoid arthritis and other inflammatory diseases.

- *Anticoagulation*—these drugs decrease coagulation by inhibiting platelet aggregation; aspirin currently is being used as a therapeutic approach to the various *thromboembolytic* diseases.
- *Uricosuria*—in high doses these drugs can increase the excretion of uric acid, but they also can antagonize other agents used in the treatment of *gout*.

Adverse Effects.   Although there are many valuable uses of these agents with relatively few problems, there are a number of side effects that can occur with the use of salicylates. Some of these are as follows:

- *GI tract*: All of the salicylates as well as the other anti-inflammatory agents are considered to be *ulcerogenic*. These agents increase gastric ulceration and bleeding by increasing acid secretion. The mechanism of action of this is thought to be a decrease in prostaglandin synthesis (the prostaglandus act as a protective mechanism in the stomach).
- *Hypersensitivity reaction (allergy)*: About 0.2–0.9 percent of the population experiences a hypersensitivity reaction resembling a true allergic phenomenon. These hypersensitivity reactions include bronchospasm, urticaria, edema, and hypotension. However, this is not a true allergic reaction because an antigen–antibody reaction has not been demonstrated.
- *Blood*: These drugs cause an anticoagulant effect as a result of a decrease in platelet aggregation. In high doses, they can cause an increase in prothrombin time by interacting with vitamin K.
- *Interactions*: Salicylates interact with and increase the effects of oral anticoagulants. Salicylates also interact with alcohol, phototoxic agents, and anti-inflammatories.
- *Salicylate Intoxication*: Toxic reactions associated with salicylates are uncommon in adults but, because pediatric flavored solutions are available over the counter, reactions can occur in young children. Toxic overdose reactions include decrease in CO_2 levels, hyperventilation by direct stimulation of the medulla, tinnitus and hearing losses, and acid–base distortions.

Nonsalicylate Nonnarcotic Drugs

Other nonsalicylate drugs that commonly are used today are substances that are classified as *para*-aminophenols. The two main drugs that belong to this group are **acetaminophen** (**Tylenol**^R) and **phenacetin**. Phenacetin has disappeared from most analgesic drugs because it has been shown to cause nephrotoxicity and neurological cancer. However, at one time it was the main constituent in substances called *APCs*. Today, the prototype of the *para*-aminophenols is acetaminophen. Acetaminophen is extremely popular and is the most widely used nonnarcotic analgesic. It has the following therapeutic effects:

- *Analgesia*—comparable to aspirin but the exact mechanism is unknown.
- *Antipyresis*—comparable to aspirin in decreasing fever; it causes the decrease in temperature probably by inhibiting prostaglandin synthesis in the hypothalamus.

(*Note*: Acetaminophen has no clinically significant anti-inflammatory property.)

TABLE 3–17   Commonly used NSAIDs

DRUG	MECHANISM OF ACTION	THERAPEUTIC USE	ADVERSE EFFECTS
Ibuprofen (Advil[R], Motrin[R])	Same as aspirin	Analgesia, antipyresis, anti-inflammatory action	Gastric irritation and renal failure
Fenoprofen (Nalfon[R])	Same as aspirin	Same as ibuprofen	GI and skin reactions
Naproxen (Naprosyn[R])	Same as aspirin	Same as ibuprofen	Same as fenoprofen plus rare bone marrow suppression
Indomethacin (Indocin[R])	Same as aspirin	Anti-inflammatory	GI distress
Phenylbutazone (Butazolidin[R])	Same as aspirin	Anti-inflammatory	Agranulocytosis
Piroxicam (Feldene[R])	Same as aspirin	Anti-inflammatory	GI reactions
Meclofenamate (Meclomen[R])	Same as aspirin	Anti-inflammatory	GI reactions
Diclofenac (Voltaren[R])	Same as aspirin	Anti-inflammatory	GI reactions

In terms of adverse effects, acetaminophen is much better than aspirin in that it causes no gastric problems, has no effect on platelets, and has fewer drug interactions. However, in high doses it can cause severe hepatic necrosis and death. It should be noted that, in cases of acetaminophen overdose, treatment often includes the use of a respiratory mucolytic agent, **N-acetylcysteine (Mucomyst**[R]**)**. The use of this drug is discussed in Chapter 12.

Nonsteroidal Anti-inflammatory Drugs

All the salicylates actually are considered to be nonsteroidal anti-inflammatory drugs (NSAIDs) but because of their historical significance they have been discussed separately in the previous sections. As a group the NSAIDs are used for the treatment of rheumatoid arthritis, osteoarthritis, acute attacks of gout, dysmenorrhea, and other inflammatory diseases. They all have mechanisms of action similar to that of aspirin because they inhibit prostaglandin synthesis. In addition, they have many side effects similar to those of aspirin. The major adverse effects of these drugs after chronic use are GI irritation and nephrotoxicity. Table 3–17 lists some of the commonly used NSAIDs.

POSTTEST: PHARMACOLOGY OF THE CENTRAL NERVOUS SYSTEM

For each of the following questions, try to select the *one* best answer from those choices given.

1. CNS drugs can alter the effects of neurotransmitters in the CNS by all of the following except:
   a. prolongation
   b. antagonism
   c. increased synthesis of neurotransmitter
   d. decreased synthesis of neurotransmitter
   e. all are correct

2. Generally a sedative drug can become a hypnotic by increasing the dose. True or False?

3. All of the following statements about benzodiazepines are true except:
   a. these agents have relatively few side effects in comparison to barbiturates.
   b. the main clinical use of these drugs is the treatment of anxiety
   c. the overall mechanism of action is to block the inhibitory effect of GABA neurotransmitters
   d. they can create additive effects when administered with alcohol and other CNS depressants

4. Although alcohol has an apparent stimulatory effect when administered in small doses, it is actually an CNS depressant. True or False?

5. The major side effect that is of greatest concern with the use of TCAs and MAO inhibitors is:
   a. hyperexcitability
   b. reduced depression
   c. hypertension
   d. allergic reactions

6. The psychostimulant drugs have a calming effect on hyeractive children. This phenomenon is called:
   a. antagonism
   b. anticholinergic
   c. idiosyncrasy
   d. hypoactivity

7. Parkinsonism is a disease caused by an imbalance between excitatory neurons and inhibitory neurons in the substantia nigra of the cerebral nuclei. True or False?

8. Because dopamine levels are low in parkinsonism, the mainstay of drug therapy is to administer dopamine. True or False?

9. All of the following general anesthetic against are volatile liquids except:
   a. chloroform
   b. nitrous oxide
   c. methoxyfluorene
   d. ether

10. What is the most important advantage in the use of injectable general anesthetics?
    a. more potent
    b. less fear by patient
    c. patient is ambulatory more quickly
    d. better analgesia
11. All of following are reasons for administering preanesthetic medication except:
    a. decrease anxiety
    b. decrease amount of general anesthetic agent needed
    c. reduce secretions
    d. reduce side effects
    e. all are true
12. All of the following are properties of acetylsalicylic acid (aspirin) except:
    a. sedation
    b. analgesia
    c. anti-inflammatory action
    d. antipyresis

REFERENCES/RECOMMENDED READING

Alfaro-LeFerve R, Blicharz ME, Flynn, NM, Boyer, MJ: *Drug Handbook: A Nursing Process Approach.* Addison-Wesley Nursing, a division of the Benjamin/Cummings Publishing Co, Inc, Redwood City, CA, 1992.

Bergman KJ, Mendoza MR, Yahr MD: Parkinson's disease and long term levodopa therapy. *Adv Neurol* 45:463–468, 1987.

Beumont A, Hughes J: Biology of opionid peptides. *Annu Rev Pharmacol* 19:203–244, 1979.

Blackwell B: Newer antidepressant drugs. In HY Meltzer (ed), *Psychopharmacology: The Third Generation of Progress.* Raven Press, New York, 1987, pp 1041–1049.

Dipalma JR, Digregorio, JG: *Basic Pharmacology in Medicine*, 3rd ed. McGraw-Hill, New York, 1990.

Graham GG, Day RO, Champion GD, Lee E, and Newton K: Aspects of the clinical pharmacology of nonsteroidal antiinflammatory drugs. *Clin Rheum Dis* 10:229–249, 1984.

Hitner H, Nagle BT: *Basic Pharmacology for Health Occupations*, 2nd ed. GlenCo Publishing Co, Mission Hills, CA, 1987.

Skolnick P, Paul SM: The mechanism of action of benzodiazepines. *Med Res Rev*, 306:401, 1982.

Williams BR, Baer HL: *Essentials of Clinical Pharmacology in Nursing.* Spring House Corporation, Springhouse, PA, 1990.

CHAPTER 4

SKELETAL MUSCLE RELAXANTS

LEARNING OBJECTIVES

After completion of this chapter and its learning activities, the student will be able to:

1. Describe the classification and mechanism of action of the peripheral-acting skeletal muscle relaxants.
2. List and describe the nondepolarizing peripheral muscle relaxants, including their therapeutic uses and adverse effects.
3. List and describe the depolarizing peripheral muscle relaxants, including their therapeutic uses and adverse effects.
4. List and describe the direct-acting peripheral muscle relaxants, including their therapeutic uses and adverse effects.
5. Describe the mechanism of action of the central-acting muscle relaxants.
6. List and describe the central nervous system (CNS) muscle relaxants, including their therapeutic uses and adverse effects.

INTRODUCTION

As described in Chapter 2 regarding autonomic nervous system drugs, the somatic motor nerves innervate nicotinic-2 receptor sites at the skeletal neuromuscular junction. When acetylcholine is released at the junction, it causes depolarization of the muscle fiber membrane and muscle contraction results. There are a number of clinical conditions that require relaxation of skeletal muscles; these may include spinal cord injury, multiple sclerosis, cerebral palsy, and pain and stiffness associated with overexertion of muscles. (*Note*: It should be pointed out that neuromuscular blocking agents are not used to treat this latter condition.) Also, there are clinical procedures that are performed during surgery, intubation, and orthopedic manipulation, and certain situations in respiratory care, wherein complete paralysis of skeletal muscles is necessary. In this chapter we discuss some common peripheral-acting and central-acting muscle relaxants that are used to control muscle contraction.

PERIPHERAL-ACTING MUSCLE RELAXANTS

These drugs interact with nicotinic-2 receptors at the skeletal neuromuscular junction and cause muscle paralysis. Both the depolarizing and nondepolarizing drugs are exclusive tools of the anesthesiologist and are used as adjuncts to various surgical procedures in order to create skeletal muscle relaxation while the patient is anesthetized. These peripheral-acting drugs also are used routinely for intubation procedures. The direct-acting drugs are used to treat conditions such as malignant hypothermia and spastic diseases that include muscle spasms associated with multiple sclerosis, cerebral palsy, and spinal cord injury. The classification and mechanisms of action of these drugs are summarized in Table 4–1.

Nondepolarizing Peripheral Neuromuscular Relaxants

These drugs are administered intravenously and produce a competitive blockade at the neuromuscular site, causing skeletal muscle relaxation within 1–2 minutes. The duration of this effect wears off slowly by diffusion and redistribution. The agents described below are used clinically during surgical procedures to obtain skeletal muscle relaxation in an anesthetized patient so that operative manipulation procedures can be performed more easily by the surgeon.

d-Tubocurarine (Curare; Curarin^R). This is an alkaloid of plant origin and an active ingredient found in poison darts used by primitive native tribes in various South American jungles. This drug was one of the original blocking agents but is now rarely used. **Therapeutic use:** skeletal muscle relaxation during surgical procedures and during intubation. **Adverse effects:** causes release of histamine with profound cardiovascular/respiratory effects, such as hypotension and respiratory arrest.

TABLE 4–1 Classification of Peripheral-Acting Muscle Relaxants

CLASSIFICATION	MECHANISM OF ACTION
Nondepolarizing neuromuscular blockers	Compete with acetylcholine for the nicotinic-2 receptor site at the neuromuscular junction
Depolarizing neuromuscular blockers	Cause a persistent depolarization at the motor/endplate so that receptors cannot react with acetylcholine
Direct-acting neuromuscular blockers	Interfere with biochemical pathways and prevent the interaction of actin and myosin in the muscle fiber; do not affect the conduction of impulses across the neuromuscular junction

TABLE 4–2   Common Peripheral-Acting Muscle Relaxants

DRUG	MECHANISM OF ACTION	CLINICAL USES
d-Tubocurarine (curare; Curarin[R])	Nondepolarizing	Surgical muscle relaxant
Atracurium (Tracrium[R])	Nondepolarizing	Same
Succinylcholine (Anectine[R])	Depolarizing	Same
Dantrolene (Dantrium[R])	Direct acting	Used as an antispasmodic in outpatients

Atracurium (Tracrium[R]).   This drug has an action similar to that of curare but does not activate the cholinergic receptors. **Therapeutic use:** same as that of curare but with fewer side effects. **Adverse effects:** same as with curare but does not release histamine (see Table 4–2). (*Note*: Both the nondepolarizing and depolarizing peripheral muscle relaxants paralyze the diaphragm when administered, and thus the anesthesiologist must breathe for the patient until the drug wears off.)

Vecuronium (Norcuron[R]).   This drug has an action similar to that of atracurium. **Therapeutic use:** same as that of atracurium. **Adverse effects:** Same as with atracurium.

Depolarizing Peripheral Neuromuscular Relaxants

The only currently used agent in this group is **succinylcholine (Anectine[R])**. This drug is similar in structure to acetylcholine and induces muscle relaxation by causing a persistent depolarization of the motor endplate area. It competes with acetylcholine, takes effect almost immediately (1–1.5 minutes), and is metabolized by plasma and liver pseudocholinesterase. It is used in the same clinical situations as curare and atracurium, but is much less potent than the other two agents.

Succinylcholine has a number of severe side effects. It releases histamine, causes cardiovascular problems, including a profound drop in blood pressure, and also can interact with general anesthetics such as halothane to cause malignant hypothermia. Initially, it may cause significant muscle fasciculation (rapid localized muscle contractions) that can lead to postoperative muscle soreness (see Table 4–2).

Direct-Acting Peripheral Neuromuscular Relaxants

The only currently used agent in this group is **dantrolene (Dantrium[R])**. This agent works directly on the actin and myosin (thin and thick myofilaments) in the skeletal muscle fiber. This is accomplished by preventing the interaction of these two proteins and their crossbridges; thus, muscle contraction is impaired. Also, this type of muscle paralysis is accomplished without affecting the normal nerve function at the neuromuscular junction. The drug can be given either intravenously or orally and should be administered under careful observation.

Dantrolene is used clinically in treatment of muscle spasms that are associated with multiple sclerosis, cerebral palsy, malignant hypothermia, and various spinal cord injuries. Adverse effects of dantrolene include dizziness, fatigue, weakness, and some liver toxicity (see Table 4–2).

CNS MUSCLE RELAXANTS

The central-acting muscle relaxants do not act peripherally but work in the CNS at the level of the spinal cord (Table 4–3). It should be noted that the exact mechanism is not understood, and many investigators believe that the main clinical effect of this group of drugs is due to their sedative properties. There are many antianxiety drugs that have the same type of muscle-relaxing properties (see Chapter 3). The value of these drugs is that they do not affect the nicotinic receptor site or the skeletal muscle fibers, so there is no danger of altering the normal function at the neuromuscular junction.

Central nervous system muscle relaxants are used in treating various types of muscle spasms and conditions in which muscles have been strained, pulled, or sprained. Supposedly the drugs interfere with the reflex nerve pathways at the level of the spinal cord, but the main effect is to cause CNS sedation, which in itself will cause some relaxation. These drugs can be given both by injection and orally. Some studies have shown that, if given by injection, they are more effective; however, the drugs more commonly are used on an outpatient basis and thus the injection route is not practical. Some of the more commonly used drugs are listed as follows:

- *Carisoprodol (Soma*R*)*—Therapeutic use: muscle relaxation of spastic contraction of skeletal muscles caused by overexertion, trauma, and nervous tension; **Adverse effects:** blurred vision, dizziness, lethargy, and mental alterations.
- *Cyclobenzaprine (Flexeril*R*)*—Therapeutic use and adverse effects: same as with carisoprodol.
- *Methocarbamol (Robaxin*R*)*—Therapeutic use and adverse effects: same as with carisoprodol.

It should be noted that, because the major effect of the CNS muscle relaxants is CNS depression, the benzodiazepines (particularly diazepam) have replaced the use of CNS muscle

TABLE 4–3 Central-Acting Muscle Relaxants		
DRUG	**MECHANISM OF ACTION**	**CLINICAL USES**
Carisoprodol (Soma R)	CNS/sedative	Muscle relaxation
Cyclobenzaprine (Flexeril R)	CNS/sedative	Muscle relaxation
Methocarbamol (Robaxin R)	CNS sedative	Muscle relaxation

relaxants. Also, all of the CNS muscle relaxants can be potentiated by other CNS depressants and therefore should not be taken with substances such as alcohol, sedatives, and tranquilizers.

POSTTEST: SKELETAL MUSCLE RELAXANTS

For each of the following questions, try to select the *one* best answer from those choices given.

1. The somatic nerve fiber innervates skeletal muscles and releases a neurotransmitter that combines with a receptor at the neuromuscular junction. The names of the neurotransmitter and receptor are:
    a. norepinephrine and nicotinic-2
    b. norepinephrine and nicotinic-1
    c. acetylcholine and nicotinic-2
    d. acetylcholine and nicotinic-1

From the following list of peripheral-acting muscle relaxants, match the corresponding mechanism of action.

2. *d*-Tubocurarine (Curare[R])   a. nondepolarizing
3. Dantrolene (Dantrium[R])   b. depolarizing
4. Succinylcholine (Anectine[R])   c. direct acting

5. The main clinical use of curare and succinylcholine is to break laryngeal spasm that sometimes occurs during intubation. True or False?
6. The mechanism of action of direct-acting peripheral muscle relaxants is to block the nicotinic-2 receptor site. True or False?
7. All of the following statements about CNS muscle relaxants are true except:
    a. these drugs work at the level of the spinal cord.
    b. these drugs do not affect normal function of the neuromuscular junction.
    c. all of these drugs cause varying degrees of sedation in the CNS.
    d. these drugs can only be given by the intravenous route and therefore have limited clinical use.
8. Because the CNS muscle relaxants work at the level of the CNS, they can be potentiated by other CNS depressants such as alcohol and other sedative hypnotic drugs. True or False?

REFERENCES/RECOMMENDED READING

Alfaro-LeFevre R, Blicharz ME, Flynn NM, Boyer MJ: *Drug Handbook: A Nursing Process Approach.* Addison-Wesley Nursing, a division of the Benjamin/Cummings Publishing Co, Inc, Redwood City, CA, 1992.

Dipalma JR, Digregorio JG: *Basic Pharmacology in Medicine*, 3rd ed, McGraw-Hill, New York, 1990.

Hitner H, Nagle BT: *Basic Pharmacology For Health Occupations*, 2nd ed. Glenco Publishing Co, Mission Hills, CA, 1987.

CHAPTER 5

CARDIOVASCULAR AND RENAL PHARMACOLOGY

LEARNING OBJECTIVES

After completion of this chapter and its learning activities, the student will be able to:

1. Describe the conduction system of the heart and relate the electrical control to a normal electrocardiogram (ECG).
2. Describe congestive heart failure (CHF) and coronary artery disease as the most common categories of heart disease.
3. Define *cardiac glycoside* and describe the overall effect of these drugs in treating CHF.
4. Describe the mechanism of action of the cardiac glycosides.
5. Describe some of the pharmacological effects of digitalis as the prototype drug of the cardiac glycosides; also explain the need for careful monitoring of adverse effects.
6. List the main cardiac glycosides used today and describe their routes of administration and duration of action.
7. List other drugs used in the treatment of CHF.
8. Define *arrhythmia* and list several types of arrhythmias.
9. List four reasons for treating or converting arrhythmias and also indicate some causes of some arrhythmias.
10. Describe four classifications of antiarrhythmic agents and indicate the overall mechanism of action of these drugs.
11. List at least one drug from each of the four classifications of antiarrhythmic agents.
12. Describe the overall effect of the antianginal drugs and explain the effects of nitrates and nitrites.
13. List some adverse effects and several methods of administering nitrates and nitrites.
14. Describe and list other categories of antianginal agents and their overall mechanism of action.
15. Define *hypertension* and list several reasons for treatment. Also define *essential* and *secondary hypertension*.

16. Describe and list the physiological factors that control hypertension and discuss the role of the kidneys in hypertension.
17. Describe the current therapeutic approach to hypertension and list the five categories of drugs used to treat hypertension.
18. Describe the basic physiology of the nephron and explain filtration, tubular reabsorption, and tubular secretion.
19. Define diuretics and list several diseases that they are used to treat.
20. List five classes of diuretics, mechanism of action of each class, and at least one example of a drug from each class.
21. List the other categories of antihypertensive drugs, describe the overall mechanism of action, and list one example of each category.
22. Briefly review the process of coagulation and list three substances produced in each of the three stages of coagulation.
23. List two classes of anticoagulants used clinically, along with various diseases for which these agents are used.
24. Compare heparin and oral anticoagulants in terms of overall action, route of administration, and adverse effects.
25. List other anticoagulants that are clinically useful.
26. Describe in a general way the relationship between cholesterol, high triglyceride level, and coronary artery disease, stroke, and hypertension.
27. List the categories and drugs generally used in controlling hyperlipidemia.

INTRODUCTION

Heart disease is the major cause of death from illness in the United States. Because respiratory problems often accompany cardiac dysfunction, it is essential that the respiratory care practitioner have some knowledge regarding drugs that are used in treating heart disease. This chapter discusses cardiac glycosides used in treating congestive heart failure, antiarrhythmic agents, antianginal drugs, and a broad group of drugs used in treating hypertension. As part of the section on antihypertensive drugs, renal function in connection with the use of diuretics is discussed. This chapter also discusses anticoagulants and hypolipidemic drugs (drugs that lower cholesterol and triglyceride levels).

CONDUCTION SYSTEM OF THE HEART

The heart is dependent on the continual contraction of the myocardium. The blood supply to the heart is carried by coronary arteries that branch from the aorta immediately after

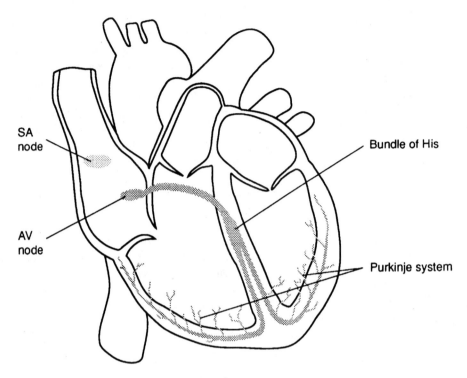

FIGURE 5-1 Conduction System of the Heart.

the aorta leaves the left ventricle. Normally the blood flow to the coronary arteries is dependent on the force of contraction of the myocardium, and any interference with normal blood flow to the heart results in a decrease of efficiency and a decrease of contraction. The constant supply of blood to the heart and the rest of the body is under control of a specialized conduction system of the heart. One of the unique characteristics of this system is that it creates and maintains its own rhythm (autorhythmicity). This characteristic enables the heart to initiate and maintain its own rate of contraction.

The normal rate of contraction is initiated by a specialized group of cells called the sinoatrial (SA) node. When the SA node depolarizes, the impulse is spread over both atria to the atrioventricular (AV) node. The AV node then causes depolarization of the ventricles. The impulse from the AV node then travels through the bundle of His, located in the intraventricular septum, through the left and right bundle branches, and into the Purkinje fibers (Figure 5-1).

It is through this conduction system that the contraction of the chambers of the heart is coordinated. Although the heart has its own conduction system, the SA node also receives nerve supply from both divisions of the autonomic nervous system. The sympathic nerves release norepinephrine, which increases heart rate (positive chronotropic effect) and increases the force of contraction (positive inotropic effect). The parasympathetic nerves

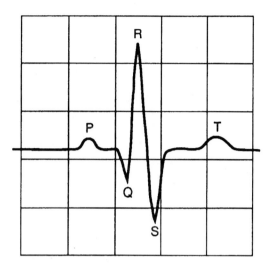

FIGURE 5–2   Normal Electrocardiogram.

release acetylcholine, causing a decrease in heart rate (negative chronotropic effect) and a decrease in force of contraction (negative inotropic effect). With the opposite effects of both autonomic divisions, the homeostatic balance of the body regarding blood supply is maintained.

Because of the electrical activity of the heart, characteristic wave forms known as the electrocardiogram can be recorded to evaluate normal as well as pathological conditions of the heart. A normal ECG is represented in Figure 5–2. The P wave represents depolarization of the atria, the QRS complex represents depolarization of the ventricles, and the T wave represents repolarization of the ventricles. The repolarization of the atria is not seen on a typical ECG because it occurs at the same time that the QRS complex is recorded. Any alteration in the wave form or shortening or lengthening of the intervals between the waves can indicate serious pathology, arrhythmias, or myocardial infarction.

HEART DISEASE

The most common diseases of the heart are congestive heart failure and coronary artery disease.

Congestive heart failure is caused by a loss of contractility of the cardiac muscle that leads to an inefficient pump. If the heart pumps less blood than it receives, the blood volume increases inside the chambers, causing enlargement. When there is less blood pumped to the rest of the body, many organs receive less blood flow. The kidneys, which are very sensitive to the amount of blood volume, react by functioning less efficiently, leading to fluid retention and a generalized edema throughout the body. When the left side of the heart fails, fluid accumulates in the lungs, causing pulmonary edema. When the right side of the heart fails, fluid accumulates in the body organs, particularly the lower extremities.

Coronary artery disease is the result of decreased flow to the coronary circulation and is associated with several cardiovascular diseases:

- *Arteriosclerosis*—hardening (fibrosis) of the arteries, which causes a narrowing of all the vessels, especially the coronary arteries. One type of arteriosclerosis is caused by accumulation of fatty plaques in the wall of the arterioles and is known as *atherosclerosis*. This eventually causes a narrowing of the vessel diameter and leads to a decrease in blood flow leading to the coronary arteries and a decrease in cardiac efficiency.
- *Angina pectoris*—a clinical term for chest pain that is the result of insufficient coronary blood flow, resulting from a decreased level of O_2 availability for cardiac contraction. Angina is often an early warning sign of decreased blood flow and/or oxygen supply to the heart.
- *Myocardial infarction*—a "heart attack" that is a result of an occlusion (coronary occlusion) of the blood supply to the cardiac muscle leading to an infarct (muscle tissue death). If the infarct involves a large area of the heart, sudden death will result. If the area of infarct is of a lesser degree, the dead tissue is replaced with fibrous connective tissue and the efficiency of the heart is greatly decreased. (Remember, cardiac cells cannot undergo mitosis and thus cannot regenerate lost tissue.)

CARDIAC GLYCOSIDES AND CHF

The cardiac glycosides are a group of drugs found in a number of plants (foxglove) and in the skin of the common toad. Because of their natural source, these drugs have been used in a variety of medicines and poisons by both ancient and modern people for hundreds of years. As early as 1785, there was published information describing the use of foxglove to treat dropsy (edema) and other diseases. In the early part of the 20th century the drug was used to treat atrial fibrillation (arrhythmia). By the end of the 20th century the drug was used as a legitimate agent in treating CHF. The glycosides are all related chemically but only digitalis, digitoxin, and digoxin are used clinically; these drugs are called cardiac glycosides.

The overall effect of the cardiac glycosides is to convert a failing pump into a more efficient organ. The beneficial effects of the cardiac glycosides in the treatment of CHF are manifested by increased cardiac output, increased efficiency of contraction, improved systemic circulation leading to an improvement in tissue perfusion, decrease in edema, and reduced peripheral resistance. In other words, the hemodynamics of the circulatory system are improved.

Mechanism of Action of Cardiac Glycosides

Cardiac glycosides combine with a receptor in the sarcolemma of the cardiac muscle fiber called sodium/potassium adenosine triphosphatase. When the drugs combine with this receptor site, the "normal cellular pump" is inhibited, which results in an increase in accumulation of intracellular sodium ions. With the increase of intracellular sodium, through a number of membrane mechanisms, there is also an increase in intracellular calcium. This increase in the amount of calcium greatly enhances the contractile apparatus and increases the strength of contraction of the myocardium (positive inotropic effect). The increase in the force of contraction occurs both in a normal and a failing heart, but the force of contraction is greatly increased in a failing heart.

Pharmacological Effects of Digitalis

Digitalis is the main drug containing cardiac glycosides, and all other cardiac glycosides are similar in action. In general, digitalis has many complex effects on the cardiovascular system, as well as effects on the autonomic nervous system. Digitalis directly affects the cardiac muscle, the conduction system, and vascular smooth muscle. It indirectly affects the autonomic nervous system and has an overall effect of increasing vagal tone. The increase in vagal tone (increase in parasympathetic stimulation of the heart) tends to decrease the frequency of firing of the AV node (pacemaker). Although there are slight differences between the effect of digitalis on a normal heart compared to that on a failing heart, the benefits in a failing heart include a drastic increase in the contractility (direct) and a decrease in heart rate (indirect). In summary, the beneficial effects of digitalis on a failing heart are:

1. Increase in stroke volume and increase in cardiac output
2. Increase in efficiency of contraction
3. Reduction of the reflex neuronal and humoral vasoconstrictor mechanisms because of the improvement of contraction, decreasing the peripheral resistance and blood pressure
4. Improvement in overall tissue perfusion, increase in renal function, and decrease of edema

Based on the overall pharmacologic effect, digitalis glycosides are the primary inotropic drugs in treating CHF and also are used in treating atrial arrhythmias such as fibrillation and flutter. Although digitalis has many therapeutic effects, it has a relatively low therapeutic index and thus the overall toxicity is high.

Adverse effects are frequent, and some of these can range from minor to severe (or even death). It is estimated that 25 percent of hospitalized patients who are treated with digitalis suffer signs of toxicity. Some of these signs include: 1) alteration of cardiac rhythm and conduction, or even complete AV block; 2) all types of arrhythmias; 3) conduction disturbances; 4) gastrointestinal effects, including nausea, vomiting, diarrhea, and abdominal pain; 5) neurological effects, including headache, muscle weakness, facial pain, delirium, hallucinations, and convulsions; 6) visual disturbances, including blurred vision and color blindness; and 7) gynecomastia (enlarged breast). Because of the severe potential side effects and toxicity, patients are given the drug orally (PO) or intravenously (IV) in a controlled sequence known as "digitalization." After the effective dose is reached, a daily maintenance dose (1/4th of the digitalization dose) is determined. The glycosides are

TABLE 5–1 Cardiac Glycosides

DRUG	ROUTE	DURATION OF ACTION
Digitalis	PO	
Digitoxin (Purodigin[R])	PO, IV	Half-life of 4–6 hr
Digoxin* (Lanoxin[R])	PO, IV	Half-life of 1–2 days

*Currently used in advanced cardiac life support drugs.

slowly metabolized and excreted; therefore, the patients blood levels are routinely checked to determine if toxic levels are present.

Main Cardiac Glycosides

Table 5–1 lists the cardiac glycosides commonly used today. All of these glycosides have the same basic therapeutic action, with the main difference being the route of administration and the duration of action.

Other Drugs Used for Treatment of CHF

Although cardiac glycosides are the main inotropic drugs used in treating CHF, diuretics and vasodilator drugs also are used. Diuretic pharmacology is discussed later in this chapter, but the main effect of diuretics in treating CHF is to decrease edema, blood volume, and congestion. Vasodilator drugs dilate the arterioles and thus decrease peripheral resistance and blood pressure. These drugs also decrease the work load on the heart and decrease oxygen consumption. The vasodilator drugs are discussed in a later section of this chapter in connection with antianginal and antihypertensive agents.

DEFINITION AND TYPES OF ARRHYTHMIAS

An arrhythmia is any sort of inappropriate electrical activity in the heart. Arrhythmias may be manifest in the diseased heart as well as a normal heart through the influence of exercise or drugs. The severity of symptoms may range from mild palpitations to complete cardiac arrest. Diagnosis of an arrhythmia is made by evaluating a combination of clinical signs and symptoms presented by the patient and confirmed by an ECG.

Both the atria and the ventricles develop arrhythmias. Generally, most arrhythmias occur when there is a defect in the AV node causing abnormal impulse formation, or a defect in conduction, or both. The automatic firing of the AV node (pacemaker) is under the influence of the proper balance between several cations, including sodium (Na^+), potassium (K^+), and calcium (Ca^{2+}). Each ion plays a significant role in the cardiac action

TABLE 5-2 Arrhythmia Characteristics

ARRHYTHMIA	LOCATION	RATE (beats/min)
Tachycardia	Atria/ventricle	150–250
Atrial flutter (supraventricular)	Atria	200–350 atrial rate
Atrial fibrillation (supraventricular)	Atria	<350 atrial rate
Ventricular fibrillation	Ventricle	<300–400 (uncoordinated contractions, no cardiac output or pulse)
Premature contractions	Atria/ventricle	Variable
Bradycardia	Atria/ventricle	<60

potential (nerve impulse). When an arrhythmia occurs, there is a disturbance in one or all of these ions. The overall action of antiarrhythmia drugs is to correct the movement or imbalance of these ions and thus restore proper function.

There are a number of types of arrhythmias that occur in the atria, the ventricles, and ectopic foci (areas other than the atria or ventricle). Arrhythmias that originate in the atria or around the AV node are referred to as "supraventricular arrhythmias" (above the ventricles). The most serious type of arrhythmia is "ventricular fibrillation," which, if not treated immediately, causes cardiac arrest and death. Table 5–2 lists some common types of arrhythmias, their location, and characteristic rates (beat/minute).

Reasons for Converting and Causes of Arrhythmias

There are many reasons for converting cardiac arrhythmias, including:

1. They may be a signal or warning of a potential problem or, more likely, a problem that already has occurred.
2. They cause extreme anxiety and fear in the patient.
3. They may indicate an infarction has occurred.
4. They can greatly decrease the efficiency of the heart.
5. They decrease O_2 delivery to heart.

Arrhythmias can occur from almost any kind of cardiovascular disease, electrolyte imbalance, or drug. They also can occur spontaneously in an apparently healthy young adult, but more predictability they occur in a debilitated or elderly individual with coronary artery disease. Thus arrhythmias can occur at any age and can be associated with a wide spectrum of diseases. The following are possible causes of arrhythmias: 1) any kind of ischemia (lack of oxygen), coronary occlusion, and myocardial infarction; 2) serious dehydration; 3) electrolyte imbalance; 4) various drugs such as digitalis; and 5) congenital and idiopathic causes.

Classification of Antiarrhythmic Drugs

Few drugs have been as well studied with regard to mechanism of action as the antiarrhythmic drugs. As a result of the intense molecular biochemical research, it is now possible for the physician to prescribe, with considerable accuracy and specificity, a specific drug for a particular arrhythmia. In general, there are four classifications of antiarrhythmic agents, and the various drugs are classified on the basis of overall mechanism of action.

Group I.   All of the drugs in this group have actions similar to those of local anesthetics. In this text, local anesthetics have not been discussed, but basically they work by blocking the influx of sodium into the nerve cell membrane. This prevents depolarization and thus prevents transmission of a nerve impulse. Contraction is initiated by depolarization with the influx of Na^+ through sodium channels in the cell membrane and the influx of Ca^{2+} through calcium channels. All of the Group I drugs block the sodium channel of the muscle cell membrane and thus decrease excitability and contraction potential.

It should be noted that many textbooks classify Group I into three subgroups based on their specificity for sodium channels. This text classifies all of the agents as Group I drugs.

Group II.   These drugs are the β blockers, and they decrease the effects of sympathetic stimulation and of endogenous catecholamines such as norepinephrine and epinephrine. The only drugs that have been released by the FDA for this purpose are propranolol and acebutolol; propranolol is the most frequently prescribed. The β blockers often are used in combination with Group I drugs.

Group III.   These agents are neuronal blockers. They decrease the release of norepinephrine from the adrenergic nerve endings and increase the refractory period of the ventricles. Generally these agents are quite toxic and are used only in treating persistent ventricular tachycardia.

Group IV.   These drugs are the most recently developed drugs and are referred to as calcium antagonists or calcium channel blockers. As do Group I drugs, they block the influx of calcium to the cardiac muscle cells and the smooth muscle cells of blood vessels. When these drugs interfere with calcium influx, several effects occur. They decrease the rate of firing of the SA and AV nodes and thus slow down the heart rate; they also relax the smooth muscles of the vasculature, leading to vasodilation. This vasodilation effect also is useful in treating angina. The main use of the Group IV agents is treating AV nodal arrhythmias and other supraventricular tachycardias.

Examples of Antiarrhythmic Drugs

Table 5–3 lists the various antiarrhythmic drugs according to group number, mechanism of action, and type of arrhythmia treated. This table is very general but emphasizes the variety of drugs available in treating various kinds of arrhythmias.

TABLE 5–3   Antiarrhythmic Drugs

GROUP AND DRUG	MECHANISM OF ACTION	TYPE OF ARRHYTHMIA
Group I	Sodium channel blockers	
Quinidine (Quinaglute[R])		Supraventricular and ventricular
Procainamide* (Pronestyl[R])		Supraventricular and ventricular
Disopyramide (Norpace[R])		Ventricular
Lidocaine* (Xylocaine[R])		Ventricular
Phenytoin (Dilantin[R])		Ventricular
Group II	β Blocker	
Propranolol (Inderal[R])		Supraventricular
Group III	Adrenergic neuronal blockers	
Amiodarone		Ventricular tachycardia
Bretylium*		Ventricular tachycardia
Group IV	Calcium channel Blockers	Supraventricular
Verapamil* (Calan[R])		

*Currently used in advanced cardiac life support.

OVERALL EFFECT OF ANTIANGINAL DRUGS AND EFFECTS OF NITRATES AND NITRITES

Angina pectoris is a painful sensation that occurs as a result of ischemia (lack of oxygen to the cardiac muscle). It usually is precipitated by anything that increases oxygen need, such as exercise, stress, excitement, or digestion of a heavy meal. This type of angina, because it is predictable, is classified as *static angina*. It usually is relieved by rest or terminating the activity that has caused it. A second type of angina, a *variant type*, is caused by vasospasm of the coronary arteries. This type of angina can occur at any time and is both unpredictable and unstable. Because the heart has no pain fibers, angina is a referred type of pain that probably is mediated through the autonomic nervous system. An individual feels the pain radiating to the left shoulder and the arm and neck, but the pain also can occur in the right shoulder and arm, depending on the site of myocardial ischemia.

The major type of drugs that improve the flow of oxygen to the myocardium, particularly in the stable type of angina, are the drugs that cause peripheral and coronary vasodilation. These drugs are called nitrates and nitrites, and their overall effect is to relax the smooth muscle of the entire vasculature. This relaxation and vasodilation occurs in the coronary vessels as well as all the vessels of the body. The vasodilation causes an overall decrease in blood pressure and a decrease in cardiac work. By decreasing cardiac work load, there is less oxygen demand on the myocardium and thus a decrease in pain. In the type of angina that is caused by vasospasm (variant type), these drugs relieve the spasm and improve blood flow.

TABLE 5–4   Nitrates And Nitrites

DRUG	DOSAGE FORM	ONSET OF ACTION	DURATION
Amyl nitrite	Ampules for inhalation	30–60 sec	10 min
Nitroglycerin*	IV	Immediate	3–5 min
Nitrol[R]	2% ointment	15 min	4–8 hr
Nitrostat[R]	Sublingual	1–3 min	10–45 min
Nitrong[R]	Extended-release tablets	30 min	8–12 hr
Nitro-Bid[R]	Extended release	30–60 min	8–12 hr
Transderm-Nitro[R]	Transdermal patch	30–60 min	24 hr
Erythrityl tetranitrate	Sublingual	5 min	3–4 hr
(Cardilate[R])	PO	30 min	3–4 hr
Isosorbide dinitrate	Sublingual	2–5 min	2–4 hr
(Isordil[R])	PO	30 min	2–4 hr
Pentaerythritol	PO	30 min	3–4 hr
(Peritrate[R])	Extended release	30 min	3–4 hr

*Currently used in advanced cardiac life support.

Adverse Effects and Methods of Administration of Nitrates and Nitrites

The nitrates and nitrites are very effective and are perhaps the most important drugs in relieving acute attacks of angina. However, certain undesirable adverse effects can occur, including throbbing headache, flushing of the face, dizziness, postural hypotension, and gastrointestinal irritation. Also, a severe hypotension (drop in blood pressure) can be dangerous for individuals who have renal failure.

There are many forms of nitrates and nitrites available and they are administered according to the patients need. It should be noted that repeated administration of these agents leads to development of tolerance, which occurs rather rapidly if the medication is used too often. In order to avoid this tolerance, some cardiologists use intermittent therapy (i.e., every other day or drug-free periods).

Table 5–4 lists examples of nitrates and nitrites along with available dosage forms, onset of action, and duration.

Other Categories of Antianginal Drugs

In addition to the nitrates and nitrites, there are two other categories of drugs used either alone or with the nitrates in treating angina. These drugs are the β blockers and the calcium channel blockers.

The β blockers decrease heart rate, reduce blood pressure, and decrease cardiac contractility without any major effect on cardiac output. These effects decrease the amount of cardiac work and, therefore decrease the oxygen demand by the myocardium. β Blockers are used in long-term treatment of angina and they are particularly effective in increasing tolerance to angina that is brought on by exercise. Although any of the β blockers can be used to treat various forms of angina, the most commonly used drug is **propranolol (Inderal^R)**.

The calcium channel blockers are newer agents used in treating angina. These drugs decrease the influx of calcium ions into the cardiac muscle as well as the vascular smooth muscle. In the vascular smooth muscle, the vasodilation decreases venous return and thus causes less cardiac work and oxygen demand. In addition, the calcium channel blockers have been shown to dilate the larger coronary arteries and decrease vasospasm. Examples of the calcium channel blockers that are used to treat angina are **verapamil (Calan^R)**, **diltiazem (Cardizem^R)**, and **nifedipine (Procardia^R)**. The most common adverse effects of these agents are similar to those of the nitrates and nitrites and include headache, facial flushing, and hypotension.

HYPERTENSION

Hypertension is a condition of elevated blood pressure and is one of the leading causes of stroke, heart attack, and kidney disease. Classification of high blood pressure is based on the diastolic pressure (Table 5–5). Generally, if the diastolic pressure is ≥100 millimeters of mercury (mm Hg), treatment is begun using antihypertensive drugs. For patients with a baseline diastolic pressure of 90–95 mm Hg or slightly lower, nondrug treatment is individualized based on such factors as heredity, overall health, diet, stress level, and sex of the patient.

Looking at Table 5–5 it can be readily seen that hypertension, if allowed to progress to an elevated level, will decrease life expectancy. The resting blood pressure of the majority of the population will remain relatively stable throughout life, with a tendency to increase only slightly with age. About 10–15 percent of the population have elevated blood pressure requiring treatment. Of the group who have an elevated blood pressure,

TABLE 5–5 Levels of Hypertension

DIASTOLIC PRESSURE (mm Hg)	DEGREE OF SEVERITY
90–104	Mild
105–114	Moderate
115–120	Serious—40% morbidity in 20 million cases
130 or above	Severe (medical emergency)

90 percent of the cases have an unknown etiology. This type of hypertension is referred to as *primary* or *essential hypertension*. The other 10 percent of hypertensive cases are called *secondary* because the elevated pressure is due to an identifiable condition (kidney disease, CHF, etc.). Although the etiology of primary or essential hypertension is unknown, there are several factors that have been implicated: genetic predisposition, stress, obesity, and excessive salt intake. In order to treat hypertension properly, these factors must be considered along with the proper selection of drugs.

Factors That Control Blood Pressure

In order to control blood pressure through proper drug therapy, as well as other methods, it is important to understand the factors that determine blood pressure. The two primary factors are cardiac output (CO) and the peripheral resistance (PR). The *cardiac output* is the amount of blood pumped by the heart per minute. Factors that makeup cardiac output are heart rate (HR) and stroke volume (SV). The formula for cardiac output is: $CO = HR \times SV$. The *peripheral resistance* is largely determined by the diameter (vasoconstriction) of the blood vessels, mainly the small arterioles, which are regulated by the sympathetic nervous system. Therefore the overall formula for blood pressure (BP) is:

$$BP = CO \times PR$$
$$= (HR \times SV) \times PR$$

By increasing any of the three factors (HR, SV, and PR), the blood pressure will increase. Antihypertensive drugs lower blood pressure by decreasing the cardiac output or reducing the total peripheral resistance by decreasing the effects of the sympathetic nervous system.

The kidneys also play a role in hypertension because, with hypertension, there is often a decrease in blood flow to the kidneys as a result of an increase in peripheral resistance. When renal blood flow is reduced, a hormone called *renin* is released into the bloodstream. Through a series of chemical reactions that are triggered by the release of renin, a substance called angiotensin II, which is a powerful vasoconstrictor, is released into the blood stream. Angiotensin II also causes the release of another hormone, *aldosterone*, from the adrenal cortex. With the release of aldosterone, there is an increase in the reabsorption of sodium and water into the bloodstream. This elevates the blood volume and, along with the increased vasoconstriction, causes the blood pressure to be elevated. Normally this renin/aldosterone/angiotensin system ensures adequate blood flow to the kidney. However, in the presence of hypertension, this normal mechanism actually makes the hypertension worse. Recently, new antihypertensive agents have been developed that inhibit this system; they are called the *angiotensin-converting enzyme (ACE) inhibitors*. These drugs are discussed later in this chapter.

Current Therapeutic Approach to Hypertension

There are currently a large number of drugs available for treating hypertension, and, as a result, it has become necessary to establish guidelines for choosing the right drug or drug combinations for a particular patient. These guidelines have led to a standard approach called "stairstep" care. This means starting with a baseline drug (usually a diuretic) and adding additional drugs or combinations of drugs in order to control hypertension. When combining drugs, a basic rule is to select drugs with different mechanisms of actions in order to enhance the antihypertensive effect while minimizing adverse effects. In addition, in some patients blood pressure can be controlled by weight management, decreasing intake of salt, and increasing exercise. The various categories of antihypertensive drugs include diuretics, adrenergic antagonists, central-acting drugs, vasodilators, and ACE inhibitors. These drugs are discussed in a later section.

Physiology of the Nephron

Urine formation is the main function of the kidney, and the functional unit of a kidney is the "nephron" or kidney tubule. Each kidney contains millions of nephrons and each nephron is composed of several segments: the glomerulus, the proximal convoluted tubule (PCT), the loop of Henle, the distal convoluted tubule (DCT), and the collecting duct (Figure 5–3). In the process of forming urine, there are three basic processes: filtration, tubular reabsorption, and tubular secretion.

Filtration.   Most of the substances in the blood are filtered through the glomerulus under the influence of blood hydrostatic pressure. The substances that are not filtered usually include the formed elements of the blood (red blood cells, white blood cells, and platelets) and the large plasma proteins.

Tubular Reabsorption.   Most of the ions and nutrients that are filtered by the glomerulus are reabsorbed back into the blood along the various segments of the nephron. The most important ion that is reabsorbed is Na^+ with 99 percent being reabsorbed. The main extracellular ion of the body is the sodium ion, and, with the absorption of large amounts of sodium, an osmotic gradient is established that attracts water. Because sodium ion concentrations are higher in the blood, water is attracted by osmosis. Therefore, the conservation of water in the body is directly related to the reabsorption of the sodium ion.

Along the length of the nephron, the reabsorption of sodium ion occurs by two mechanisms: 1) cation exchange between sodium ion, hydrogen ion, and potassium ion, and 2) anion transport by chloride ion. The exchange between sodium and hydrogen occurs in the PCT and in the DCT. The exchange between sodium and potassium occurs in the DCT. In the loop of Henle, chloride ion is actively reabsorbed and sodium follows the chloride ion. When the renal tubules reabsorb the sodium ions by the described mechanisms, an osmotic gradient is established with a high concentration of sodium in the blood. Because of the higher concentration of sodium in the blood, water also is reabsorbed. In addition to being reabsorbed by osmosis, water is reabsorbed in the collecting duct under the influence of *antidiuretic hormone* (ADH) and *aldosterone*. It is important to understand reabsorption mechanisms of sodium and water because diuretics increase urine volume by inhibiting or altering these mechanisms.

Tubular Secretion.   The main secretory functions of the nephron already have been mentioned regarding the cation exchange between sodium, hydrogen, and potassium. In addition to hydrogen and potassium exchange, weak acids and weak bases also are secreted into the renal tubules. These substances are the product of normal cell metabolism and

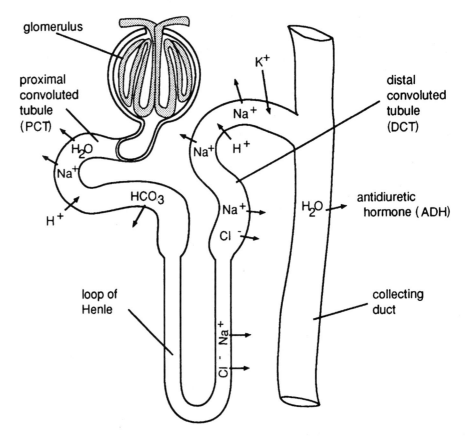

FIGURE 5–3   The Nephron of the Kidney.

are delivered to the kidney for excretion. As mentioned in Chapter 1, many drugs that are weak acids and weak bases also are secreted through the kidneys. The secretion of hydrogen ion should be emphasized as another major function of the tubular secretion. By secreting excess hydrogen ion in the urine, the kidney becomes a major organ controlling blood pH. The probable source of hydrogen for secretion can be seen in the following equation:

$$CO_2 + H_2O \quad \overset{(CA)}{\longrightarrow} \quad H_2CO_3 \quad \longrightarrow \quad H^+ + HCO_3^-$$

This reaction occurs in the renal tubule cells and is under the control of the enzyme carbonic anhydrase (CA). If the CO_2 level in the blood is elevated, the above reaction shifts to the right and hydrogen ion is excreted in exchange for sodium. The reabsorbed sodium then is paired with bicarbonate ion (HCO_3^-), which is part of the important sodium bicarbonate buffer system of the blood (see Figure 5–3).

CATEGORY	DRUG	MECHANISM OF ACTION
Osmotic	Mannitol (Osmitrol^R)	Osmosis
Carbonic anhydrase inhibitor	Acetazolamide (Diamox^R)	Block CA
Thiazide and Thiazide-like	Chlorothiazide (Diuril^R)	Prevent Na$^+$ reabsorption
	Hydrochlorothiazide (Hydropres^R)	
	Chlorthalidone (Hygroton^R)	
	Metolazone (Zaroxolyn^R)	
Loop	Ethacrynic acid (Edecrin^R)	Block reabsorption of chlorine in loop
	Furosemide (Lasix^R)	
Potassium sparing	Spironolactone (Aldactone^R)	Block aldosterone
	Triamterene (Dyrenium^R)	
	Amiloride (Midamor^R)	

TABLE 5–6 The Diuretics

Diuretics and Their Therapeutic Role

Diuretics can be defined as agents that increase urine volume. As long as the kidneys are capable of normal function, diuretics can be administered to increase urine formation by increasing glomerular filtration or, more commonly, by preventing reabsorption of sodium and water. Diuretics are used in the treatment of hypertension to reduce blood volume and peripheral edema. In addition, diuretics can be used for pathological conditions involving edema, such as glaucoma, CHF, and obesity.

Classes of Diuretics

As mentioned earlier, diuretics are the main first-line agents in the treatment of hypertension. There are five classes of diuretics available, and the classifications are based on the mechanism of action (Table 5–6). The following discussion lists the classes of diuretics along with the mechanism of action and examples of drugs. These classes include osmotic diuretics, CA inhibitors, thiazide and thiazide-like diuretics, and loop diuretics.

Osmotic Diuretics. The osmotic diuretic **mannitol** (Osmitrol^R) is used as an adjunct in treating oliguria and anuria (scanty or no urine formation). It is filtered by the glomerulus but not reabsorbed by the renal tubules. Mannitol is a large molecule and, by the process of osmosis, attracts water into the tubules, causing a mild diuresis that does not affect electrolyte and acid–base balance. In addition, mannitol is used in treating cerebral edema (that is not secondary to head injury) and glaucoma. The drug has relatively few side effects, but can cause an increase in plasma volume and can cause CHF.

Carbonic Anhydrase Inhibitors.   These drugs create a diuretic action by inhibiting the enzyme CA in the equation:

$$CO_2 + H_2O \xrightarrow{\text{(CA)}} H_2CO_3 \longrightarrow H^+ + HCO_3^-$$

By inhibiting the enzyme CA, there is less hydrogen available to exchange with sodium; therefore, less sodium is reabsorbed. Thus, water remains in the tubule and is excreted, which produces a moderate diuresis. These diuretics are used in the treatment of edema and glaucoma. The main adverse effects include problems with acid–base balance and, because these drugs are related to sulfonamides, various allergic reactions and blood dyscrasias. An example of a CA diuretic is **acetazolamide (Diamox[R])**.

Thiazide and Thiazide-Like Diuretics.   These agents comprise the largest and most widely used group of diuretics. They are all related chemically to sulfonamides and have similar mechanisms of action regarding diuresis. These diuretics prevent reabsorption in the DCT of the nephron, causing a relatively potent diuresis. The main adverse effects of these drugs include hypotension, dizziness, lightheadedness, and an increase in potassium and chloride loss. The potassium loss occurs because the increase in sodium in the DCT and collecting ducts is so much greater due to the diuretic that there is an increase in secretion of potassium. This decrease in potassium can be a particular problem in a patient taking digitalis for CHF because the low potassium causes a stronger binding of the digitalis and increases its toxicity. In the past this group of diuretics provided one of the mainstays in treating hypertension. With the discovery of the ACE inhibitors, which often are employed as first-line agents now, the thiazide and thiazide-like drugs are used less commonly. Examples of the thiazide diuretics are **chlorothiazide (Diuril[R]), hydrochlorothiazide (Esidrix[R], Hydropres[R])**, and **hydrodiuril**. Examples of thiazide-like diuretics are **chlorthalidone (Hygroton[R])** and **metolazone (Zaroxolyn[R])**.

Loop Diuretics.   These are the most potent of the diuretics and can cause a tremendous water loss by preventing the reabsorption of sodium and chloride in the loop of Henle (loop diuretics). They are organic acids but are unaffected by acid–base balance. Because of their extreme potency, these drugs are used for short periods of time and usually are administered when thiazide diuretics are ineffective. In addition to their effectiveness in treating hypertension, they also are useful in treating peripheral edema, pulmonary edema, and acute attacks of glaucoma. The adverse effects of these drugs are similar to those of the thiazides except that, in high doses, they can cause ototoxicity (damage to the eighth cranial nerve). Examples of loop diuretics are **ethacrynic acid (Edecrin[R])** and **furosemide (Lasix[R])**.

Potassium-Sparing Diuretics.   As the name implies, these agents cause a diuresis by promoting sodium excretion in the collecting tubules. This is accomplished by inhibiting the effects of aldosterone. Potassium is not exchanged for sodium, and sodium is not reabsorbed and thus stays in the tubule along with water. These agents create a mild diuresis and are used as adjuncts to therapy with other thiazide diuretics. These potassium-sparing diuretics also are used in patients who are taking digitalis in order reduce digitalis toxicity. Examples of potassium-sparing diuretics are **spironolactone (Aldactone[R])**, **triamterene (Dyrenium[R])**, and **amiloride (Midamor[R])**.

TABLE 5–7   Other Antihypertensive Drugs

CATEGORY	DRUG	MECHANISM OF ACTION
Adrenergic antagonist	Prazosin (Minipress[R])	α Blocker
	Propranolol (Inderal[R])	β Blocker
	Atenolol (Tenormin[R])	β Blocker
	Guanethidine (Ismelin[R])	Neuronal blocker
Central-acting	Clonidine (Catapres[R])	CNS (cardiovascular center)
	Methyldopa (Aldomet[R])	
Vasodilator	Hydralazine (Apresoline[R])	Direct vasodilator
	Minoxidil (Loniten[R])	Direct vasodilator
	Diazoxide*	Vasodilator
	Sodium nitroprusside*	Vasodilator
	Calcium channel blockers	
	Nifedipine (Procardia[R])	Block Ca^{2+} influx
	Verapamil (Calan[R])	
	Diltiazem (Cardizem[R])	
ACE inhibitor	Captopril (Capoten[R])	ACE inhibition
	Enalaprilat (Vasotec[R])	
	Lisinopril (Prinivil[R])	

*Currently used in advanced cardiac life support.

Other Categories of Antihypertensive Drugs

In addition to the diuretics, there are a number of other categories of drugs that are used to treat hypertension. Many of these drugs have been included in other sections of this text, but they will be presented here in the context of treating hypertension. The categories include adrenergic antagonists, central-acting drugs, vasodilators, and ACE inhibitors (Table 5–7).

Adrenergic Antagonists.   This group of drugs lower blood pressure by reducing sympathetic activity to the heart and/or blood vessels, thus reducing cardiac output and/or peripheral resistance. They include:

- Prazosin (Minipress[R])—an α blocker that causes vasodilation and a profound drop in blood pressure.
- **Propranolol (Inderal[R]), metoprolol (Lopressor[R]), nadolol (Corgard[R]), and atenolol (Tenormin[R])**—β blockers that decrease blood pressure by decreasing heart rate, which in turn decreases cardiac output.
- **Guanethidine (Ismelin[R])**—a neuronal blocker that causes blood pressure to drop by decreasing the release of norepinephrine; thus, it controls both cardiac output and peripheral resistance.

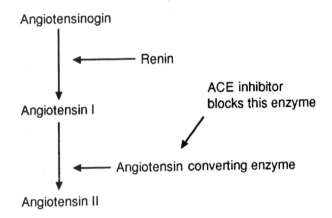

FIGURE 5–4 Mechanism of Action of ACE Inhibitors.

Central-Acting Antihypertensive Drugs. These drugs lower blood pressure by depression of sympathetic outflow from the central nervous system. They include:

- Clonidine (Catapres[R])—works on the cardiovascular regulatory center in the brain and decreases sympathetic outflow.
- Methyldopa (Aldomet[R])—mechanism is similar to that of clonidine; it is a precursor to α-methylnorepinephrine.

Vasodilator Drugs. These agents work by causing vasodilation of the arterioles. They include:

- Hydralazine (Apresoline[R])—causes direct vasodilation of arterioles.
- Minoxidil (Loniten[R])—same mechanism as hydralazine.
- Diazoxide and sodium nitroprusside—both used as IV vasodilators and are used only in severe hypertensive situations.
- Calcium channel blockers: nifedipine (Procardia[R]), verapamil (Calan[R]), and **dilti-azem (Cardizem[R])**—block the entry of calcium into the vascular smooth muscle membranes, causing vasodilation and a decrease in blood pressure.

ACE Inhibitors. These drugs block the effect of angiotensin II, which is formed when renin is released from the kidney. Examples of these drugs are **captopril (Capoten[R])**, **enalaprilat (Vasotec[R])** and **lisinopril (Prinivil[R])**. Figure 5–4 describes how ACE inhibitors work.

COAGULATION PROCESS

Coagulation is a normal function that occurs when trauma causes injury or severance of a blood vessel. The clot forms in order to prevent further loss of blood from the area.

This protective mechanism is called hemostasis and is an important mechanism in maintaining the homeostatic balance in the body. Occasionally the clotting mechanism (coagulation) becomes too active or, as a result of a narrowing of a blood vessel lumen, a clot is formed and a *thrombus* occurs. If the thrombus completely occludes or partially impairs the blood flow to the local tissue, it can lead to an infarct or necrosis. If the thrombus becomes dislodged, an *embolus* is released into the bloodstream and can travel to various organs of the body, occluding other vessels. Tissues that are particularly prone to thrombus and embolism damage are the heart, lungs, and brain. Anticoagulant drugs are administered to control the formation of thrombi or emboli by preventing clot formation.

In order to understand how anticoagulant drugs function, a brief review of the process of coagulation is presented. It is not necessary to memorize all of the factors and pathways included in the clotting mechanism. In this text, the mechanism is reduced to three stages (Figure 5–5). At the end of each stage, three important substances are formed: *thromboplastin*, *thrombin*, and *fibrin*. The anticoagulant drugs work at the various stages by affecting the formation of one of these three substances and thus prevent clotting.

Anticoagulant Drugs

The most frequently used anticoagulant drugs are the oral anticoagulants (coumarin like) and heparin. The main therapeutic effect of these drugs is to prevent the formation of venous thrombosis. The diseases that result from thrombosis include stroke, thrombophlebitis, and myocardial infarction. It is important for the respiratory care practitioner to recognize these drugs and their effects, particularly if a patient on anticoagulant therapy requires arterial blood gas sampling (extra precautions must be taken to avoid or minimize hematoma formation at the site of an arterial puncture).

Comparison of Heparin and Oral Anticoagulants

The following discussion briefly compares heparin and oral anticoagulants with regard to general action, route of administration, and adverse effects. Table 5–8 lists the comparison between heparin and coumarin-like oral anticoagulants. It is not necessary to memorize these factors but one should be aware of the overall differences.

Heparin.   This drug is a natural occurring substance found primarily in mast cells. It is commercially available from bovine intestine and lung tissue. When administered in the blood, it combines with various circulating clotting factors; however, heparin mostly inhibits thrombin activity so that fibrinogen cannot be converted to fibrin. In addition, it affects the formation of thromboplastin and also prevents the aggregation of platelets. **Route of administration:** because heparin is broken down in the stomach by hydrochloric acid, it is administered by injection (subcutaneous or IV). As a result, heparin almost always is administered in a hospital setting or an inpatient facility, where it can be monitored carefully. **Adverse effects:** the major toxic reaction of heparin is hemorrhage. During the administration of heparin through the IV route, if the level becomes too high, it can cause bleeding in the mucosa (petechiae) and gastrointestinal bleeding, resulting

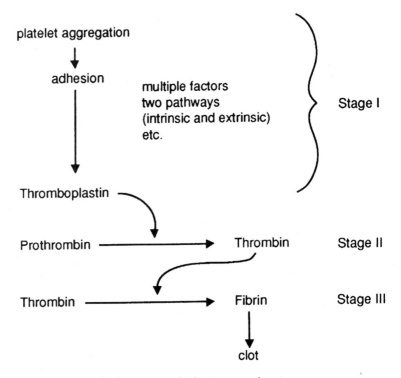

FIGURE 5–5 Simplified Version of Clotting Mechanism.

in a drop in both the hematocrit and blood pressure. Other side effects include hypersensitivity, alopecia (loss of hair), osteoporosis, and thrombocytopenia.

Oral Anticoagulants (Coumarin Like).   All of the oral anticoagulants used today are derivatives of a substance called bishydroxycoumarin, which is a substance that was isolated from spoiled sweet clover. In the 1920s a number of cattle grazing in a field that contained spoiled clover developed hemorrhagic disease, as did some humans who drank milk from these cows. Oral anticoagulants are significantly different from heparin because they can be administered by mouth. The overall action of these agents is to prevent the synthesis of a number of clotting factors, including prothrombin. The coumarins, which include **dicoumarol, phenprocoumon,** and **warfarin sodium,** all resemble vitamin K in their structure. Vitamin K is essential in forming normal clotting factors in the liver, and these agents compete with vitamin K by forming incomplete molecules that are biologically inactive. Because of this antagonism with vitamin K, anything that decreases vitamin K levels will enhance the anticoagulant properties of the coumarin. **Route of Administration:** all of these agents can be taken by mouth and, unlike heparin, are not absorbed in the gut. However, the onset of action is rather slow and it takes 12–36 hours for the drug to reach its peak effect. **Adverse effects:** like heparin, the main adverse effect is hemorrhage, and the action of the coumarin derivatives cannot be reversed as

TABLE 5-8 Comparison of Heparin and Oral Anticoagulants

	HEPARIN	ORAL ANTICOAGULANTS
Prototype	Heparin (several trade names)	Bishydroxycoumarin (dicumarol); warfarin sodium (other trade names)
Source	Cattle lung & liver; mast cells	Synthetic
Route of administration*	IV (continuous or intermittent); SC or IM; ineffective by mouth	PO; IV
Onset of action	Immediate, IV; 1–2 hr, SC or IM	12–24 hr
Peak action	10 min, IV; 2–4 hr, SC or IM	48–72 hr
Offset of action	1–3 hr, IV; 12–24 hr, SC or IM	4–7 days
Mechanisms of action	Several, but mainly inhibits formation of thrombin	Several, but mainly inhibits hepatic synthesis of prothrombin
Coagulation time	Markedly prolonged	Moderately prolonged
Prothrombin time	Slightly prolonged	Markedly prolonged
Antagonists	Protamine; whole blood or plasma	Vitamin K; fresh whole blood or plasma
Variations in response	Slight	Marked; influenced by many dietary, drug, disease, & other factors
Laboratory control	Lee & White blood coagulation time; keep time twice control	Prothrombin time; keep time twice control
Toxic effects	Hemorrhage (prolonged therapy: alopecia, osteoporosis)	Hemorrhage
Drug interactions	Few; rare	Many, varied, important; exert care!
Therapeutic uses	Prophylaxis and therapy of thromboembolic disorders	Prophylaxis & therapy of thromboembolic disorders

*IM = intramuscular, SC = subcutaneous.

rapidly. Other side effects include nausea, diarrhea, urticaria, and alopecia. Also, oral anticoagulants should never be used in individuals who have a vitamin K deficiency.

Other Anticoagulant Drugs

There are a number of other drugs that are used as anticoagulants. These agents can be used in various combinations and prevent other illnesses that are not discussed in this text. However, as mentioned in the section on aspirin in Chapter 3, there are a number

TABLE 5–9 Other Anticoagulants

CATEGORY	DRUG	MECHANISM OF ACTION
Chelator	Ethylenediaminetetraacetic acid	Binds calcium so clotting cannot occur
Dipyridamole like	Dipyridamole (Persantine^R)	Prevents aggregation of platelets
Acetylsalicylic acids	ASA, aspirin	Prevents aggregation of platelets

of clinicians who are placing patients on one-a-day acetylsalicylic acid therapy in order to decrease platelet aggregation and decrease the chance of thromboembolic disease. Table 5–9 lists some of the other medications that are used as anticoagulants.

EFFECTS OF HIGH LIPIDS IN BLOOD

Even though a balanced diet requires proteins, carbohydrates, and lipids (fats), it has been well established that certain disease processes are clinically related to high lipid levels in the blood. The important dietary lipids include fatty acids, triglycerides, and cholesterol. Even though these lipids are essential for the formation of cell membranes, nerve tissue, and lipoproteins, when they occur in sufficiently high levels they permit the formation of fatty deposits in the walls of arterial blood vessels. These plaques, called *atherosclerosis*, can lead to coronary artery disease, stroke, and hypertension. Although cholesterol has been implicated as the main positive agent in the formation of plaque, triglycerides also are important. The American diet is particularly high in these kinds of fat because of the high consumption of cholesterol-rich food such as meat, eggs, and dairy products. In addition to the high cholesterol levels, there are high-density (HDL) and low-density (LDL) lipoproteins that carry cholesterol and fats in the blood.

It is generally acknowledged that, as a goal, all individuals maintaining normal nutrition should maintain a cholesterol level below 200 mg/dL, and increase the proportion of HDL relative to LDL. This text will not discuss these various interrelationships and the complex mechanisms that affect these substances, but will discuss the overall approach to the treatment of *hyperlipidemia*. The primary treatment includes dietary restriction of saturated fats, cholesterol, and carbohydrates. When proper diet does not control the levels of the lipids, several drugs are used to lower fats; they are called *hypolipidemic* agents.

Drugs Used in Treatment of Hyperlipidemia

There are currently many drugs available that lower blood lipids. There is a great amount of interest in this area of drug therapy, and many new drugs are continually being developed. It is not the intent of this text to present all these agents in great detail, but the following discussion lists some of the more commonly used hyperlipidemic drugs, with a brief description of their mechanism of action and adverse effects.

Cholestyramine (Questran^R*).*   **Mechanism of action:** binds with bile salts in the small intestine. The bile salts are products of cholesterol breakdown and normally are reabsorbed in order to synthesize new cholesterol. Cholestyramine is an inert resin that is not absorbed into the bloodstream, and, because it prevents the reabsorption of bile salts, there is a 20–30 percent decrease in overall body cholesterol. **Adverse effects:** because cholestyramine is not absorbed into the bloodstream, there are very few side effects besides minor nausea and vomiting.

Colestipol (Colestid^R*).*   **Mechanism of action:** Similar to that of cholestyramine. **Adverse effects:** Same as cholestyramine.

Niacin (Nicolar^R*).*   **Mechanism of action:** in the form of nicotinic acid, this drug lowers the level of LDL, which carries cholesterol and triglycerides in the blood. **Adverse effects:** nausea, vomiting, diarrhea, and vasodilation. The vasodilation causes extreme flushing in the face. Also, niacin can increase uric acid levels in the blood and may cause symptoms of gout.

Clofibrate (Atromids^R*).*   **Mechanism of action:** interferes with the synthesis of cholesterol and lowers some of the lipoproteins in the blood. **Adverse effects:** nausea, headaches, diarrhea, and skin rash; also can alter liver function.

Gemfibrozil (Lopid^R*).*   **Mechanism of action:** Similar to that of colestipol; also used as a specific agent in lowering triglyceride levels.

Probucol (Lorelco^R*).*   **Mechanism of action:** lowers cholesterol without affecting triglyceride levels. **Adverse effects:** gastrointestinal disturbances; has been shown to cause arrhythmias.

Lovastatin (Mevacor^R*).*   **Mechanism of action:** a newer drug that lowers cholesterol levels by interfering with synthesis in the liver and also lowers the lipoproteins, specifically LDL. Lovastatin's effectiveness exceeds that of all the other agents. **Adverse effects:** severe liver toxicity and a condition called myositis (inflammation of the muscles).

D-Thyroxine (Choloxin^R*).*   **Mechanism of action:** an isomer of thyroxin; although it does not have a major effect on the metabolic rate, it does lower cholesterol. **Adverse effects:** similar to those of thyroxin.

POSTTEST: CARDIOVASCULAR AND RENAL PHARMACOLOGY

For each of the following questions, try to select the *one* best answer from those choices given.

1. All of the following statements about cardiac glycosides are true except:
   a. these drugs cause a decrease in intracellular calcium.
   b. these drugs cause an increase in force of contraction.
   c. these drugs cause an increase in stroke volume and cardiac output.
   d. these drugs cause an increase in peripheral edema.

2. An arrhythmia can cause symptoms ranging from mild palpitations to cardiac arrest. True or False?

The following statements describe the mechanism of action of various antiarrhythmic drugs. From the list of drugs on the right, match the appropriate drug with the appropriate mechanism of action.

3. Calcium channel blocker   a. quinidine
4. β Blocker   b. propranolol (Inderal[R])
5. Adrenergic neuronal blocker   c. bretylium
6. Sodium channel blocker   d. verapamil (Calan[R])

7. Adverse effects of the nitrates and nitrites include all of the following except:
   a. severe headache
   b. dizziness
   c. hypertension
   d. hypotension

8. Treatment of hypertension is usually begun when the diastolic pressure is:
   a. 80–85 mm Hg
   b. less than 90 mm Hg
   c. 85–90 mm Hg
   d. 110 mm Hg

9. Which of the following conditions are not treated by diuretics?
   a. congestive heart failure
   b. glaucoma
   c. hypertension
   d. edema
   e. all are treated with diuretics

10. All of the following are drugs used in the treatment of hypertension except:
    a. α-adrenergic
    b. β blockers
    c. vasodilators
    d. ACE inhibitors

11. The main therapeutic use of anticoagulant drugs is the prevention of stroke, thrombophlebitis, and myocardial infarction. True or False?

12. The primary nondrug treatment of atherosclerosis is the dietary restriction of unsaturated fats, cholesterol, and carbohydrates. True or False?

REFERENCES/RECOMMENDED READING

Alfaro-LeFerve R, Blicharz ME, Flynn NM, Boyer MJ: *Drug Handbook: A Nursing Process Approach.* Addison-Wesley Nursing, a division of the Benjamin/Cummings Publishing Co, Inc, Redwood City, CA, 1992.

Braunwald E: Mechanism of action of calcium channel blocking agents. *N Eng J Med* 307: 1618, 1982.

Canner PL, et al: Fifteen year mortality in coronary drug project patients: Long term benefits with niacin. *J Am Coll Cardiol* 8:1245–1255, 1986.

Dipalma JR, Digregorio, JG: *Basic Pharmacology in Medicine*, 3rd ed. McGraw-Hill, New York, 1990.

Hamer J: Antiarrhythmic drugs. In J Hamer (ed), *Drugs for Heart Diseases*, 3rd ed. Chapman and Hall, London, 1987.

Hitner H, Nagle BT: *Basic Pharmacology for Health Occupations*, 2nd ed. GlenCo Publishing Co, Mission Hills, CA, 1987.

Kaplan NM: Non-drug treatment of hypertension. *Ann Intern Med* 102:359–373, 1985.

Marder, VJ, Sherry S: Thrombolytic therapy: Current status 1; *and* Thrombolytic therapy: Current status 2. *N Eng J Med* 318:1512–1520; 1585–1595, 1988.

Nordlander R: Use of nitrates in the treatment of unstable and variant angina. *Drugs* 33(suppl. 4):131–139, 1987.

Schocken DD, Holloway JD: Vasodilators in the management of congestive heart failure. *Rational Drug Ther* 22:1–7, 1988.

Smith TW: Digitalis, mechanisms of action and clinical use. *N Eng J Med* 307:1357–1362, 1988.

Williams BR, Baer HL: *Essentials of Clinical Pharmacology in Nursing*. Spring House Corporation, Springhouse, PA, 1990.

CHAPTER 6

PHARMACOLOGY OF THE GASTROINTESTINAL TRACT

LEARNING OBJECTIVES

After completion of this chapter and its learning activities, the student will be able to:

1. Briefly describe the process of digestion and the roles of hydrochloric acid and pepsin; also indicate the role of mucus as a protective agent.
2. Define ulcers and list the overall cause of ulcer disease, its location, and its prognosis.
3. Describe the overall treatment of ulcer disease.
4. List the two broad categories of drugs used to treat ulcers and, within each category, list the subgroups with at least one drug example for each group.
5. Describe the overall function of the lower bowel and define the terms *diarrhea* and *constipation*.
6. List some of the causes of diarrhea and indicate some of the overall treatments.
7. List the four categories of antidiarrheal drugs, with two examples of each category.
8. List some of the causes of constipation and indicate some of the overall treatments.
9. Define the terms *laxative* and *cathartic*.
10. List four categories of laxatives/cathartics and give one example of each category.

INTRODUCTION

The gastrointestinal (GI) system is responsible for digestion and absorption of nutrients, and the upper GI tract also is responsible for absorption of drugs. This chapter discusses the general process of digestion, the treatment of ulcers, and drugs that affect intestinal motility, including antidiarrheal drugs and laxatives. In general, most ulcers occur in the upper GI tract, and thus the antiulcer drugs have their main effect in the stomach and small intestine. Intestinal motility problems (diarrhea and constipation) are primarily associated with the lower GI tract (which includes the large intestine and the rectum).

ROLE OF HYDROCHLORIC ACID AND PEPSIN IN DIGESTION

The process of digestion actually begins in the mouth with the secretion of salivary amylase. The stomach and the small intestine play a major role, with most of the important enzymes necessary for digestion being released into the duodenum. The main secretions of the stomach are released from specialized cells (parietal cells) that secret hydrochloric acid (HCl) and the proteolytic enzyme pepsin. These two products help break down food substances into absorbable forms, and most of the absorption occurs in the small intestine. The secretion of gastric juice (HCl and pepsin) is stimulated by several factors that include sight and smell of food (through the parasympathetic nervous system [vagus nerve], the presence of food in the stomach (through the parasympathetic nervous system), and the secretion of the hormone *gastrin*. The secretion of HCl causes the contents of the stomach to reach a pH of 1–2, which is necessary to activate pepsin. Eventually the digestive mass leaves the stomach and passes into the duodenum, where the final phase of digestion occurs with the secretion of pancreatic enzymes and bile.

In the final phase of digestion, the duodenum secretes an inhibitory enzyme that stops gastric flow. With the low pH of the gastric and duodenal mucosa, it is obviously necessary that a mucus barrier remains intact in order to protect the mucosal lining of these organs from *autodigestion*. Therefore, if any product or drug alters or interferes with the production of mucus, the lining of the GI tract becomes vulnerable to the formation of ulcers.

ULCER DISEASE

An ulcer is an open sore or break in the lining of the mucosa. Generally, in the GI tract, ulcers occur in the lower area of the stomach (pyloric area) and the first part of the small intestine (duodenum). These are collectively called peptic ulcers.

The overall cause of ulcer disease is a change in the balance between two factors: 1) an increase in the "attack factors," which include HCl and pepsin, and 2) a decrease in the "resistance" or "defense" factors, which include the intact mucosal barrier and the secretion of mucus. The balance between the attack factors and the resistance factors can be influenced by some of the following: excessive secretion of HCl, nonproduction of mucus, nonsecretion of the inhibitory enzyme, emotional stress, increased parasympathetic activity, ingestion of alcohol, consuming large amounts of nonsteroidal anti-inflammatory drugs (aspirin, etc.), use of steroids (inhibit secretion of mucus), and a genetic predisposition.

Generally, the prognosis of ulcer disease is positive if proper treatment is begun early. The major symptom that occurs is pain, usually centered in the epigastric area, that usually is relieved following the ingestion of food. If the patient ignores the recurrence of pain and treatment is not instituted, ulcers can begin to bleed. Severe hemorrhage can occur, requiring hospitalization and often blood transfusion. If the ulcer perforates the stomach or intestinal lining, severe cases of *peritonitis*, and in some instances death, can occur.

Treatment of Ulcers

The overall goal in the management and treatment of ulcers is to decrease the secretion of HCl and pepsin. This can be accomplished by altering the patient's life-style and controlling various nonmedicinal factors such as emotional stress, alcohol intake, intake of spicy foods, and heavy use of anti-inflammatory drugs. In addition to these factors, which are under the control of the patient, there are a number of available drugs that can decrease the attack factors and increase the resistance factors.

DRUGS USED IN TREATMENT OF ULCERS

As mentioned earlier, drug therapy for ulcers can be divided into two broad categories: drugs that decrease the attack factors (HCl and pepsin) and drugs that increase the resistance or defense factors. The following discussion describes the drugs used in decreasing secretion of HCl and pepsin, along with their mechanism of action and adverse effects. Drugs that increase resistance factors also are discussed along with their mechanism of action and adverse effects.

Drugs That Decrease Attack Factors

Drugs that decrease attack factors include histamine-2 (H_2) blockers, antacids, antimuscarinic drugs, and proton pump inhibitors.

H_2 Blockers. Most of the HCl that is secreted in the GI tract occurs as a result of stimulation of the H_2 receptor site located in the gastric mucosa. Histamine, which is released by mast cells, not only combines with H_1 receptor sites in other parts of the body (bronchial smooth muscle) but it also combines with H_2 receptor sites present in the gastric mucosa. When this occurs there is an increase in HCl secretion from the parietal cells. Although H_2 blockers do not totally prevent the release of HCl, they have become the mainstay of ulcer therapy. The following drugs are H_2 blockers:

- Cimetidine (Tagamet[R])—one of the first H_2 blockers developed; will decrease the basal HCl secretion by 70 percent. It also decreases stimulation of secretion of acid created by food at a level of about 50–70 percent. It does not affect HCl secretion that is affected by gastrin and has no direct effect on gastric motility. **Adverse effects:** mild diarrhea, headache, and tremors; also, in males it can cause gynecomastia.
- **Ranitidine (Zantac[R])**—effects are similar to those of cimetidine, but ranitidine is 10 times more potent. This allows higher doses and, because ranitidine has a higher therapeutic index, more effective doses can be administered over long periods of time. **Adverse effects:** similar to cimetidine but to a lesser degree.
- **Famotidine (Pepcid[R])**—a newer H_2 blocker that is approximately 10–30 times more potent than either ranitidine or cimetidine. **Adverse effects:** similar to those of the other two drugs.

Antacids. These substances tend to neutralize the hydrogen ion concentration, but true neutralization (raising the pH to 7.0) rarely is accomplished. Today these drugs are not considered first-line agents although they can be effective if used properly and are sometimes used in combination with the H_2 blockers. The following agents are antacids:

- **Sodium bicarbonate (baking soda)**—very effective but, because of its systemic absorption, it can cause severe alkalosis (high pH).
- **Calcium carbonate (Tums^R, Tempo^R)**—relatively effective in neutralizing acid, but acid rebound (more acid secretion than before the drug is taken) and kidney stone formation are common.
- **magnesium hydroxide (Milk of Magnesia^R)**—has rather poor neutralizing capacity.
- **Aluminum hydroxide (Amphojel^R)**—has poor neutralizing property when used alone.
- **Simethicone**—not an antacid but a silicone substance that breaks up foam formation when excessive gas is present.

All of these agents except sodium bicarbonate are used in combination with each other in order to obtain a reasonable and effective antacid effect. All these agents have the following potential **adverse effects:** sodium retention and alkalosis (sodium bicarbonate), kidney stone formation (calcium carbonate), constipation (aluminum compounds), and diarrhea (magnesium compounds). This text does not discuss all of the problems associated with antacid use, but they all should be used with care and for short periods of time. Also, many drug interactions are possible when these drugs are used.

Table 6–1 summarizes the contents and acid-neutralizing capacities of some of the more common over-the-counter (OTC) antacids.

Antimuscarinic Agents. These agents inhibit the parasympathetic activity that causes release of HCl and pepsin through the vagus nerve. The inhibition of the parasympathetic

TABLE 6–1 Antacids

PRODUCT*	CONTENTS (mg/5 mL)				
	$Al(OH)_3$	$Mg(OH)_2$	$CaCO_3$	Simethicone	ANC†
Maalox TC^R	600	300	0	0	27
Mylanta-II^R	400	400	0	40	25
Celusil-II^R	400	400	0	30	25
Milk of Magnesia^R	0	390	0	0	14
Maalox^R (reg.)	225	200	0	0	13
Mylanta^R	200	200	0	20	13
Celusil^R	200	200	0	25	12

*All of these agents are liquid preparations; however, many are available in tablet form.
†ANC = acid-neutralizing capacity.

nervous system also decreases gastric motility and intestinal motility. In order for these drugs to reach high enough levels actually to decrease gastric secretion, they must be given in doses that also create undesirable side effects, such as dry skin, dry mouth, blurred vision, constipation, and urinary retention. When taken at night, they may reduce gastric secretion and reduce night pain. Since the introduction of the H_2 blockers and other drugs, the antimuscarinics are used less frequently. Examples of some of these agents are **atropine** and **scopolamine (belladonna alkaloids), propantheline (Pro-Banthīne^R),** and **dicyclomine (Bentyl^R).**

Proton Pump Inhibitors. The proton pump inhibitors represent the newest drugs available for the treatment of ulcer disease. There is a potassium/hydrogen adenosine triphosphatase pump in the parietal cell of the stomach. This mechanism pumps hydrogen ion into the stomach in exchange for potassium ion. This appears to be a system unique to the GI tract, and not found in other cells of the body. Because of this high degree of localization, there are very few side effects caused by these drugs. To date the only drug that is used clinically is **omeprazole (Prilosec^R).** Clinical trials of this drug have shown that full doses result in a continuous higher gastric pH, which provides excellent results in preventing ulcers. One serious negative effect of this drug is that, in animal studies, it has been shown to cause tumor growth in the GI tract. This observation has not been shown to occur in humans.

Drugs That Increase Defense Factors

Drugs that increase the defense factors of the GI tract and increase healing and enhance mucus production include sucralfate, misoprostol, and the bismuth subsalicylate compounds.

Sucralfate (Carafate^R). This agent is a very nonreactive substance that combines with the proteins that exude from the surface of an ulcer. This produces a protective coating that is impenetrable to HCl, pepsin, and bile acids. It also has some *antispasmodic* activity and binds with bile salts. It is about as effective as cimetidine and accelerates the healing of an ulcer. **Adverse effects:** minimal but may include constipation, diarrhea, and nausea.

Misoprostol (Cytotec^R). This is a synthetic drug related to prostaglandins; it inhibits gastric acid secretion and has a cytoprotective effect (protects cells of the GI tract). The exact mechanism of protection is not clear, but it probably increases synthesis of mucosa cells and mucus, increases mucosal blood flow, and increases secretion of sodium bicarbonate. The drug has been extensively used to protect ulcers in patients receiving nonsteroidal anti-inflammatory drugs for rheumatoid arthritis. **Adverse effects:** diarrhea is the most common; also, some studies have linked the use of this drug with an increase in abortion rate.

Bismuth subsalicylate compounds. Bismuth compounds are perhaps one of the most highly used OTC agents for a number of GI problems. With regard to their protection and healing ability, they have been shown to coat ulcers and perhaps promote a protective barrier against HCl and pepsin. The exact mechanism is unknown, but bismuth compounds have been shown to be bacteriocidal against the GI organism *Helicobacter pylori*. Some authorities believe that this organism plays a role in peptic ulcer disease. **Adverse effects:** Minimal, but long-term use can cause constipation.

OVERALL BOWEL FUNCTION

The overall function of the lower bowel (large intestine) is to absorb some nutrients and eliminate waste material. The intestinal contents are moved along the length of the GI tract by rhythmic contractions known as peristalsis. In the small intestine, nutrients and water are absorbed, but, as the material moves into the large intestine, very little nutritional material is absorbed and most of the remaining water is finally absorbed. As the contents move into the lower bowel, the final process of defecation is initiated in the rectum. The movement of the fecal material and final defecation of the material can be affected by such factors as emotional stress, other changes in the nervous system, and changes in the autonomic nervous system. The process of defecation is under control of two divisions of the autonomic nervous system. The parasympathetic division generally increases intestinal motility and peristalsis, and the sympathetic division inhibits or decreases intestinal motility.

Occasionally normal bowel function can be altered, as is manifested by a change in motility. If the motility is increased, the contents move through the bowel more rapidly, creating inadequate time for water absorption and thus producing a watery stool (diarrhea). If the motility is decreased so that contents remain in the bowel, too much water is absorbed and a hard formed stool results, creating difficult defecation (constipation).

CAUSES AND TREATMENT OF DIARRHEA

Diarrhea is a symptom of increased intestinal motility and can either be acute (2 weeks or less) or chronic (lasting several weeks to several months). Acute diarrhea can occur very quickly and can be caused by infection, drugs, toxins, or diet. Acute diarrhea generally does not necessarily occur from any kind of organ pathology, but chronic diarrhea usually is accompanied by weight loss, muscle weakness, and electrolyte imbalance. Regardless of the type, if diarrhea is allowed to progress for long periods of time, it can lead to dehydration and electrolyte imbalance. If the dehydration and electrolyte imbalances are not treated, serious difficulties and even death can occur.

There are many causes and treatments of diarrhea, and Table 6–2 summarizes some of these. The overall treatment of diarrhea includes proper diagnosis of causative agents or conditions, followed by proper selection of an appropriate antidiarrheal agent. Sometimes an accurate diagnosis is very difficult in the management of diarrhea because there are over 50 diseases producing chronic diarrhea, and they can involve the kidney, liver, heart, thyroid glands, and other organs. Regardless of the choice of an appropriate drug,

TABLE 6–2 Causes and Treatments of Diarrhea

CAUSES	TREATMENT
Agents	
Microorganisms	Antibiotics
Drugs	
Antiacids	Discontinue drug use
Antibiotics	Discontinue drug use
Parasympathomimetics	Discontinue drug use
Laxatives	Discontinue drug use
Medical problems	
Chronic increase in intestinal motility	
Anemia	Antidiarrheal drugs
Carcinoma	Antidiarrheal drugs
Diabetes	Antidiarrheal drugs
Various forms of colitis	
Ulcerative colitis	Antidiarrheal drugs
Emotional stress	Antidiarrheal drugs

fluid loss cannot be tolerated, and the overall goal in the treatment of any diarrhea should be the replacement of fluids and electrolytes.

Categories of Antidiarrheal Drugs

There is some overlap in the various categories of antidiarrheal drugs. In order to simplify the learning of these drugs, they will be classified as absorbants, antimuscarinics, narcotics, and antimicrobials. Table 6–3 summarizes the categories and gives examples of antidiarrheal agents.

Absorbants. These drugs are intended to absorb the causative agents or substances such as bacterial, virus, and toxins. Also, some of these agents tend to decrease the fluid content of the stool. Most of these agents are classified as OTC drugs, but many clinicians hold these in low esteem. One major problem with some of these agents is their tendency to absorb nutrients and various drugs that many patients may be taking chronically. Some of the common absorbant drugs that are used include **kaolin** and **pectin** (Kaopectate[R]), **activated charcoal, bismuth salts** (Pepto-Bismol[R]), and **ion exchange resins.**

Antimuscarinics. These agents have been used for many years because they tend to decrease intestinal motility by blocking the parasympathetic nervous system. However, in order to have a significant effect, these drugs must be given in relatively high doses, and there is little evidence that suggests they are effective in treating diarrhea. Also, with higher doses antimuscarinic drugs can cause severe side effects such as dry mouth, blurred vision, and urinary retention. Examples of these agents are **atropine** and **scopolamine.**

TABLE 6–3 Antidiarrheal Agents	
CATEGORY	**DRUGS**
Absorbants	Bismuth subsalicylate (Pepto-Bismol[R])
	Kaolin and pectin (Kaopectate[R])
	Kaolin and pectin, atropine, scopolamine, and hyoscine (Donnagel[R])
Antimuscarinics	Atropine
	Scopolamine
Narcotic agents	
Natural	Opium
	Tincture of opium
	Paregoric
	Codeine
Synthetic	Diphenoxylate-atropine (Lomotil[R])
	Loperamide (Imodium[R])
Antimicrobials	Doxycycline
	Sulfamethoxazole-trimethoprim (Bactrim[R])

Narcotic Derivatives. This group of drugs represents the most effective group of antidiarrheal agents used today. The drugs that are clinically effective are all opioids, including naturally occurring opioids or synthetic derivatives. These drugs decrease intestinal motility by several mechanisms. First, they decrease emptying time of the stomach and, second, they act on the small intestine smooth muscle by causing localized spasms that break up the normal propelling activity of peristalsis. It is thought that this effect occurs by inhibiting acetylcholine release by the parasympathetic nerves and combining with opioid receptors. The opioids that are used most often include **tincture of opium, (paregoric),** and **codeine** (naturally occurring) and **diphenoxylate-atropine (Lomotil[R])** and **loperamide (Imodium[R]).** In general, the naturally occurring agents are used much less because of their potential central nervous system effects, such as analgesia, respiratory depression, and potential addiction. The synthetic agents are much less addicting, and particularly loperamide has far fewer central nervous system effects with a longer duration of action. It should be noted that there is some controversy regarding the use of any of these agents, but loperamide is probably the safest.

Antimicrobial Agents. Although a large number of diarrhea cases are caused by various microbial infections, in a normally healthy individual they usually are self-limiting and generally do not require antimicrobial therapy. It is generally believed that these agents should not be used unless the patient has a high fever or bloody diarrhea, or the infection is persistent. If an antibiotic is necessary, it should be remembered that some of the antimicrobials themselves can cause diarrhea, and great caution should be used in selecting a drug. Some effective antimicrobials that have been used in the treatment of diarrhea include **doxycycline** and **sulfamethoxazole-trimethoprim (Bactrim**^{R}**)**. Also, sometimes these agents are used in combination with loperamide.

CONSTIPATION AND ITS TREATMENT

Constipation is described as a decrease in frequency of fecal elimination and is characterized by difficult passage of hard, dry stools. It often is difficult to determine whether or not a patient is truly constipated because the so-called normal frequency varies anywhere from 3 per day to 3 per week. Treatment of constipation includes the use of some type of *laxative* or *cathartic* that stimulates defecation.

There are a number of conditions that can cause constipation, including poor bowel habits, lack of normal fiber in the diet, inadequate fluid intake, the use of narcotic drugs, and emotional stress. In addition, there can be some underlying medical and pathophysiological problems, such as metabolic and endocrine disorders, neurogenic problems, and defects in bowel structure.

In the overall treatment of constipation, one should realize that constipation is a symptom and not a disease. Therefore, before using a laxative/cathartic, a number of preliminary steps should be taken:

1. Eliminate any constipating drugs
2. Deal with any underlying pathological problem
3. Use nondrug therapy, such as adequate fiber in the diet, physical exercise, and adequate fluid intake
4. Reduce emotional stress
5. Teach patient to respond to the urge to defecate (this is especially true in children)

There are four recognized medical indications for laxative use: 1) treatment of patients who have had long-term bed confinement, 2) preparation for diagnostic procedures, 3) to ensure soft stools following certain surgical and medical problems, and 4) treatment of patients with anal–rectal disorders.

LAXATIVES AND CATHARTICS

These two terms are used when describing a drug effect rather than the drug itself. In other words, the same drug, depending on the dose that is used, can result in a laxative effect or a cathartic effect. A laxative facilitates the elimination of a soft but firm stool, whereas a cathartic is used to produce a fluid stool. Also, the cathartic effect is more rapid and acts with a great deal more intensity.

Categories of Laxatives/Cathartics

There are many categorizations of laxatives/cathartics that have been used based on the site of action, chemical substance, intensity, and mechanism of action. Because there is so much overlap in all of these categories, the categories used in this text are bulk-forming agents, saline cathartics, contact cathartics, and others. Table 6–4 summarizes the categories and lists some of the commonly used laxatives.

Bulk-Forming Agents.   These are inert, nonabsorbable substances that absorb and retain water, increase fecal mass, and increase rate of defecation. These agents are the most gentle types of agents and are most desirable for elderly patients, who may have *diverticulosis* problems. These drugs are not rapid in terms of onset of action and take 1–3 days for clinical results. The agents that are included in this group are: **methylcellulose, carboxy methylcellulose, dietary fiber, psyllium,** and **polycarbophil.**

Saline Cathartics.   These are very potent relatively nonabsorbable inorganic salts. They osmotically pull water into the bowel, creating watery stools within 1–3 hours. These agents primarily are used to evacuate the bowel for *endoscopic* examination procedures, for elimination of drugs, and in preparation for bowel surgery. These agents include **magnesium sulfate, hydroxide,** or **citrate, sodium phosphate** or **sulfate,** and **potassium salts.**

Contact Cathartics.   These are chemical substances that are absorbed and act as irritants or stimulants to the bowel, causing a rather rapid onset of action, usually within 2 hours. These agents are commonly available over the counter but should never be consumed for more than 1 week at a time. These drugs can be particularly dangerous if used when symptoms of appendicitis are present. These agents include **phenolphthalein, bisacodyl, senna, danthrarim,** and **castor oil.**

Other Laxatives and Cathartics.   This miscellaneous group act as lubricants and *emollients* by coating the stool to make it soft and reducing water absorption. These agents include **docusate, mineral oil,** and **olive oil.**

TABLE 6–4 Commonly Used Laxatives	
CATEGORIES	**DRUGS**
Bulk forming	Dietary foods—prunes, bran
	Carboxylcellulose (Bu-lak[R])
	Psyllium (Metamucil[R])
Saline cathartics	Magnesium hydroxide (Phillips Milk of Magnesia[R])
	Magnesium citrate
	Sodium biphosphate and Sodium phosphate (Fleet Enema[R])
	Sodium phosphate, carbonate and citrate (Sal Hepatica[R])
Contact cathartics	Phenolphthalein (Ex-Lax[R])
	Bisacodyl (Dulcolax[R])
	Danthron (Dorbane[R])
	Senna (Fletcher's Castoria[R])
	Castor oil
Other cathartics	Mineral oil (Haleys MO[R])
	Phenolphthalein, docusate, and olive oil

POSTTEST: PHARMACOLOGY OF THE GASTROINTESTINAL TRACT

For each of the following questions, try to select the *one* best answer from those choices given.

1. All of the following stimulate the secretion of gastric juice except:
   a. vagus nerve
   b. sympathetic nervous system
   c. parasympathetic nervous system
   d. gastrin
2. Any drug or secretion that alters the production of mucus in the lining of the GI tract has the potential of causing ulcers. True or False?
3. All of the following are nonmedicinal factors in the management of ulcer disease except:
   a. decreasing emotional stress
   b. avoiding the use of nonsteroidal anti-inflammatory drugs
   c. increasing intake of high protein food
   d. limiting alcohol intake
4. Which of the following drugs do not decrease the attack factors in the treatment of ulcer disease?
   a. H_2 blockers
   b. antacids
   c. bismuth compounds
   d. antimuscarinics
5. Which of the following drugs do not increase the defense factors in the GI tract?
   a. sucralfate (Carafate[R])
   b. ranitidine (Zantac[R])
   c. bismuth compounds
   d. misoprostol (Cytotec[R])
6. Even though narcotics are powerful stimulants of smooth muscle, they are excellent antidiarrheal agents. True or False?

REFERENCES/RECOMMENDED READING

Dipalma JR, Digregornio JG: *Basic Pharmacology in Medicine*, 3rd ed. McGraw-Hill, New York, 1990.

Handbook of Nonprescription Drugs, 9th ed. American Pharmaceutical Association, Washington, DC, 1990.

Hitner H, Nagle BT: *Basic Pharmacology for Health Occupations*, 2nd ed. Glenco Publishing Co, Mission Hills, CA, 1987.

Physicians' Desk Reference for Nonprescription Drugs, 12th ed. Medical Economics Company, Montvale, NJ, 1991.

Tortora GJ, Anagnostakus NP: *Principles of Anatomy and Physiology*, Harper & Row, New York, 1990.

CHAPTER **7**

PHARMACOLOGY OF THE ENDOCRINE SYSTEM

LEARNING OBJECTIVES

After completion of this chapter and its learning activities, the student will be able to:

1. Describe the relationship between the pituitary gland and the hypothalamus as the regulatory mechanism of hormones of the body.
2. Describe negative feed back as a example of an endogenous control mechanism of hormones, using thyroxin as an example.
3. Describe the structure and location of the adrenal glands and list the hormones produced by the adrenal cortex, along with effects of the corticosteroids.
4. List the overall effects, therapeutic uses, and side effects of the glucocorticoids; also list some of the synthetic glucocorticoids.
5. List the overall effects, therapeutic uses, and side effects of the mineralocorticosteroids.
6. Describe the overall function of the thyroid gland hormones and contrast hyperthyroidism and hypothyroidism.
7. Describe the symptoms of hypothyroidism and list the various drugs used in treatment of this condition.
8. Describe the symptoms of hyperthyroidism and list the various drugs used in treatment of this condition.
9. Describe the structure and location of the parathyroid gland and list the two hormones that control calcium levels.
10. Describe the symptoms of hypoparathyroidism and list the drugs used in the treatment of this disease.
11. Describe the overall function of the pancreas and list the functions of insulin and glucagon.
12. Describe the pathogenesis of diabetes mellitus and describe two types of this disease.
13. Describe the overall treatment of diabetes mellitus and emphasize the role of proper diet.
14. List the drugs used to treat type I diabetes mellitus and describe the general mechanism of action and side effects of these drugs.

120

15. List the drugs used to treat type II diabetes mellitus and describe the general mechanism of action and side effects of these drugs.
16. Describe the relationship between antigen–antibody reactions, mast cells, and histamine
17. Describe the overall effects of histamine and list the locations and types of histamine receptors.
18. Define the terms *antiallergic* and *antihistamine*.
19. Describe the clinical effects of antihistamines and list several commonly used antihistamine drugs, along with potential side effects.
20. List uses of antihistamines other than the treatment of allergies.

INTRODUCTION

Like the nervous system, the endocrine system regulates various functions of the body. This is accomplished by the release of chemicals (hormones) directly into the bloodstream from various endocrine glands located throughout the body. In contrast to nervous control of the body functions, hormones have a slower onset and a longer duration of action. Hormones are regulatory and are an intricate part of the body's control mechanisms. They differ from drugs in the following ways:

1. In general they have a higher therapeutic index.
2. Unlike most drugs, many have an endogenous control mechanism called *feedback control*.
3. Many hormones have a very broad effect on various organ systems.
4. The effects of one hormone can be *additive*, *nonreactive*, or *antagonistic* with those of a second hormone.

In terms of therapeutics, hormones and related compounds have the following uses: replacement therapy, reduction of endogenous hormone synthesis, reduction of the effects of endogenous hormones, and diagnosis of endocrine pathophysiology. In addition, some are used in the treatment of nonendocrine diseases.

This chapter discusses a selected group of hormones that commonly are used therapeutically along with some disease entities that are treated by these hormones. The hormones included are adreno-corticosteroids, thyroid and parathyroid hormones, insulin, and glucagon. The antihistamines also are discussed in this chapter because histamine is an endogenous substance that is released into the bloodstream by mast cells and, like hormones, has a broad effect throughout the body.

PITUITARY GLAND AND HYPOTHALAMUS

The pituitary gland often is referred to as the "master endocrine" gland of the body. It is located in the cranial cavity attached to an inferior portion of the brain called the hypothalamus (Figure 7–1).

The hypothalamus is the part of the central nervous system that controls the autonomic nervous system as well as the pituitary gland. It is the close association between the hypothalamus and the pituitary gland that establishes a direct anatomical relationship between the two systems of the body responsible for involuntary control of *homeostatic* mechanisms (i.e., the autonomic nervous system and the endocrine system). We have already discussed the autonomic nervous system in Chapter 2; this chapter discusses how the hypothalamus controls the pituitary gland. Whereas the autonomic nervous system controls functions of the body by direct innervation through parasympathetic and sympathetic nerves, the endocrine system controls body functions by secreting hormones directly into the bloodstream.

The pituitary gland is composed of two lobes: the anterior lobe (adenohypophysis) and the posterior lobe (neurohypophysis). Each of these lobes contains different hormones that can be released into the systemic circulation. Each lobe is controlled by the hypothalamus by two different mechanisms. The hormones of the adenohypophysis are controlled by hormones produced in the hypothalamus called *releasing hormones*. These hormones are secreted by the hypothalamus and travel through a *portal* blood system to the anterior lobe and cause release of the various hormones produced in the anterior lobe. The hormones of the adenohypophysis include human growth hormone (hGH), adrenocorticotropic hormone (ACTH), follicle-stimulating hormone (FSH), prolactin (Prl), luteinizing

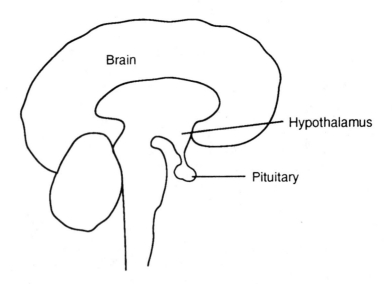

FIGURE 7–1   Relationship of Pituitary Gland and Hypothalamus.

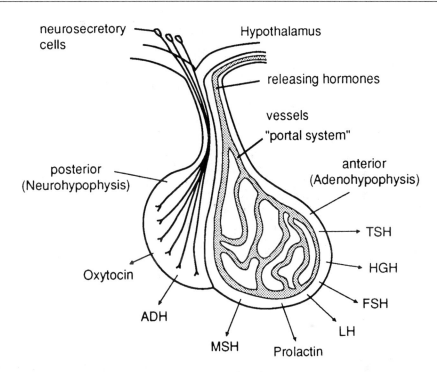

FIGURE 7–2   Hormones of the Pituitary Gland.

hormone (LH), thyroid-stimulating hormone (TSH), and melanocyte-stimulating hormone (MSH). Most of the hormones in the anterior lobe have an effect on other endocrine glands located throughout the body. (Hormones that affect other endocrine glands are called *tropic* hormones.)

The hormones of the neurohypophysis are synthesized in the hypothalamus and travel through the nerve axons of neurosecretory cells to the posterior lobe, where they are stored until released. The hormones secreted by the neurohypophysis include antidiuretic hormone (ADH) and oxytocin. In summary, there are actually three types of hormones that function in the endocrine system: the releasing hormones produced in the hypothalamus, the tropic hormones released from the anterior lobe that affect other endocrine glands, and the hormones released from each of the individual endocrine glands. Figure 7–2 represents the structure of the pituitary gland and the hormones that are released from both lobes.

CONTROL OF HORMONE RELEASE

With the release of the various hormones throughout the body, there is need for some type of control mechanism. Although several different mechanisms exist, the main type

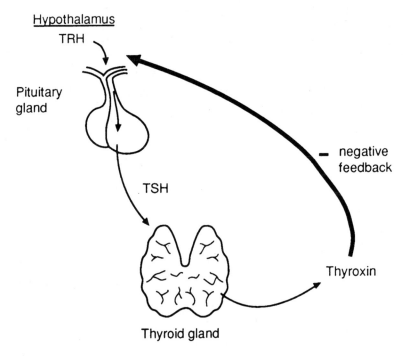

FIGURE 7–3   Negative Feedback Control of Thyroxin.

of control mechanism is known as negative feedback. The term *negative feedback* does not mean that the feedback is in someway harmful, but essentially means that, once a hormone is released and reaches a certain blood level, this appropriate blood level inhibits any further release by negative feedback. Figure 7–3 shows an example of this negative feedback with the control of thyroxin release.

As seen in Figure 7–3, when thyroxin levels are low or there is a physiological need to increase these levels, the hypothalamus releases thyrotropin-releasing hormone (TRH). This hormone travels through the portal system to the adenohypophysis and causes the release of TSH. TSH then travels to the thyroid gland through the systemic circulation and causes the thyroid gland to release thyroxin. When thyroxin reaches normal levels, the elevated hormone concentration feeds back to the hypothalamus and shuts off the release of TRH. Thus, the increased level of the hormone feeds back and decreases its own release.

CORTICOSTEROIDS AND OVERALL EFFECTS

The adrenal glands (*suprarenal*) are located on the superior surface of each kidney. Each gland is composed of an outer cortex and an inner medulla. (Figure 7–4). The medulla

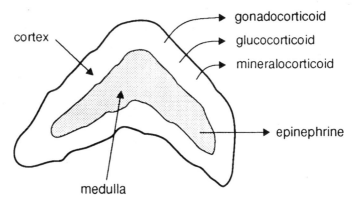

cortex

gonadocorticoid

glucocorticoid

mineralocorticoid

epinephrine

medulla

FIGURE 7–4 The Adrenal Gland.

is responsible for the secretion of epinephrine and is innervated by the sympathetic nervous system. When the body is in a "fight or flight" condition, epinephrine is secreted into the blood by the adrenal medulla. The adrenal cortex is divided into three zones, each of which produces a different hormone. These hormones are the glucocorticoids, the mineralocorticoids, and the gonadocorticoids, collectively known as corticosteroids. All of the corticosteroids have specific functions and effects on the body, but the effects of the gonadocorticoids are not as significant or as completely understood as those of the glucocorticoids and the mineralocorticoids. Therefore, this text will only mention the general function of the gonadocorticoids. Table 7–1 summarizes the overall effects of corticosteroids.

Glucocorticoids

The glucocorticoids are responsible for carbohydrate and protein metabolism, particularly during periods of stress. When the body is stressed, there is a need for glucose, particularly in tissues undergoing repair. Also, the brain as well as other tissue needs glucose as an

TABLE 7–1 Function of Corticosteroids

CORTICOSTEROIDS	OVERALL FUNCTION
Glucocorticoids	Regulate metabolism of carbohydrates and proteins by gluconeogenesis and protein catabolism; also have a potent anti-inflammatory effect
Mineralocorticoids	Sodium and potassium balance: controlled by reabsorption of sodium in the kidney
Gonadocorticoids	Major/minor effect on the function of the sex glands; overall function not clearly understood

TABLE 7–2 The Glucocorticoids	
DRUG	**GENERAL ANTI-INFLAMMATORY DOSE (per kg)**
Naturally occurring	
Hydrocortisone	20 mg
Cortisone	25 mg
Synthetic	
Prednisone	5 mg
Triamcinolone	4 mg
Betamethasone	0.60 mg
Dexamethasone	0.75 mg

energy source, and high levels are needed, particularly in periods of stress. Thus, the overall effect of the glucocorticoids is to replenish body stores of glucose through *gluconeogenesis* and protein *catabolism*. Therapeutic uses of glucocorticoids include replacement therapy for adrenal gland insufficiency, as seen in Addison disease; also, the glucocorticoids often are used clinically as potent anti-inflammatory agents.

Usually inflammation is a normal reaction of the healing process, but there are many pathological conditions wherein inflammation itself becomes the disease process. Some of these are rheumatoid arthritis, asthma, systemic lupus erythematosus, and various chronic allergies. Clinically, the naturally occurring glucocorticoids originally were used as therapeutic agents, but today newer synthetic agents are administered because of their longer duration of action and generally fewer side effects. Table 7–2 lists the naturally occurring and some of the synthetic glucocorticoids, along with their comparative anti-inflammatory doses.

A major problem with the clinical use of glucocorticoids is that, when they are used for long periods of time and particularly in high doses, a condition known as Cushing Syndrome can occur (symptoms are listed in Table 7–3). Also, with long-term use adrenal suppression can occur and, if withdrawal is abrupt, adrenal shutdown will occur, causing severe shock and even death. Table 7–3 lists some of the adverse side effects that can occur with long-term glucocorticoid use.

Mineralocorticoids

The mineralocorticoids are responsible for maintaining a balance between sodium and potassium and help to maintain fluid–electrolyte balance. The mineralocorticoid aldosterone is the main substance that controls sodium reabsorption. This occurs in the distal convoluted tubal of the nephron in exchange for potassium (refer to Figure 5–3 in Chapter 5). Because of the reabsorption of sodium, water is also reabsorbed and thus normal sodium and water balance is maintained.

TABLE 7-3   Adverse Effects of Glucocorticoids

DRUG EFFECT	SYMPTOMS
Increased gluconeogenesis	Obesity and diabetes mellitus
Increased protein catabolism	Muscle weakness, osteoporosis, decreased growth in children, poor wound healing, increase in infection, peptic ulcer formation, Cushing syndrome (edema, moon face, buffalo hump, etc.)
Miscellaneous effects	Glaucoma, cataract formation, euphoria, addiction, depression

The mineralocorticoids are used clinically only when there is some type of adrenal failure causing hyposecretion of aldosterone. This occurs when the adrenal gland is removed or as the result of some type of tumor. Also, the mineralocorticoids are used as replacement therapy in Addison disease. The main adverse effects that occur with mineralocorticoid use are sodium and water retention and loss of potassium. The symptoms associated with high levels of mineralocorticoids include edema, hypertension, and muscle weakness from the potassium loss. There are very few commercially available mineralocorticoids; Table 7-4 lists some of these along with their route of administration.

OVERALL FUNCTION OF THYROID GLAND

The thyroid gland is located anterior to the trachea just below the larynx. It produces three hormones that are responsible for growth and development of body tissue: triiodothyronine (T_3), thyroxine (T_4), and thyrocalcitonin (TCT). The designations T_3 and T_4 represent the number of iodine atoms attached to the central molecule. Iodine is absolutely essential in the synthesis of these two hormones, and this is one of the reasons that iodine is added to our normal source of salt (iodized salt) in order to ensure adequate amounts in our diet.

TABLE 7-4   Mineralocorticoids

MINERALOCORTICOIDS	ROUTE
Aldosterone	Not available
Desoxycorticosterone (Percorten[R])	Intramuscular
Fludrocortisone acetate (Florone[R])	Oral

TABLE 7–5 Thyroid Hormones	
DRUG	**TRADE NAME**
Levothyroxine sodium	Levothroid[R], Synthroid[R]
Liothyronine sodium	Cytomel[R]
Liotrix	Euthroid[R]
Thyroglobulin*	Proloid[R]
Thyroid hormone (desiccated)	Armour Thyroid[R], Thyrar[R]

*This substance is the globulin that stores thyroxin in the thyroid gland.

The secretion of T_3 and T_4 is under the control of TSH from the anterior pituitary gland. The secretion of TCT is controlled by calcium levels in the blood and is discussed in the section covering the parathyroid gland. When T_3 and T_4 are released into the bloodstream they are responsible for stimulation of protein synthesis, increase in levels of blood glucose, increase in circulation of fatty acids, and decrease in serum cholesterol. All of these substances are necessary and essential for cell repair and energy. Also, when there is an increase in T_3 and T_4, cellular metabolism increases and results in an elevation of the basal metabolic rate. Thus, these hormones are important in the generation of heat.

There are two disease entities or conditions of the thyroid gland that are treated by drugs: hyposecretion of T_3 and T_4 leading to hypothyroidism, and hypersecretion leading to hyperthyroidism. Hyposecretion can be caused by excessive exposure to radiation, lack of iodine, lack of secretion of TSH from the pituitary, or surgical removal of a thyroid gland. Hypersecretion can be caused by tumors or *autoimmune* disease (Graves' disease).

Treatment of Hypothyroidism

When hypothyroidism occurs, it is manifested differently in children and adults. In children and infants, hyposecretion can lead to mental and physical retardation and dwarfism, called *cretinism*. In adults, hyposecretion leads to a clinical condition called myxedema and nontoxic goiter. Symptoms of myxedema include lethargy, low blood pressure, and sensitivity to cold, and the patient has an appearance of *senility* and *dementia*.

Hypothyroidism is treated by hormonal replacement, and these hormones are extracted from various animal sources or are produced synthetically. Although the various preparations are effective, they must be given on a gradual and carefully monitored basis in order to meet the patients needs. Table 7–5 lists several of the currently used thyroxine preparations along with their trade names.

Adverse effects that are associated with overdose of thyroid hormones can include symptoms similar to hyperthyroidism, such as psychic disorders, diarrhea, increased blood pressure, weight loss, menstrual irregularities, and sweating. Also, elevated levels of these hormones can have a profound effect on the cardiovascular system, causing angina, hypertension, and cardiac arrhythmias.

Treatment of Hyperthyroidism

When hyperthyroidism occurs, it is the result of increased secretion or release of T_3 and T_4. This excessive secretion usually is caused by a glandular tumor of the thyroid or pituitary gland or a malignancy of the hypothalamus. In addition, an autoimmune disease (Graves disease) produces effects similar to chronic thyroid stimulation. The overall effects of excessive thyroid secretion cause symptoms that resemble excessive stimulation of the sympathetic nervous system. The hypersecretion may cause a condition of exophthalmic goiter, hypertension, weight loss, and *thyroid storm* (potentially fatal).

The treatment of hyperthyroidism is accomplished by three approaches: use of antithyroid drugs, radiation, and surgical removal. Often a combination of these three methods is used in treatment of this disease. The drugs used in the treatment of hyperthyroidism have a very complex mechanism of action and basically interfere with various methods of absorbing iodine. This text will not go into details of the mechanism of action and will only summarize the main mechanisms that are pertinent to the various drugs mentioned. Table 7–6 lists some of the commonly used antithyroid drugs with a brief description of mechanism of action.

The adverse effects of the antithyroid drugs include rash, fever, myalgia, jaundice, nausea, and bone marrow suppression. Occasionally patients using radioactive iodine become hypothyroid and have to use replacement therapy throughout life. Also, high doses of iodine (high doses inhibit the thyroid gland from incorporating iodine) should be used only for short-term treatment because eventually the suppression is overcome by the gland and there is an immediate surge in T_3 and T_4, causing a hyperthyroid crisis.

STRUCTURE AND FUNCTION OF PARATHYROID GLAND

The parathyroid gland is made up of four islands of tissue located in the two lobes of the thyroid gland. Because of their location, when the thyroid gland is surgically removed, the parathyroids are sometimes removed also. The hormone that is secreted by the parathyroid gland is called parathyroid hormone (PTH). As mentioned earlier, it is one of two hormones that control blood levels of calcium. The other hormone controlling blood calcium levels is calcitonin, which is secreted by the thyroid gland. The effects of the two hormones are summarized in Table 7–7.

The secretion of the two hormones is controlled by blood calcium levels. When the blood calcium drops (*hypocalcemia*), PTH is released and stimulates osteoclastic activity, which increases resorption of bone. In addition, PTH increases the absorption of calcium in the intestinal tract as well as the kidney, and these two reabsorption processes require the presence of vitamin D. When the blood calcium level increases (*hypercalcemia*), TCT

TABLE 7–6 Antithyroid Drugs

DRUGS	MECHANISM OF ACTION
Potassium iodide and sodium iodide (Lugol Solution[R])	Excessive iodine doses inhibit the incorporation of iodine into the gland
Radioactive iodine (Iodotope I-131[R])	Emits radioactive particles to the glandular cell and destroys the gland
Methimazole (Tapazole[R])	Interferes with synthesis of T_3 and T_4
Propylthiouracil	Interferes with synthesis of T_3 and T_4

is released and directly inhibits PTH and also inhibits bone resorption. Vitamin D is not necessary for the action of TCT.

Hypoparathyroidism

The main disease associated with calcium balance is hypoparathyroidism. Because of this condition, PTH is not available and hypocalcemia results. This causes hyperexcitability of the neuromuscular junction, leading to *spastic* and *tetanic* muscle contraction. Contrary to most endocrine disorders in which a hormone deficiency exists, PTH is not adminis-

TABLE 7–7 Hormones Controlling Blood Calcium

HORMONE	SOURCE	EFFECT ON BLOOD CALCIUM	MECHANISM
Parathyroid hormone	Parathyroid gland	Increases blood calcium	Increases calcium and magnesium absorption in gastrointestinal tract, stimulates osteoclastic activity, and, along with vitamin D, increases calcium absorption in the kidney
Thyrocalcitonin	Thyroid gland	Decreases blood calcium	Accelerates calcium absorption by bone

TABLE 7–8 Drugs Used in the Treatment of Hypoparathyroidism	
DRUG	**USE**
Calcium chloride	Increases blood calcium
Calcium gluconate	Increases blood calcium
Calcium lactate	Increases blood calcium
Vitamin D	Increases absorption of blood calcium
Ergocalciferol (Vit D_2^R)	
Dihydrotachysterol (Hytakerol^R)	

tered. This hormone is available for injection but causes severe allergic reactions, and drug resistance usually develops within a short period of time.

The normal treatment for hypoparathyroidism is the administration of oral calcium salts along with vitamin D supplements. Table 7–8 lists some of the substances used in the treatment of hypoparathyroidism.

It should be noted that the use of calcium salts and vitamin D are not without problems. Excessive use can lead to kidney stone formation and excessive vitamin D can lead to *hypervitaminosis* problems.

Hyperparathyroidism and hypercalcemia are rather rare disorders and they will not be discussed in this text.

OVERALL FUNCTION OF THE PANCREAS

The overall function of the pancreas is to produce important digestive enzymes plus two hormones, insulin and glucagon. Therefore, the pancreas functions as both an *exocrine* gland for digestion and an endocrine gland for the control of blood glucose levels. This text will not mention the digestive functions but will discuss the endocrine function of the two hormones.

Located throughout the body of the pancreas are islands of cells (islets of Langerhans) that secrete the two hormones. A type of cell called an alpha cell secretes glucagon and another cell called a beta cell secretes insulin. Insulin levels are controlled in response to blood glucose levels. When the blood glucose level increases, insulin is released and has the following functions:

1. Increases glucose absorption into tissues that cannot absorb glucose without a special mechanism (i.e., skeletal muscle, cardiac tissue, and fat)
2. stimulates the storage of glycogen
3. stimulates the storage and synthesis of fat and protein.

Glucagon is released in response to a drop in blood glucose levels and has the following functions: 1) stimulates breakdown of glycogen to glucose (*glycogenolysis*), and

2) stimulates the breakdown of protein through the conversion of amino acids to glucose (*gluconeogenesis*). Thus, insulin and glucagon maintain a homeostatic balance of blood glucose.

DIABETES MELLITUS

Diabetes mellitus is a common disease of endocrine cell dysfunction of the pancreas caused by a failure of the beta cells to produce adequate insulin. In diabetic patients the production may be totally absent or partial. If the disease is due to total insulin insufficiency, the patient is said to be insulin dependent or to have type I disease. This type of diabetes has an early onset in life and also is called *growth onset*. If the circulating insulin is ineffective as a result of a number of factors, the patient is said to be insulin resistant or to have type II diabetes. Also, type II diabetes can result from a low level of insulin secretion. This type of diabetes has an onset after the age of 40 and therefore is called *maturity-onset* diabetes. The exact cause of diabetes mellitus is unknown, but it is probably an autoimmune disorder with genetic factors implicated in the growth-onset type. In the maturity-onset type, aging, obesity, and improper diet control with a corresponding genetic background are involved.

The symptoms of both types are caused by lack of insulin, and thus there is a lack of glucose in the cells of the body. Some of the classic characteristics of lack of glucose absorption in tissues and cells of the body are *hyperglycemia*, *glucosuria*, *ketosis*, *polyphagia*, *polydipsia*, and dry mouth. Table 7–9 summarizes some of the symptoms of diabetes mellitus.

Overall Treatment of Diabetes Mellitus

When diabetes is first diagnosed, the overall objective is to control the metabolic balance and return fluids and electrolytes to the body. If symptoms are severe, immediate insulin administration rapidly reduces hyperglycemia and eliminates ketoacidosis. Depending on whether a patient has type I or type II diabetes, therapy generally is aimed at regulating glucose levels through diet control and/or drug administration. In terms of diet control, carbohydrate intake is limited so that a constant challenge for insulin release is decreased. In addition, it is important to maintain an adequate exercise program to burn excess glucose and thus decrease hyperglycemia. Also, it should be noted that, when diabetes is diagnosed, regardless of whether or not treatment and diet control have begun, only the symptoms of hyperglycemia and acidosis can be controlled by proper therapy. Insulin use is not a cure and will not prevent some of the long-term effects of the disease, but proper medication and diet can greatly reduce severity of the long-term effects.

Treatment of Type I Diabetes

Type I diabetics (growth onset) usually will require the use of insulin throughout life. In addition to proper control of dosage of insulin at proper intervals, the patient must

TABLE 7–9 Symptoms of Diabetes Mellitus

SYMPTOM	CAUSE
Hyperglycemia	Elevated glucose levels caused by lack of insulin to transport glucose into the tissues
Glucosuria	Glucose is increased in the urine because so much glucose is in the blood and the kidney cannot reabsorb it
Ketosis*	Because the cells cannot access glucose, the body breaks down protein and fats as source of energy, causing ketone bodies and ketone acidosis in the urine. (ketonuria) and metabolic acidosis (ketosis)
Polyphagia	A desire to eat or "hunger" because the cells are starving, causing a desire for increased food intake
Polydypsia	Extreme thirst because the glucose molecules in the kidney act as an osmotic diuretic, causing an increase in urine volume (dehydration)
Polyuria	Same as for polydypsia
Dry mouth	Caused by loss of excess amounts of water from the body, dehydration

*It should be noted that ketosis is more common with type I than type II diabetes.

continually watch carbohydrate intake, maintain a healthy life-style, and maintain a good exercise program. The main problem with insulin use is that the drug must be given parenterally (intravenously, subcutaneously, or by intramuscular injection). In addition to the problem of administration, most insulins are active *polypeptide* substances that are extracted from various animal sources (beef and pork). Because of this animal source, they often cause allergic reactions necessitating a change of medication in order to find a less allergenic substance. Also, many diabetics eventually experience various tissue reaction problems at the site of the injection. In order to minimize problems in the subcutaneous tissue, the patient must keep records of the site of injection and rotate the site to alternative areas of the body. The most common adverse effects of insulin include blurred vision. The most severe effect is when the insulin dose is too high, causing a sudden drop of blood glucose (insulin shock). When this occurs, the patient will experience hunger, headache, fatigue, anxiety, nervousness, and *paresthesia*. If the hypoglycemia is severe enough, fainting, unconsciousness, and convulsions may occur. If the patient is awake and coherent, this can be counteracted by administration of fruit juice, candy bars, or some other type of oral glucose preparation. If the patient is unconscious and in a coma, intravenous (IV) glucose or some type of IV dextrose solution can be administered.

Insulin is available in many different forms with various onsets of action. Also, human insulin, which has fewer complications, is now available. Table 7–10 lists a few

TABLE 7–10   Characteristics of Commercially Available Insulin Preparations

DRUG	DURATION
Regular insulin, crystalline zinc insulin (Humulin[R], Iletin I[R])	Short acting
Globin zinc insulin (Globin Zinc Insulin Injection*)	Intermediate
Isophane insulin suspension (Humulin N[R], NPH Iletin I[R], NPH Iletin II[R])	Intermediate
Protamine zinc insulin suspension (Protamine, Zinc & Iletin I[R])	Long
Prompt insulin zinc suspension (Semilente Iletin I[R], Semilente Insulin[R], Semitard[R])	Short
Insulin zinc suspension (Lentard[R], Lente Iletin I[R], Lente Insulin[R], Monotard[R])	Intermediate
Extended insulin zinc suspension (Ultralente Iletin I[R], Ultralente Insulin[R], Ultratard[R])	Long

of the commonly available insulin preparations, which are listed according to the drug name and length of action.

It should be noted that a human insulin preparation has been synthesized by recombinant DNA technology but is not as readily available and is extremely expensive.

Treatment of Type II Diabetes

This type of diabetes occurs later in life and can be treated with diet control, insulin, and a group of drugs called oral hypoglycemic agents. This type of diabetes usually is easier to control and often can be controlled by careful monitoring of diet without any drug therapy. If the pancreas is still functioning and the beta cells are able to release insulin, type II diabetes can be controlled with the oral hypoglycemic drugs. These drugs have no "insulin-like" activity but are able to stimulate the release of insulin from the intact beta cells in the pancreas. These drugs are not effective in type I diabetes because the beta cells in these individuals usually are nonfunctional. The biggest advantage of these drugs is that no trauma or complication at an injection site occurs; however, if the patient suffers from acidosis, insulin will need to be added to the regimen. This group of drugs stimulate the beta cells to release insulin and are called sulfonylureas. There are four first-generation drugs and two second-generation drugs currently available. Table 7–11 lists the names and duration of action of some of the commonly used oral hypoglycemic agents. The major adverse effect of these drugs is that they can cause hypoglycemia. In addition, other adverse effects include gastrointestinal (GI) irritation, muscle weakness, fatigue, and dizziness. Also, various kinds of hypersensitivity reactions, such as photosensitivity, rashes, and jaundice, can occur.

TABLE 7–11 Oral Hypoglycemic Agents	
DRUG	**DURATION**
First Generation	
Acetohexamide (Dymelor[R])	12–24 hr
Chlorpropamide (Diabinese[R])	60 hr
Tolazamide (Tolinase[R])	24 hr
Tolbutamide (Orinase[R])	6–12 hr
Second Generation	
Glipizide (Glucotrol[R])	10–24 hr
Glyburide (Micronase[R])	24 hr

ANTIGEN–ANTIBODY REACTIONS

Allergic reactions in the body are manifested by various symptoms that commonly are associated with symptoms, such as nasal congestion, sneezing, runny eyes, and itching. If a severe reaction occurs (antigen–antibody), more serious complications can occur, such as severe drop in blood pressure, bronchial constriction, and cardiovascular collapse. This type of reaction is termed *anaphylactic shock*. The substance that triggers an allergic or anaphylactic reaction is called an antigen. Antigens are usually protein in structure but can include a number of substances, such as animal products, mold, dust, and drugs.

When antigens enter the body, they stimulate the formation of antibodies in both the blood and tissues. When the body has become sensitized and an antigen is introduced or reintroduced, an antigen–antibody reaction occurs that can lead to severe allergic symptoms. Allergic reactions that occur in asthmatics or patients with chronic obstructive pulmonary disease can be very serious and greatly affect the ability of the patient to breath. When an antigen–antibody reaction occurs, certain cells (mast cells) release a number of active substances into the blood. The most important substance released is histamine, and it is histamine that is responsible for most of the symptoms of an allergic reaction.

Overall Effects of Histamine

In order to understand the effects and mechanism of action of antihistamines, it is necessary to know the overall physiological effects of histamine. Histamine is produced by mast cells and certain *basophil* white cells throughout the body. The largest concentrations of mast cells are found in the lungs, GI tract, and skin. When histamine is released into the bloodstream, it produces a number of physiological effects, particularly in the vascular and nonvascular smooth muscle and the heart. These effects are summarized in Table 7–12.

TABLE 7–12 Effects of Histamine	
SYSTEM/TISSUE	**HISTAMINE EFFECT**
Blood pressure	Decreased
Heart rate	Increased
Bronchial	Constriction
Intestine	Contraction
Small vessels and capillaries	Dilation

Vascular Effects. The main effect of histamine on the vascular tissue is on the smooth muscles of blood vessels and capillaries. The smooth muscle relaxation causes vasodilation that also, in the presence of large amounts of histamine, can cause a profound drop in blood pressure and cardiovascular collapse. When the vasodilation occurs in the skin, it causes erythremia (redness). When the vasodilation occurs in the brain, it causes a headache (histamine headache). In addition to the vasodilation, the capillary membranes become "leaky" and fluids diffuse into the extravascular space, causing congestion in the nasal and upper airway mucosa and edema and/or hives on the skin. Also, histamine stimulates small nerve endings, causing extreme itching and in some cases pain. In summary, the vascular effects of histamine cause the symptoms commonly associated with allergic reactions: swelling, itching, headaches, redness, and a drop in blood pressure.

Nonvascular Smooth Muscle. There are two main areas of nonvascular smooth muscle that are affected by histamine: the smooth muscle of the GI tract and the smooth muscle of the bronchial tree. In the GI tract, histamine causes smooth muscle contraction and the release of hydrochloric acid. In the bronchial tree, histamine causes bronchial smooth muscle constriction, which can severely impair respiratory function. In humans, the bronchial smooth muscle effect of histamine is much stronger than the GI effect, and people with chronic respiratory disease (asthma) are unusually sensitive to it.

Heart Effects. Histamine usually causes an increase in heart rate and, when larger amounts are present, arrhythmias and cardiac collapse can occur.

Histamine Receptors

In order for histamine to create its physiological action, it combines with two different types of receptors. These receptors are know as the H_1 and H_2 receptors. The most important receptors, as far as allergic reactions are concerned, are the H_1 receptors, which are located in the blood vessels, bronchioles, and smooth muscle. When these receptors are stimulated, the clinical effects of allergic reactions are seen. The H_2 receptors are located in other blood vessels and in the GI tract. The main response that occurs when these receptors are stimulated is an increase in hydrochloric acid secretion (this was discussed in Chapter 6).

TABLE 7–13 Antihistamine Drugs

DRUG	DEGREE OF SEDATION
Diphenhydramine (Benadryl^R)	High
Chlorpheniramine (Chlor-trimeton^R)	Intermediate
Tripelennamine (PBZ^R)	Intermediate
Promethazine (Phenergan^R)	High
Dimendhydrinate (Dramamine^R)	High
Terfenadine (Seldane^R)	None
Meclizine (Antivert^R)	Low

Antihistamines and Antiallergic Agent Definitions

Antihistamines are substances that block the action of histamine in various tissues throughout the body. They are called *competitive antagonists*, meaning they occupy the histamine receptor without causing any drug effect (see Chapter 1—definition of antagonist and agonist).

Antiallergic drugs are substances that block the release of histamine from mast cells. These agents are discussed in Chapter 14.

Antihistamine Drugs

The main clinical effect of currently used antihistamines is to counteract the effect of histamine on the H_1 receptor sites. They are most effective when administered prophylactically as an antagonist against histamine that has already been released. They are of little value in a rapidly developing or acute antigen–antibody reactions such as anaphylaxis. Most are administered orally and therefore some time (30 minutes to 1 hour) must elapse before clinical effects can be observed. All of the various antihistamines have similar properties but differ in onset of action and intensity of side effects. Also, many antihistamines that are effective in one individual may not be effective in another, thus requiring a change of medication in order to find an appropriate antihistamine that is effective. Table 7–13 lists some of the more commonly used antihistamines along with their degree of sedation.

The main side effects of all antihistamines are similar but differ in intensity. The clinically important side effects include sedation and drying of secretions in the nasal lining and mouth (*xerostomia*). In recent years a new antihistamine, **terfenadine** (**Seldane**^R), has been developed with very little sedative effects.

Other Uses of Antihistamines

Antihistamines have many uses other than treating allergies. Many antihistamines have side effects that, in some instances, are used therapeutically. Because of their sedative action, they are often used as main ingredients in over-the-counter sleep aides. Many of the antihistamines also are used in cold medications to decrease secretions, and another common use of antihistamine is in the control of *vertigo* and motion sickness. Drugs that are most commonly used for motion sickness are **dimenhydrinate (Dramamine^R)** and **meclizine (Antivert^R).**

     Finally, antihistamines potentially can cause interaction with other drugs. The most important interaction occurs when they are combined with CNS depressants, such as alcohol, barbiturates, phenothiazines, and tranquilizers. With any of these drugs, antihistamines can potentiate or increase CNS depression.

POSTTEST: PHARMACOLOGY OF THE ENDOCRINE SYSTEM

For each of the following questions, try to select the *one* best answer from those choices given.

1. In addition to an anatomical relationship between the hypothalamus and the pituitary gland, the hypothalamus controls homeostasis through the autonomic nervous system and the pituitary gland controls homeostasis through the release of hormones. True or False?

2. The anterior lobe of the pituitary gland is synonymous with the neurohypophysis and the posterior lobe in synonymous with the adenohypophysis. True and False?

3. The most important adrenocortical hormones in terms of clinical use are:
    a. mineralocorticoids
    b. glucocorticoids
    c. gonadocorticoids
    d. none of the above

4. Which of the following symptoms are not associated with long-term glucocorticoid use?
    a. poor wound healing
    b. edema
    c. Addison disease
    d. Cushing disease

5. All of the following hormones are produced by the thyroid gland except:
    a. parathyroid hormone
    b. thyroxin
    c. thyrocalcitonin
    d. thyroid hormone

6. The treatment of hyperthyroidism is accomplished by all of the following except:
    a. administration of radioactive iodine
    b. surgical removal
    c. radiation
    d. administration of corticosteroids

7. Growth onset or type I diabetes mellitus is always treated by:
   a. control of diet
   b. administration of insulin
   c. use of oral hypoglycemic agents
   d. none of the above
8. In addition to problems associated with the administration of insulin, allergic reactions also are quite prevalent. True or False?
9. When an antigen–antibody reaction occurs in the body, histamine can be released by:
   a. plasma cells
   b. white blood cells
   c. erythrocytes
   d. mast cells
10. Antihistamines are excellent drugs in treating acute anaphylactic reactions. True or False?

REFERENCES/RECOMMENDED READING

Arnaud CD: Calcium homeostatis: Regulatory elements and their integration. Fed. Proc. 37:2557–2560, 1978.

Cader Asmal A, Marble A: Oral Hypoglycaemic agents: Update. *Drugs* 28:62–78, 1984.

Cooper DS, Ridgway, EC: Clinical management of patients with hyperthyroidism. *Med Clin North Am* 69:953–971 1985.

Dipalma, JR, Digregorio JG: *Basic Pharmacology in Medicine*, 3rd ed. McGraw-Hill, New York, 1990.

Fainer, AS, Dale DC, Balow JE: Glucocorticoid therapy: Mechanisms of action and clinical considerations. *Ann Intern Med* 84:304–315 1976.

Hitner H, Nagle BT: *Basic Pharmacology for Health Occupations*. Harper & Row, New York, 1990.

Seltzer HS: Efficacy and safety of oral hypoglycemic agents. *Annu Rev Med* 31:261–272, 1980.

Thorn GW, Lawler DP: Clinical therapeutics of adrenal disorders. *Am J Med* 53:673–684 1972.

Tortora GJ, Anagnostakus NP: *Principles of Anatomy and Physiology*. Harper & Row, New York, 1990.

CHAPTER 8

ANTIMICROBIAL PHARMACOLOGY

LEARNING OBJECTIVES

After completion of this chapter and its learning activities the student will be able to:

1. Discuss general concepts in the use of antimicrobial agents and define the terms *antibacterial, antibiotic, antimicrobial, bacteriostatic, bacteriocidal, gram negative, gram positive,* and *spectrum.*
2. List and describe principles in the wise use of antibiotics.
3. List and describe various causes of failure in the use of antibiotics.
4. List the classification and categories of antibacterial drugs presented in this text.
5. Describe the basic mechanism of action of the beta-lactam antibiotics and list some characteristics of the four categories of the beta-lactam drugs, including examples, spectrum, and adverse effects; also explain the use of beta-lactamase inhibitors.
6. List and describe some miscellaneous antibiotics used in the treatment of gram-positive and gram-negative infections, including examples, spectrum, and adverse effects.
7. List and describe broad-spectrum antibiotics, including examples and adverse effects.
8. Describe the overall clinical use and mechanism of action of the sulfonamides and related drugs, along with examples, spectrum, and adverse effects.
9. List two categories of antifungal drugs, along with examples and adverse effects.
10. Describe the overall approach to the treatment of viral infections and list examples of antiviral drugs, along with therapeutic uses and adverse effects.

INTRODUCTION

Antimicrobial pharmacology has become very extensive and includes many categories frequently used in clinical medicine and dentistry. This chapter discusses the more traditional and established areas of antimicrobial therapy, and it is not the intent of the author to present a comprehensive discussion. This chapter covers some general definitions and concepts and some general principles in the use of antimicrobial drugs, and presents a few examples of mechanism of action and adverse effects of the following categories: antibacterial drugs, antifungal drugs, and antiviral drugs.

ANTIMICROBIAL AGENTS AND DEFINITIONS

Antimicrobial agents elicit their effect on various microscopic organisms by being selectively toxic to them. Basically this is accomplished by interfering with the growth of organisms or killing the organism outright. Therefore, most clinically effective agents are selectively toxic to the organisms without causing damage to host cells or tissues. The degree of selectivity determines the ultimate usefulness of the drug in terms of side effects.

Generally the antimicrobial agents exert their effects through one of the following mechanisms: inhibition of cell wall synthesis, inhibition of protein synthesis, inhibition of nucleic acid function, and inhibition of certain cell membrane functions. Throughout the following discussion of various antimicrobial substances, the overall mechanism that is appropriate to each drug group will be indicated. Before discussing antimicrobial substances, it is necessary to define the following terms:

- *Antimicrobial*—any substance that kills or inhibits the growth of any microorganism.
- *Antibacterial*—any substance that inhibits the growth of or destroys bacteria.
- *Antibiotic*—compound that is produced by other living organisms that kill or inhibit the growth of bacteria. This term thus distinguishes between substances that are naturally occurring and those that are synthetic. The difference is rather academic, and the term *antibiotic* now is used to incorporate both groups of drugs, naturally occurring and synthetic.
- *Bacteriostatic*—an antibiotic that inhibits or retards the growth of bacteria.
- *Bacteriocidal*—an antibiotic that kills bacteria.
- *Gram positive*—an agent that kills or inhibits bacteria and stains a dark color as a result of the Gram staining technique.
- *Gram negative*—an agent that kills or inhibits the growth of bacteria and stains a lighter color as a result of the Gram staining technique.
- *Spectrum*—the specificity or selectivity of antibiotics regarding whether they are gram positive, gram negative, or both. Some antibiotics are effective against gram-positive organisms, some are effective against gram-negative organisms, and some are effective against both gram-positive and gram-negative organisms (broad-spectrum antibiotics).

PRINCIPLES IN THE WISE USE OF ANTIBIOTICS

When using antibiotic therapy, it is obviously important to identify the organism involved and select the most appropriate drug. Also, in the course of treatment, many antibiotics become ineffective, usually because the organism develops a resistance to that drug. In order to minimize these problems, the following steps should be considered when selecting and administering antibiotic therapy:

1. Identify the causative organism if at all possible.
2. Determine the in vitro sensitivity of the organism to candidate antibacterial agents and their combinations. Remember, in vitro sensitivity does not guarantee in vitro efficacy.
3. Obtain a history regarding previous sensitization to and intoxication by antibacterial drugs and test for sensitivity where appropriate.
4. Know the course of the disease, its prognosis with and without antibacterial treatment, and possible adverse effects of such treatment. Weigh the risks of therapy against its advantages.
5. Select the appropriate drug(s) according to the identified organism and its sensitivities, the history or presence of drug allergy, general clinical experience with single-drug and combination-drug treatment, and cost.
6. In an urgent situation in which you cannot afford to wait for bacteriological diagnosis and determination of sensitivities or when an organism cannot be identified:
   a. Apply an educated intuition as to the offending organism and its probable susceptibility to antibacterial drugs.
   b. Begin bacteriological tests before giving any antibacterial drugs.
   c. Begin therapy with a likely drug combination while waiting for laboratory tests. **Remember that such hurried therapy may interfere with subsequent diagnosis.**
   d. Regard initial therapy as trial only, to be altered according to laboratory findings or disappointing response.
7. Aim for vigorous antibacterial therapy:
   a. Start treatment promptly to:
      – prevent irreversible damage
      – discourage secondary infection
      – give body defense a chance
      – minimize the probability of resistant mutants in the invading population
   b. Employ supraeffective doses sufficiently high to suppress most first-stage resistant organisms.
   c. Continue therapy for an appropriate time after apparent disappearance of the infection.
8. Constantly monitor and evaluate antibacterial therapy with respect to identity and sensitivity of the organism, effectiveness of control of bacterial population, secondary infection and superinfection, and toxicity, and alter therapy when indicated.

9. Render other treatment with the same concerns as though there were no antibiotics available.
    a. Apply appropriate surgical means.
    b. Apply supportive and symptomatic treatment.
    c. Remember fluid and electrolyte control.
10. Avoid topical therapy with systematically useful antibacterial agents to which resistance or sensitivity can develop. Where such topical therapy appears necessary, employ concomitant systemic therapy.
11. Individualize treatment.
12. Avoid trivial and promiscuous use of antibacterial drugs.
    a. They are not universal antipyretics.
    b. They are not necessary in clean surgical cases.
    c. There was a preantibiotic era with good survival in many diseases.
    d. Resist pressures by your patients to use a drug when it is not indicated.
13. Discontinue therapy when toxins present themselves, except where experience disavows danger.
14. Know the advantages and dangers of chemoprophylaxis.
15. Know and avoid causes of failure.

CAUSES OF FAILURE IN ANTIBACTERIAL THERAPY

The cause of failure in the use of antibacterial therapy are as follows:

1. Organism originally insensitive to drug
    a. No bacterial diagnosis and determination of sensitivity
    b. Error in bacteriological diagnosis
    c. Futile prophylaxis
2. Mixed infection
3. Failure to select appropriate drug or drug combination
4. Development of resistance
5. Superinfection
6. Inadequate regimen
    a. Therapy begun late
    b. Dose too small
    c. Inappropriate route of administration
    d. Therapy not continued long enough after subsidence of signs and symptoms
7. Drug not able to penetrate into site of infection
8. Failure to use adjuvant surgical and supportive measures
    a. Drainage
    b. Topical installation
    c. Enzymatic liquefaction of pus and débridement in infected area
    d. Immunological

    e. Fluid and electrolyte

    f. Nutritional

9. Supervention of toxicity or hypersensitivity

CATEGORIES OF ANTIBIOTIC DRUGS

The categories of antibiotics discussed in this text include the following: the beta-lactams, miscellaneous antibiotics against gram-positive and gram-negative organisms, broad-spectrum antibiotics, and sulfonamides and related drugs.

BETA-LACTAM ANTIBIOTICS

The beta-lactam antibiotics include the penicillins, cephalosporins, carbapenems, and monobactams. These substances all have a four-member beta-lactam ring as part of their chemical structure (Figure 8–1). It is this chemical structure (beta-lactam ring) that is responsible for the antibacterial activity of all four groups. Figure 8–2 presents the general structural formulas of the currently used beta-lactam drugs. They all have in common the beta-lactam ring, with various substitutions made as indicated by the letter R. It is not necessary to memorize the individual structures, but they are presented in order to show how all of the beta-lactam antibiotics are related.

The basic mechanism of action of the beta-lactams is the inhibition of bacterial cell wall synthesis. This action causes *autolytic* enzymes in the bacterial cell wall to be activated, causing lysis of the cell. The bacterial cell wall is very unique in microbial organisms, and is made of substances called *peptidoglycans*. The beta-lactam antibiotics interfere with the synthesis of these peptidoglycans; because this substance does not occur in human or mammalian cells, most antibiotics are not toxic for human cells.

One of the major problems associated with the use of beta-lactam antibiotics is the development, by various bacterial species, of resistance to the drug. There are a number of mechanisms that are operational in the development or resistance, but the most important one is that some bacteria produce enzymes that inactivate various drugs. These enzymes are called beta-lactamases, and they cleave the carbon–nitrogen bond in the beta-lactam ring, which destroys the antibacterial activity. There are several beta-lactamases

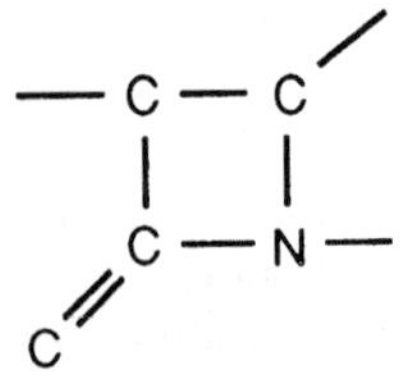

FIGURE 8–1 The Beta-Lactam Ring.

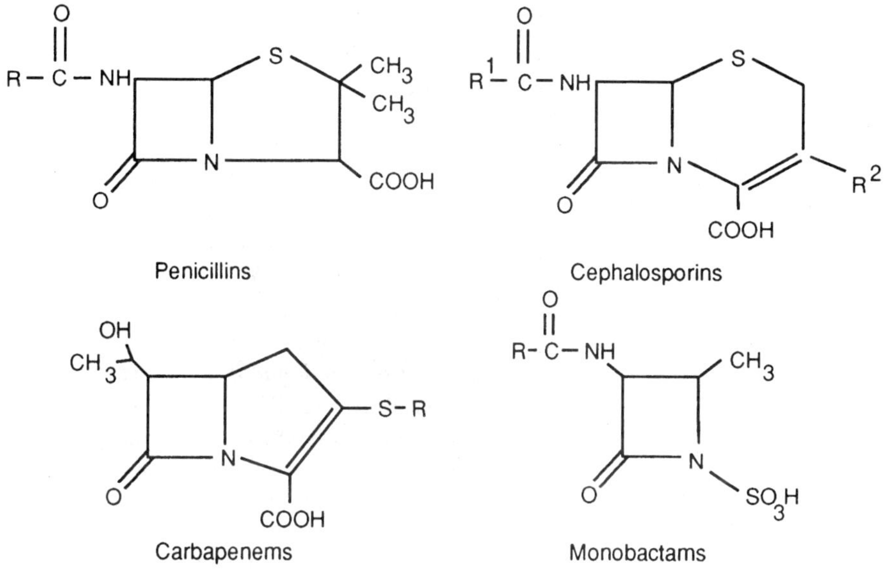

FIGURE 8–2   The Beta-Lactam Antibiotics.

that are produced by various gram-positive and gram-negative organisms, and this phenomenon has necessitated the development of new-generation beta-lactams that are effective against the beta-lactamase–producing bacteria. As the various beta-lactam antibiotics are discussed, the antibiotics that are resistant to the effects of beta-lactamases are identified. In addition, the beta-lactamase inhibitors, used in combination with the penicillins, are described.

Penicillins

The discovery of penicillin in 1928 by Alexander Fleming was one of the most important events in medical history. Because the original natural penicillins came from a mold (a living organism), the penicillins are considered true antibiotics. All of the various penicillins have the same basic structure, and the different categories are determined by modifications made at the R side chain (see Figure 8–2).

Most penicillins are effective by the oral route, but there is some variability in absorption (e.g., penicillin G is unstable in the low-pH environment of the stomach and penicillin V is acid stable). Most penicillins are bound to plasma proteins, which creates an equilibrium between bound and free drug. The bound form serves as a constant reservoir that releases more free drug as the penicillin is metabolized. Most penicillins are rapidly eliminated from the body by the kidney in an unchanged form; however, some penicillins are metabolized by the liver. The major adverse effect of the penicillins is the high incidence of allergic reactions. These can range from an acute anaphylactic reaction to a milder delayed reaction, but, regardless of the extent of the allergy, there is a high incidence of cross-allergenicity between all penicillins (i.e., allergy to one penicillin probably means allergy to all). The categories of penicillins include natural penicillins, penicillinase-resistant penicillins, amino penicillins, and extended-spectrum penicillins. The following discussion includes for the various categories examples, spectrum, and adverse effects.

Natural Penicillins.   These penicillins include **penicillin G (benzylpenicillin)** and **penicillin V (phenoxymethylpenicillin)**. Because penicillin G is not stable in an acid environment, it is most often given by injection. Penicillin V is acid stable and is given orally. *Spectrum:* gram-positive streptococci, gonococcic, meningococci, non–beta-lactamase-producing anaerobes, syphilis, diphtheria, rat bite fever, and anthrax. **Adverse effects:** most common are allergic reactions, both immediate and delayed.

Penicillinase-Resistant Penicillins.   These penicillins include **methicillin, nafcillin, oxacillin, cloxacillin,** and **dicloxacillin.** Methicillin is only available by injection; nafcillin is better absorbed by injection and the other three can be given orally. **Spectrum:** gram-positive penicillinase-producing staphlococcus organisms; also effective against streptococcus organisms A, B, C, and G and pneumococci. **Adverse effects:** allergic reactions and some kidney damage (methicillin).

Amino Penicillins (Broad Spectrum).   These drugs include **ampicillin** and **amoxicillin.** Ampicillin is not as stable as amoxicillin when give orally and therefore should be taken on an empty stomach. **Spectrum:** considered to be extended, and they are effective against some gram-negative organisms but are no more effective against gram-positive than penicillin G or V. **Adverse Effects:** With ampicillin, skin rashes or diarrhea are common; amoxicillin has fewer side effects but both can cause allergic reactions.

Extended-Spectrum Penicillins.   This group of drugs includes **carbenicillin, ticarcillin, mezlocillin, azlocillin,** and **piperacillin.** None of these agents are absorbed from the gastrointestinal (GI) tract and therefore must be given by injection. **Spectrum:** as the name implies, these agents are effective not only against gram-positive organisms but also against a number of gram-negative aerobic organisms. Because of rapidly developing resistance, these agents often are administered in combination with aminoglycosides. **Adverse effects:** allergic reactions and the occurrence of superinfection. (*Note*: A superinfection is one that occurs when the normal flora is interrupted or destroyed, allowing a second organism to become dominant. The most common organism responsible is *Candida albicans* [fungal infection].)

Beta-Lactamase Inhibitors

The production of beta-lactamase by bacteria is one of the main methods that bacteria use in creating resistance. To prevent this resistance, there are two agents that are specific beta-lactamase inhibitors: **clavulanic acid** and **sulbactam.** These substances have no antibacterial action themselves, but are used in combination with other beta-lactam drugs to broaden their antibacterial spectrum. Clavulanic acid is available by oral route in combination with **amoxicillin (Augmentin[R])** and combined with **ticarcillin (Timentin[R])** for intravenous (IV) use. Sulbactam is available in combination with **ampicillin (Unasyn[R])** for parenteral use.

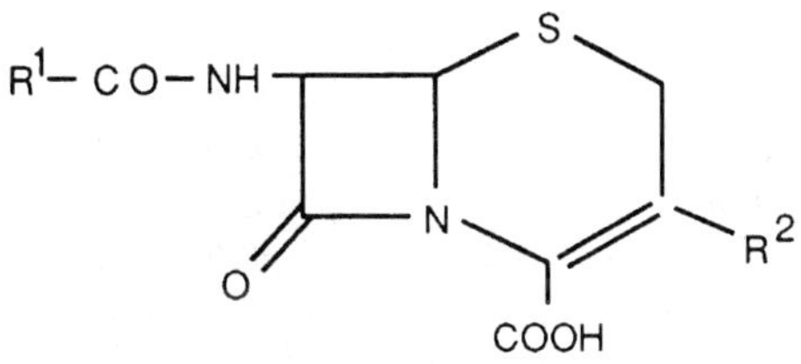

FIGURE 8–3   Structure of Cephalosporins.

Cephalosporins

The structure of the cephalosporins is very similar to that of penicillin except that the cephalosporin nucleus is more resistant to beta-lactamase (see Figure 8–3 for basic structure). The two R positions provide sites for a variety of modifications to the basic structure, and there are presently 21 different drugs available in this group. The cephalosporins are classified into three groups or generations, and their classification is based on their activity against gram-negative organisms. Table 8–1 lists examples of each generation with its route of administration and spectrum.

The mechanism of action is similar to that of penicillin, and the drugs have similar adverse effects in terms of allergy. It is estimated that about 5–10 percent of the patients allergic to penicillin also are allergic to cephalosporins. In general, the cephalosporins are

TABLE 8–1   Cephalosporins

CATEGORY	ROUTE	SPECTRUM
First generation Cephalexin (Keflex^R) Cephalothin (Keflin^R)	Oral IV, IM*	Greater effectiveness against gram-negative organisms than penicillin G and more effective against a wider variety of gram-positive agents
Second generation Cefaclor (Ceclor^R) Cefoxitin (Mefoxin^R)	Oral	Increased effectiveness against gram-negative organisms and against beta-lactamase producers; less effective against gram-positive organisms
Third generation Cefotaxime (Claforan^R) Moxalactam (Moxan^R)	IV	Broader gram-negative and decreased gram-positive spectrum, less resistant to beta-lactamase, and effective against some hospital gram-negative infections

*IM = intramuscular.

fairly nontoxic except for cross-sensitivity with penicillin, superinfections, and potential renal damage when used in combination with aminoglycosides. They are generally very expensive, and the newer generations have problems with development of bacterial resistance. Regarding clinical use, the cephalosporins have been overutilized when less expensive antibiotics are adequate. They are the drugs of choice in serious *Klebsiella* infections and meningitis, and are alternatives for streptococci and staphlococci, some resistant gonorrhea, and serious gram-negative infections that are resistant.

Carbapenem

This category of beta-lactams is similar in structure to penicillins but, with modification of the chemical structure, it has a marked resistance to beta-lactamase produced by resistant bacteria. Only one drug in this group is available for clinical use—**imipenem.** The drug is partially broken down in the kidney and often is administered with cilastatin to block tubular metabolism. This drug has the broadest spectrum of all the beta-lactam antibiotics and is effective against 90 percent or more of all the clinically significant bacteria. It is resistant to most penicillinase- and beta-lactamase–forming bacteria. The drug is not effective orally and must be given IV or intramuscularly (IM). **Adverse effects:** painful injection, allergies, nausea and vomiting, superinfections, diarrhea, and some blood disorders. The main clinical use of this drug is in the treatment of *nosocomial* (hospital-acquired) infections. The drug should be used conservatively primarily because of high cost (patient charge per dose is $90 and for 10-day therapy is $3600).

Monobactam

This drug group has only a single ring in its structure, hence the name *monobactam*. It is a synthetic antibiotic and is effective against facultative aerobic gram-negative bacteria. The spectrum is similar to the aminoglycosides, which makes this drug unlike other beta-lactams. It is less toxic than the aminoglycosides (as discussed in the next section) but has a potential for causing penicillin-resistant gram-positive superinfections. The only monobactam currently available in the United States is **aztreonam (Azactam**[R]**),** which is not absorbed by the oral route and must be given IV.

Summary

The beta-lactams are very popular drugs, particularly the penicillins and cephalosporins. The newer beta-lactams are very limited in their use, must be given IV and are very expensive. Table 8–2 summarizes the currently used beta-lactam antibiotics.

MISCELLANEOUS ANTIBIOTICS

This group of drugs includes agents that are primarily effective against gram-positive organisms, anaerobic organisms, and gram-negative organisms. Although there are other antibiotic groups used in treating the infections listed, these drugs provide important

TABLE 8–2 The Beta-Lactams

CATEGORY	SUBCATEGORY	ROUTE OF ADMINISTRATION
Penicillins	Natural penicillins	
	Penicillin G	Oral, IM
	Penicillin V	Oral
	Penicillinase resistant	
	Methicillin	IV
	Nafcillin	Oral
	Oxacillin	Oral
	Cloxacillin	Oral
	Dicloxacillin	Oral
	Amino penicillins (Broad spectrum)	
	Ampicillin	Oral
	Amoxicillin	Oral
	Extended spectrum	
	Carbenicillin	IV
	Ticarcillin	IV
	Mezlocillin	IV
	Azlocillin	IV
	Piperacillin	IV
Beta-Lactamase inhibitors	Clavulanic acid and amoxicillin (Augmentin[R])	Oral
	Sulbactam and ampicillin (Unasyn[R])	IM
	Calvulanic acid and ticarcillin (Trimenton[R])	
Cephalosporins	First Generation	
	Cephalexin (Keflex[R])	Oral
	Cephalothin (Keflin[R])	IV, IM
	Second generation	
	Cefaclor (Ceclor[R])	Oral
	Cefoxitin (Mefoxin[R])	IM
	Third generation	
	Cefotaxime (Claforan[R])	IV, IM
	Moxalactam (Moxam[R])	IV, IM
Carbapenem	Imipenem (Primaxin[R])	IV
Monobactam	Aztreonam (Azactam[R])	IV

alternative therapies. As in other sections of this chapter, only brief information is presented. Discussion of the following groups includes examples, clinical use, general mechanism of action, spectrum, and adverse effects.

Agents for Gram-Positive Infections

Erythromycin (E-Mycin[R]).   This drug is a large (*macrolide*) antibiotic that is a good alternative for patients allergic to penicillin. It is also the drug of choice for *Mycoplasma pneumoniae*, Legionnaire disease, and whooping cough. The mechanism of action is the inhibition of protein synthesis and the drug is bacteriostatic. **Spectrum:** good against gram-positive cocci that are susceptible to penicillin. **Adverse effects:** GI irritation; certain individuals may develop *cholestatic* hepatitis, and allergic reactions occasionally occur but are very rare.

Vancomycin (Vancocin[R]).   This drug has a *microprotein* structure, its mechanism of action is inhibition of cell wall synthesis, and it is bacteriocidal. This drug is used as an alternative for penicillinase-resistance staphylococci and, because of poor oral absorption, usually is given IV. **Spectrum:** gram-positive cocci and particularly staphlococci organisms that are resistant to penicillin or cephalosporins. **Adverse effects:** include *ototoxicity* (toxic to the eighth cranial nerve) and *nephrotoxicity*. Also, this drug can cause *thrombophlebitis* when used IV.

Agents for Anaerobic Infections

Clindamycin (Cleocin[R]).   This drug has a unique structure called a lincosamide. It is a synthetic derivitive of lincomycin and is used as an alternative in treating penicillin- and erythromycin-susceptible infections. It is an inhibitor of protein synthesis and therefore is bacteriostatic. It also can be used topically for acne infections. It usually is administered orally but can be given by injection for serious anaerobic infections not involving the central nervous system. **Spectrum:** similar to that of erythromycin and penicillin: gram-positive cocci, in particular *Staphlococcus aureus*; also is very active against many anaerobic bacteria. **Adverse effects:** include high incidence of diarrhea and, in some individuals, antibiotic-associated colitis. Local thrombophlebitis can occur when administered IV.

Metronidazole (Flagyl[R]).   This drug is a synthetic agent that is effective against both parasitic and bacterial infections. The general mechanism is to inhibit DNA synthesis and the drug generally is *mutagenic* to bacteria. It is effective orally with good GI absorption and is distributed to tissues and fluids such as vaginal secretions, seminal fluid, saliva, breast milk, and cerebrospinal fluid. It is used IV for various anaerobic infections and orally for prostatic infections. **Spectrum:** effective against anaerobic bacteria and antiparasitic against *Trichomonas*, amebiasis, and giardiasis. **Adverse effects:** include GI disturbances, metallic taste, dizziness and vertigo, and blood dyscrasias; definitely not recommended during pregnancy because of teratogenic effects.

Agents for Gram-Negative Organisms

Aminoglycosides (Gentamicin, Tobramycin, Amikacin, and Netilmicin). There are a number of aminoglycosides, such as streptomycin, neomycin, and kanamycin, that now are rarely used because of their severe ototoxicity and other toxic effects. These antibiotic substances were derived from various *Streptomyces* species in 1943. They are very important in treating gram-negative hospital infections and patients with *Pseudomonas* infections. The mechanism of action is the inhibition of protein synthesis, and these drugs are bacteriostatic. They are poorly absorbed orally and are given IM or IV. They have a low therapeutic index and must be monitered carefully in terms of plasma concentration. **Spectrum:** effective against most gram-negative bacilli, *Staphlococcus aureus*, and myco-bacteria. They are ineffective against anerobic organisms and *Rickettsia*. **Adverse effects:** primarily result from accumulation of drug in the middle ear, causing ototoxicity, which is quite common (and irreversible in 3–5 percent of the population). The toxicity can include hearing loss, vertigo, and ataxia. Nephrotoxicity and renal disfunction also are quite common (8–14 percent of the population). These drugs sometimes are administered in combination with other drugs, and all aminoglycosides are capable of causing neuro-muscular blockade, resulting in respiratory paralysis.

Fluoroquinolones: Ciprofloxacin (Cipro^R) and Norfloxacin (Noroxin^R). This group of drugs were synthesized in the 1960s and primarily are used in the treatment of urinary tract infections. In the 1980s, the drugs were changed by adding fluorine to the molecule, creating fluoroquinolones. These agents decrease DNA synthesis in bacteria but cause no effect on normal host cells. They are effective by the oral route but develop rapid resistance when used long term. **Spectrum:** effective against gram-negative organisms, particularly those causing urinary tract infections. **Adverse effects:** generally infrequent, but they can cause GI disturbances, allergic responses, and central nervous system problems involving headache, dizziness, and visual disturbances.

BROAD-SPECTRUM ANTIBIOTICS

Although there are several antibiotics that have a fairly broad spectrum, the traditional classification "broad-spectrum" antibiotics includes chloramphenicol and the tetracyclines. These agents both were isolated from different species of soil *Actinomycetes* organisms in 1947 and 1948. Since that time, the drugs that presently are used are synthetically produced.

Chloramphenicol

This drug orginally was used to treat thyphoid fever. In the 1950s it was used as a broad-spectrum drug but can cause (severe) *aplastic* anemia, which can be fatal. In recent years it has been used in the treatment of brain abscess associated with *meningitis*. The mechanism of action is the inhibition of protein synthesis, and the drug is bacteriostatic. Also, it can cause some inhibition of protein synthesis in the host cells and there is a fair amount of bacterial resistance to this drug, particularly by staphylococci. The drug is given orally and is readily absorbed in the GI tract. **Spectrum:** effective against a variety of gram-positive and gram-negative organisms. **Adverse effects:** main effect is bone marrow suppression, which can be fatal. Prolonged use should be avoided when patients are taking this drug, and blood levels should be monitored frequently.

Tetracyclines: Chlortetracycline, Demeclocycline, and Doxycycline

The tetracyclines are a family of related compounds that were introduced in the late 1940s, and there have been several modifications of these drugs up through the 1970s. Although some of the drugs have differences in terms of absorption and distribution, they all have similar properties. The overall mechanism of action is to interfere with protein synthesis, and they are bacteriostatic. These drugs are effective orally but some are *chelated* with calcium and therefore should not be taken with drug products that contain aluminum hydroxide, dairy products, and other substances containing calcium, magnesium, and iron. These drugs have a good ability to penetrate certain tissues, particularly bones and teeth. Although the tetracyclines have a broad spectrum, they are used for a fairly limited number of infections that include *Rickettsia*, *Chlamydia*, Lyme disease, acne, and brucellosis. **Spectrum:** effective against a wide range of gram-positive and gram-negative organisms. **Adverse effects:** include rash and renal, hepatic, and skin toxicity. Also, superinfections are very common, particularly from opportunistic *Candida albicans* (thrush). These drugs should not be used in pregnant patients and are contraindicated in children under age 12.

SULFONAMIDES AND RELATED DRUGS

Sulfonamides are antibiotics that have been available for many years. Today the main clinical use of these drugs is the treatment of uncomplicated urinary tract infections. They are synthetic derivatives of sulfanilamide, which is an *analog* of *para*-aminobenzoic acid (PABA). PABA is a precursor to folic acid, which is an essential substance in the DNA synthesis of bacterial cells. Because the structure of PABA and sulfa drugs is very similar, sulfa competes with PABA in the formation of folic acid, thus causing a decrease in growth of bacteria. The drugs interfere with cell growth and are bacteriostatic. The sulfonamides are readily and competely absorbed in the GI tract but they also have the ability to penetrate the cerebrospinal fluid as well as the placental barrier. Sulfonamides include a large number of drugs and are categorized as rapidly absorbed (e.g., **sulfisoxazole [Gantrisin^R]**, poorly absorbed (e.g., **succinylsulfathiazole [Sulfasuxidine^R]**), and various other compounds. **Spectrum:** wide range of activity against gram-positive and gram-negative organisms; however, resistance is quite common with many strains of bacteria. **Adverse effects:** most sulfonamides cause various allergic reactions, including rash, photosensitivity, and drug fever. Occasionally renal and liver damage is reported and, rarely, blood dyscrasias.

In addition to the standard sulfonamides mentioned, the following are special examples and combination drugs:

- *Sulfaninylacetamide (Sulamyd^R)*—used topically for various eye infections.
- *Sulfasalazine (Azulfidine^R)*—used in treating ulcerative colitis.
- *Silver sulfadiazine (Silvadene^R)*—used in treating burn patients with bacterial infection.
- *Trimethoprim-sulfamethoxazole (Bactrim^R and Septra^R)*—an excellent drug that is effective against gram-positive and gram-negative organisms as well as resistant staphylococci; effective against urinary tract infections, prostatic infections, travelers diarrhea, and bacterial meningitis.

ANTIFUNGAL DRUGS

Mycotic or fungal infections can occur in superficial areas of the body, including the skin and mucous membranes, as well as systemically. Fungal infections of the skin are the most common and infections of mucous membranes the second most common. Systemic fungal infections occur much less frequently but, when present, are very severe and difficult to treat. Also, the drugs that are used to treat systemic fungal infections are extremely toxic. The following discussion describes two categories of fungal infections and includes agents used in treatment, along with examples and adverse effects of each drug.

Superficial Fungal Infections

Nystatin (Mycostatin^R).   Nystatin is similar to the drug amphotericin B and is available for topical and oral administration. It has a fairly broad spectrum, including yeasts and many fungi, and is used in treatment of topical *Candida* infections. **Adverse effects:** include nausea, vomiting, some diarrhea.

Griseofulvin (Fulvicin^R).   This drug prevents reccurrence of mycotic infections and also has an anti-inflammatory effect. It is not useful against systemic infections but is effective against difficult dermatological infections. **Adverse effects:** include headache and superinfection caused by *Candida albicans*, and can be carcinogenic and teratogenic in experimental animals.

Miconazole (Monistat^R) and clotrimazole (Lotrimin^R).   These agents cause leakage of small molecules in the fungal cells that are exposed to the drug. They are broad-spectrum agents active against most superficial fungal infections and are very good against vaginal candidiasis. **Adverse effects:** minimal when used topically.

Ciclopirox (Loprox^R).   Broad-spectrum agent that penetrates the dermis but is not systemically absorbed.

Over-the-Counter Agents.   Over-the-counter agents used in treatment of fungal infections include **miconazole (Micatin^R)**, **clotrimazole (Lotrimin^R)**, **tolnaftate (Aftate^R)**, and **undecylenic acid (Desenex^R)**.

Systemic Fungal Infections

Amphotericin B (Fungizone^R).   This drug increases fungal cell permeability, inhibiting growth at low concentrations, and is *fungicidal* at high concentrations. This drug is not absorbed orally and is given IV. **Adverse effects:** extremely toxic to most individuals, with symptoms that include nausea, vomiting, and diarrhea. In some cases it causes extreme *nephrogenic* toxicity, which greatly limits it use.

Flucytosine (Ancobon^R).   This drug has a narrower spectrum against fungi than amphotericin B and is fungostatic. Can be given orally and often is given in combination with amphotericin B. **Adverse effects:** include nausea, rashes, diarrhea, and hepatic diseases; some bone marrow suppression also can occur, which can be fatal.

Ketoconazole (Nizoral^R).   This drug has a broad spectrum against most infections in chronic suppressive therapy. It is very effective in treating chronic candidiasis. **Adverse effects:** include nausea, vomiting, and diarrhea; also has an antitestosterone effect, causing gynecomastia and impotence. This drug usually is given orally.

ANTIVIRAL AGENTS

Because viruses are intracellular obligate parasites requiring an intact host cell for their reproduction, they are not affected by antibiotics. Therefore, the treatment of viruses has been approached by three basic modalities: immunization, use of interferon, and the development of antiviral drugs.

Immunization has been the most effective approach for the treatment of most viral infections. Effective vaccines are available against such diseases as measles, mumps, polio, and rubella. Interferon has been successful in certain diseases, but its overall usefulness has not been established. The development of effective antiviral drugs has occurred in recent years, but because drugs that inhibit viral replication also affect the host cells, clinical usefulness is somewhat limited. The general mechanism of action of antiviral drugs is basically the same—they work by inhibiting viral cell replication by altering DNA synthesis. A few of the more effective antiviral drugs are listed below, along with their main therapeutic uses and adverse effects.

Amantadine (Symmetrel^R)

Therapeutic uses: has a very narrow spectrum and is well absorbed orally, and its main use is in the treatment of viral influenza A. It also is used as an adjunct in the treatment of parkinsonism. **Adverse effects:** fairly well tolerated but can cause central nervous system difficulties, such as confusion, ataxia, sleep disorders, and hallucinations.

Acyclovir (Zovirax^R)

Therapeutic uses: has had some success in the treatment of many herpes simplex viruses. It also has been effective against varicella zoster, Epstein-Barr virus, and sometimes cytomegaloviruses. It is effective in the membranous lesions of genital herpes and also in other herpetic diseases. It can be applied topically in ointment form, or orally as a pro-phylactic agent. The drug does not appear to be a cure, but it can decrease healing time and duration of the illness when used early. In addition to oral and topical forms it can be given IV. **Adverse effects:** include local reactions such as mild pain, burning, and stinging; with oral use, nausea, vomiting, and headache and, with IV use, inflammation and thrombophlebitis.

Ribavirin (Virazole^R)

Therapeutic uses: effective against respiratory syncytial virus (RSV), herpes simplex, and influenza A and B. It is approved for aerosol treatment in infants and young children. Also, it has been used experimentally in acquired immunodeficiency syndrome (AIDS) patients. **Adverse effects:** include rash, headache, and fatigue.

Other Antiviral Agents

Other antiviral agents include **vidarabine (Vira-A^R), idoxuridine (Herplex^R)**, and **zidovudine (Retrovir^R)** (formerly AZT, used in the treatment of AIDS virus).

POSTTEST: ANTIMICROBIAL PHARMACOLOGY

For each of the following questions, try to select the *one* best answer from those choices given.

1. The difference between an antibacterial and an antibiotic is that the term *antibiotic* means that the drug is synthetic. True or False?
2. Which of the following principles is more important in preventing the development of resistant bacterial strains?
   a. know the course of the disease.
   b. continually monitor and evaluate effectiveness.
   c. aim for vigorous therapy and continue for appropriate length of time.
   d. individualize treatment.
3. The most important cause of failure in the use of antibiotic therapy by an outpatient is not continuing therapy long enough after the signs and symptoms disappear. True or False?
4. Which of the following antibiotics is not a beta-lactam?
   a. cephalosporin
   b. erythromycin
   c. penicillin
   d. carbapenems
5. Which of the following is not a penicillin?
   a. nafcillin
   b. amoxicillin
   c. cloxacillin

      d. ampicillin

      e. all are penicillins

6. A superinfection is an infection that no antibiotics are effective against. True or False?

7. Which of the following is a third-generation cephalosporin?

      a. cefotaxime (Claforan^R)

      b. cefaclor (Ceclor^R)

      c. cephalothin (Keflin^R)

      d. cephalexin (Keflex^R)

8. Which of the following drugs often is used as the drug of choice for patients who are allergic to penicillin?

      a. vancomycin (Vancocin^R)

      b. erythromycin (Erythrocin^R)

      c. clindamycin (Cleocin^R)

      d. metronidazole (Flagyl^R)

9. The most serious side effect of the aminoglycosides is severe ototoxicity. True or False?

10. Although tetracyclines are broad-spectrum antibiotics, they are the drugs of choice against:

      a. staphylococcus infections

      b. streptococcus infections

      c. *Rickettsia* infections

      d. urinary infections

REFERENCES/RECOMMENDED READING

Appel GB, Neu HC: Antifungal agents of systemic mycoses; Antiviral agents. In *AMA Drug Evaluations*, 6th ed. 1986, pp 1553–1564; 1615–1631.

Dipalma JR, Digregorio JC: *Basic Pharmacology in Medicine*, 3rd ed. McGraw-Hill, New York, 1990.

Framcle EL, Neu, HC: Chloramphenicol and tetracyclines. *Med Clin North Am* 71:1155–1168, 1987.

King K: Antifungal chemotherapy. *Med J Aust* 143:287–290, 1985.

Leitman PS, Smith CR: Aminoglycoside nephrotoxicity in humans. *Rev Infect Dis* 5(suppl. 2):S284–S293, 1983.

Salter AJ: Trimethoprim-sulfamethoxazole: An assessment of more than 12 years of use. *Rev Infect Dis* 4:196–236, 1982.

CHAPTER 9

PHARMACOLOGY OF CHEMOTHERAPY

LEARNING OBJECTIVES

After completion of this chapter and its learning activities, the student will be able to:

1. Describe the general characteristics of cancer cells and define the terms *neoplasia*, *malignant*, *benign*, and *metastasis*.
2. Describe various approaches to the treatment of cancer, including surgery, radiation, and chemotherapy.
3. Describe the rationale for the use of chemotherapy and its effectiveness as one modality in the treatment of cancer.
4. List two categories of chemotherapeutic agents and describe their general mechanism of action.
5. List examples of the alkylating drugs and the antimetabolites, along with examples, mechanism of action, and clinical use.
6. List some miscellaneous drugs used in the treatment of cancer, along with examples and clinical uses.

INTRODUCTION

The term *chemotherapy* can have many meanings, such as the treatment by drugs of various illnesses such as infections, any type of physiological imbalance, and the treatment of tumor growth in cells. Today the term more commonly is used in reference to the treatment of *neoplasia*. Therefore, in this chapter, the term *chemotherapy* is used to describe antineoplastic or anticancer drugs. This chapter first reviews some characteristics of cancer cells along with appropriate definitions and types of cancers. Second, the general approach to treatment of neoplasia is presented, including chemotherapy. Finally, the effectiveness of chemotherapy is discussed, with a few examples of chemotherapeutic agents along with their overall mechanism of action and representative examples.

CANCER CELLS AND DEFINITIONS

Most normal cells in the body have the ability to reproduce themselves (mitosis or meiosis); the exceptions are muscle cells and nerve cells. Generally, mitotic activity occurs at a steady or normal rate, with the reproduction of daughter cells that are exactly the same as the original cell. Unfortunately, normal mitosis does not always occur, and abnormal cells can develop along with an accelerated rate of mitosis. When abnormal cells emerge, they are referred to as cancer cells. As these abnormal cells develop, they usually occupy space or develop neoplasms (tumors) that are localized, or they develop a more diffuse type of neoplasm such as leukemia or other blood- and lymph-related cancers. In order to understand characteristics of cancer, the following terms must be defined:

- *Neoplasia*—literally means "new growth"; also implies an abnormal increase in mitotic rate and the production of abnormal cells.
- *Malignant*—implies that the new growth of cells is spreading into the immediate area (local invasiveness) or groups of cells are spreading via the blood and lymph system to other sites in the body.
- *Benign*—means that there is overgrowth of new cells, but implies that this new growth is slower and usually does not have the property of invasiveness or spreading to other areas of the body.
- *Metastasis*—means the spreading of abnormal cells to distant sites via the bloodstream and lymphatics.

In order to understand the overall process of cancer formation, one needs to understand two characteristics all cancers have in common: 1) regardless of whether the neoplasia is localized or diffuse, the cells show loss of normal structure and function; and 2) the rate of cellular mitosis always is increased in both benign and malignant alterations, and, in the case of a malignant neoplasm, the mitotic rate is greatly increased or uncontrolled.

If the neoplasm is stationary or is localized, as in breast, prostate, and lung cancer, it often can be *palpitated* (manually felt) or seen on various types of diagnostic images. This is true for both benign and malignant neoplasias. In the localized state, the neoplasm is called the "primary site." If the neoplasm is a diffuse type and metastasis has occurred to various secondary or distant sites of the body, diagnosis and treatment approaches are more complex.

Regardless of the type of neoplasm present, normal body tissues are affected and the new cancer cells rob the normal cells of nutrition or, in the case of invasiveness, destroy surrounding tissue.

TREATMENT OF CANCER

The treatment approach is dependent on several factors: 1) early diagnosis, 2) whether or not the cancer is benign (usually localized), 3) whether or not the neoplasm has metastasized, and 4) if metastasis has occurred, whether the neoplasm in the early or late stage of development. With these factors in mind, there are generally three approaches to the treatment of cancer:

- *Surgery*—If the neoplasm is well localized and is in an area that is accessible, early surgical removal can be very effective. This is particularly true if the neoplasm is diagnosed early and treatment is begun immediately.
- *Radiation*—If the neoplasm is inaccessible or inoperable (such as certain brain tumors) and was not diagnosed early, radiation treatment can be given over a period of time in order to destroy the tumor cells.
- *Chemotherapy*—the administration of drugs to destroy cancer cells; most often used in treating the more diffuse types of cancer, such as leukemia and Hodgkin disease.

It should be noted that no single method is totally effective in arresting or suppressing a neoplasim. Often various combinations of all three are used in order to increase the chance of total cure. The overall success of any treatment modality is directly dependent on early diagnosis and instigation of therapy.

CHEMOTHERAPY

As mentioned earlier, chemotherapy in this text refers to the use of antineoplastic drugs that interfere with the growth and mitotic rate of cancer cells. The biggest problem with the use of these agents is that the drugs cannot differentiate between cancer cells and normal cells; therefore, these drugs are very toxic. The ultimate goal of chemotherapy is to destroy more cancer cells than normal cells and thereby control the neoplasm. This generally is possible with these agents because they attack cells with the highest mitotic and metabolic rates, and cancer cells generally are more susceptible because they are fast growing.

This selectivity for cells with a high growth rate is the basis for the extreme toxicity of these drugs; normal body cells with a high growth rate, such as bone marrow, gastrointestinal tract, and skin cells, also are affected. As a result, toxic effects often include bone marrow suppression, stomatitis (sores in the mouth), gastrointestinal ulceration, and alopecia. In order to minimize these toxic effects, the chemotherapeutic agents usually are given in a series at scheduled intervals, so that the patient has time to recuperate during drug-free periods.

Categories of Chemotherapeutic Agents

There are a number of antineoplastic drugs available, but the most commonly used are the alkylating drugs and the antimetabolites. As noted earlier, all chemotherapeutic agents cause varying degrees of toxicity, and thus both categories generally have similar adverse effects, such as nausea, vomiting, bone marrow suppression, gastrointestinal ulceration, hair loss, liver toxicity, and diarrhea.

Alkylating Drugs. These drugs also are known as nitrogen mustards and originally were developed for chemical warfare during World War I. These agents were observed to

TABLE 9–1   Chemotherapy Agents

CATEGORY	MECHANISM OF ACTION	CLINICAL USE
Alkylating drugs	Alkylation of DNA	
Mechlorethamine (Mustargen^R)		Hodgkin disease
Busulfan (Myleran^R)		Leukemia and Hodgkin disease
Cyclophosphamide (Cytoxan^R)		Leukemia and Hodgkin disease
Nitrosureas	Alkylation of DNA	
Carmustine (BiCNU^R)		Brain tumors and Hodgkin disease
Semustine (Methyl-Ccnu^R)		
Cisplatin (Platinol^R)		Testicular and ovarian cancer
Antimetabolite drugs		
Methotrexate (Methotrexate^R)	Folic acid antagonist	Leukemia
Mercaptopurine (Purinethol^R)	Purine antagonist	Leukemia
Fluorouracil (Adrucil^R)	Pyrimidine antagonist	Various neoplasms
Cytarabine (Cytosar^R)	Pyrimidine antagonist	Leukemia

cause inhibition of growth of bone marrow and other body cells. The overall mechanism is one of inhibition of cell reproduction by binding with DNA. This type of binding is known as *alkylation*.

Antimetabolites.   These drugs are similar in structure to normal metabolites that cells use in normal cell growth and function. Because of their similarity in structure, they compete with the metabolites needed by the cells and are incorporated into normal synthesis pathways, causing blockage of growth and normal reproduction.

Alkylating and Antimetabolite Drugs

Table 9–1 lists some examples of the drugs used either in the past or currently as chemotherapeutic agents. They all have various complex mechanisms of actions and specific adverse effects. Only a few are presented here in order to provide representative examples. The table lists chemotherapy agents according to category, mechanism of action, and clinical use.

TABLE 9–2 Miscellaneous Cancer Drugs	
CATEGORY	**EXAMPLES**
Plant extracts	Vinblastine (Velban^R)
	Vincristine (Oncovin^R)
Antibiotics	Bleomycin (Blenoxane^R)
	Dactinomycin (Cosmegen^R)
Radiation isotopes	Iodine (I-131)
	Phosphorus (P-32)
Others	Asparaylnase
	Hydroxyurea
Hormones	Estrogen, adrenocorticoids

Miscellaneous Cancer Drugs

There are a number of drugs used in cancer treatment other than alkylating and anti-metabolite drugs. They include plant extracts, radioactive isotopes, and other drugs. Table 9–2 lists some of these drugs according to category and examples.

POSTTEST: PHARMACOLOGY OF CHEMOTHERAPY

For each of the following questions, try to select the *one* best answer from those choices given.

1. All of the following characteristics usually apply to malignant neoplasia except:
   a. new growth
   b. invasiveness
   c. metastases
   d. localized
2. Which one of the following treatment approaches to cancer is effective in the early stages if the location is accessible?
   a. chemotherapy
   b. surgery
   c. radiation
   d. none of the above
3. The major problem with chemotherapy is that antineoplastic drugs cannot differentiate between abnormal and normal cells. True or False?
4. All of the following types of cells are highly susceptible to toxicity of chemotherapy agents except:
   a. muscle cells
   b. skin

   c. bone marrow

   d. gastrointestinal tract

  5. All of the following chemotherapeutic agents are antimetabolites except:

   a. mercaptopurine (Purinethol[R])

   b. cytarabine (Cytosar[R])

   c. busulfan (Myleran[R])

   d. Fluorouracil (Adrucil[R])

REFERENCES/RECOMMENDED READING

Calabrese P, Schein PS, Rosenberg SA: *Medical Oncology: Basic Principles and Clinical Management of Cancer.* Macmillan, New York, 1985.

Devita, VT, Hellman S, Rosenberg SA: *Cancer Principles and Practice of Oncology.* JB Lippincott, Philadelphia, 1985.

Dipalma JR, Digregorio JG: *Basic Pharmacology in Medicine*, 3rd ed. McGraw-Hill, New York, 1990.

Hinter H, Nagle BT: *Basic Pharmacology for Health Occupations*, 2nd ed. Glencoe Publishing Co, Mission Hills, CA, 1987.

PART II
RESPIRATORY CARE
PHARMACOLOGY

CHAPTER 10

PRINCIPLES OF AEROSOLIZED AND INSTILLED MEDICATION ADMINISTRATION

LEARNING OBJECTIVES

After completion of this chapter and its learning activities, the student will be able to:

1. List four advantages of drug administration by the aerosol route.
2. Describe the disadvantages and limitations of drug administration by the aerosol route.
3. Describe the equipment used for aerosol administration of drugs by small-volume nebulizer and the procedure that should be followed.
4. Describe patient instructions for taking an effective small-volume nebulizer treatment.
5. Describe equipment used for aerosol administration of drugs by metered dose inhaler.
6. Describe patient instructions for taking an effective dose of medication by metered dose inhaler, including the use of a spacer.
7. List two drugs that currently are administered by powder aerosol, including the devices used for this administration.
8. Define drug administration by instillation.
9. List three indications (or clinical settings) for drug administration by instillation.
10. Describe the disadvantages or hazards of drug administration by instillation.

INTRODUCTION

Respiratory care practitioners deliver medications by two primary routes, aerosolization and instillation. Each route has its advantages, disadvantages, and limitations. State licensure for respiratory care practitioners may allow drug adminstration by other routes, or may allow infiltration for procedures such as local anesthesia for the insertion of indwelling arterial catheters. This chapter discusses the rationale for administering medications by aerosol or instillation, as well as the appropriate equipment and techniques to optimize these routes of delivery.

AEROSOLIZED MEDICATIONS

There are several advantages to the delivery of medications directly to the mucosal membrane by aerosol:

1. Immediate onset of drug action at desired site
2. Reduced side effects from systemic absorption
3. Smaller doses of potent drugs (e.g., bronchodilators) may provide comparable therapeutic benefits
4. Patients may be taught to self-administer medications

Aerosol administration of many drugs provides a convenient and rapidly effective route while minimizing side effects. Drugs that are administered by aerosol include bronchodilators, decongestants, antibiotics, anti-inflammatory agents (e.g., steroids), mucolytics, wetting agents, surface-active agents (e.g., ethyl alcohol), and anti-asthmatic agents (i.e. cromolyn sodium). Chapters 11–15 will provide specific information about drugs in each of these categories.

Recent studies have investigated the use of aerosol delivery of other drugs to take advantage of its *noninvasive* route, ease of self-administration, and broad mucosal membrane for drug absorption. A small but significant study utilizing aerosolized insulin demonstrated excellent deposition and absorption of the insulin, with good therapeutic blood levels achieved in this group of nonsmoking, non–insulin-dependent diabetics. Studies such as these have broad implications for the future use of aerosolized medications and the role of the respiratory care practitioner in drug administration.

Disadvantages and Limitations of Aerosol Delivery

The primary disadvantage of drug administration by aerosol route is the inability to determine the absolute amount of the drug that is deposited in the lung. When a drug is inhaled, some inevitably rains out in the oropharynx and upper airways, some is swallowed, some is deposited on the mucosal membrane, and some is exhaled. Studies have shown that as little as 10 percent of the drug may actually be deposited in the lung, although the proportion increases when the variables mentioned below are controlled.

Other variables include the breathing pattern of the patient and the type of nebulizer used to aerosolize the drug. If the nebulizer operates continuously, rather than during inspiration only, much of the drug may be lost during exhalation and the pause between respiratory cycles. If the patient is unable to perform an optimal breathing pattern during the treatment (slow, deep inspiration with an end-inspiratory pause), very little of the drug is deposited in the smaller airways and lung periphery. If the type of nebulizer used to aerosolize the drug produces a particle size that is outside the therapeutic range, the aerosol may be unstable (rains out in upper airway/pharynx) or too stable (very little of the drug deposits). When a drug is swallowed rather than being deposited on the mucosal membrane, it typically is broken down and metabolized instead of providing its intended therapeutic effect.

Factors in Aerosolized Drug Delivery

Medications for aerosol delivery typically are nebulized in a *small-volume nebulizer* (SVN) (maximum volume about 10 mL), in contrast to large-volume nebulizers used for high output and humidification. The Bird micronebulizer and Bennett twin-jet nebulizers originally were incorporated into intermittent positive pressure breathing circuits but have since provided the prototypes for the development of small hand-held nebulizers that can be powered by a gas source (i.e., oxygen or compressed air) or a small compressor (i.e., PulmoAide and MicroStat). Ultrasonic nebulization of medications also can be accomplished with the use of specially designed equipment such as the Aerosonic and UltraAir nebulizers.

The single most important variable in providing effective aerosol administration of medications is the patient's breathing pattern. Often the practitioner is in the position to improve the outcome of a course of therapy by exercising good clinical assessment skills. Most institutions establish some *appropriateness* criteria for the selection of patients who can benefit from aerosol administration of drugs (in addition to or instead of some other route). These criteria usually are based on several patient factors:

1. The patient's willingness and ability to cooperate with the treatment
2. The patient's ability to generate a deep breath and perform a brief "breath-hold" at end-inspiration
3. The responsiveness of the patient's pulmonary disease to the drug being used.

Standardizing such criteria would improve patient selection and ultimately improve the cost-effectiveness of therapy. Professional organizations such as the American Association for Respiratory Care (AARC) are currently developing such Practice Guidelines with input from practitioners and physicians.

There is much controversy regarding whether the most appropriate vehicle for delivering aerosolized medication is the SVN or the metered dose inhaler (MDI). Some studies have shown equivalent therapeutic outcomes with both devices, suggesting that the more cost-effective method (MDI) should be adopted for routine use. Other studies have demonstrated that, because SVN treatments require more time (and more respiratory cycles), drug delivery to the lung may be enhanced. It is likely that some balance between the two methods will emerge, perhaps establishing MDI as the primary method and allowing practitioner discretion when specific patients do not respond to therapy or are unable to master the coordination to take an effective treatment by MDI.

There also is significant evidence that currently used disposable SVNs may vary widely in the quality of aerosol produced. The selection of SVNs to be purchased for an institution ideally should be based on both cost-effectiveness and the quality and consistency of aerosol produced. Aerosolized medications are deposited in the major airways when the mean (average) particle diameter size is in the 5–10-micron range. The *therapeutic range* is considered to be 1–5 microns; aerosol particles in this range tend to deposit in small airways and the lung periphery. Aerosol particles less than 1 micron in diameter tend to stay in suspension and be exhaled.

Taking into account all of the factors mentioned and the results of recent studies about aerosol therapy, the following general guidelines should be observed when administering a SVN treatment:

1. A range of 2.5–4.0 mL of solution should be used (e.g., 0.50 mL of medication and 2.50 mL of diluent).
2. Flow rates of 6 L per minute have been shown to produce the optimal particle size for most disposable SVNs.
3. Nebulization should occur on inspiration only; this usually is accomplished through the use of a Y-adaptor in the power line or a "thumb-port" on the nebulizer.
4. The patient should be instructed to inhale slowly and deeply (at least double the normal tidal volume) and to hold at end-inspiration for 3–5 seconds before exhaling.

Metered Dose Inhalers

Metered dose inhalers frequently are used by patients at home and are becoming increasingly common as part of the inpatient care provided in many hospitals. MDI delivery of bronchodilators long has been the standard used during pre- and postdilator pulmonary function testing. However, proper use of these devices (to achieve the desired results) requires a cooperative and coordinated patient and conscientious instruction and supervision by a practitioner. Because MDI aerosols have been available as over-the-counter drugs for decades, the critical nature of proper patient use and instruction has not been appreciated until recent studies showed the variability in medication delivery by this method.

Ideal medication deposition by MDI occurs when the patient uses the following procedure:

1. Remove cap and vigorously shake the cannister to evenly distribute the medication.
2. Open mouth wide and hold cannister about 1 inch in front of mouth.
3. Exhale normally, then squeeze MDI at the beginning of a slow, deep inspiration.
4. Inhale fully, and hold breath for about 5 seconds at end-inspiration.
5. Exhale normally, wait 1–2 minutes, and repeat procedure for second inhalation.

Although these instructions seem rather simple, many patients have difficulty in successfully following them. Studies have shown that patients frequently squeeze the can-

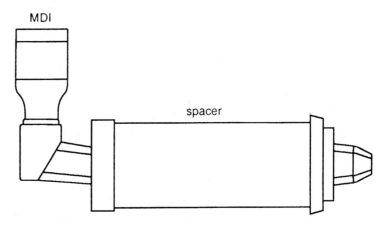

FIGURE 10–1   MDI with Spacer/Chamber.

nister at the wrong time (at end-inspiration or during exhalation), they interrupt or stop inhalation when the cannister is squeezed (causing most of the medication to impact in the mouth and be swallowed), they inhale too rapidly, or they fail to hold their breath when their lungs are fully inflated.

Because of these factors, devices (such as spacers or chambers) have been developed to provide a reservoir of aerosol to improve medication delivery by MDI (Figure 10–1). A wide variety of spacers and chambers are available, their primary purpose being to hold the aerosol in suspension for a longer period of time. They are particularly helpful for patients who have difficulty in coordinating the MDI and their breathing patterns.

MDI use has not been considered appropriate for infants, but the AeroChamber[R] (spacer) with an infant mask currently is being used successfully for infant MDI therapy. MDI therapy also may be effective for pediatric patients when a spacer or chamber is used. It is still essential, however, that a patient (or family member) receive good instructions and practice while supervised by a practitioner until the procedure has been mastered.

If a patient is receiving more than one type of medication by MDI (such as an asthmatic who may take both a bronchodilator and an anti-inflammatory agent), the bronchodilator always should be taken first. It also is suggested that, for administration of corticosteroid drugs such as **beclomethasone (Vanceril[R])**, which may make the patient more vulnerable to oral infections such as candidiasis, the technique should be slightly modified. For MDI treatment with corticosteroids, the patient should be instructed to wait 1–2 minutes after taking the bronchodilator and then hyperextend the neck when inhaling. This modification (having the patient look toward the ceiling during inhalation) will reduce the amount of the drug that is deposited in the mouth and pharynx.

A full MDI cannister should provide about 200 puffs of medication. A simple method to determine approximately how much medication remains in the cannister is to float it in a bowl of water. If the cannister sinks, or completely submerges with the nozzle down, it is full. If the cannister does not fully submerge but floats with the nozzle down,

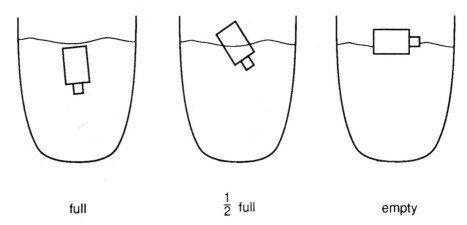

full $\frac{1}{2}$ full   empty

FIGURE 10–2   Method to Determine MDI Contents.

it is about half-full. If the cannister floats on its side on the surface of the water, it is almost empty (or empty) (see Figure 10–2).

Powder Aerosols

Two drugs frequently administered by respiratory care practitioners are available in *powder aerosol capsules* that are activated by the patient's breath. **Cromolyn sodium (Intal[R])** and **albuterol (Ventolin)[R]** currently are marketed in capsules that must be administered by specific devices manufactured for these drugs.

Intal[R] is an anti-asthmatic drug that is described in detail in Chapter 14. This drug is effective only when administered by aerosol and originally was marketed only in the powder aerosol form. It is now available in solution, MDI and powder; the powder capsules are administered by use of the Spinhaler[R] (Figure 10–3).

Ventolin[R] is a bronchodilator that is described in detail in Chapter 11. It is available in solution, MDI, and powder capsules (**Rotacap[R]**). The powder aerosol is administered by use of the Rotahaler[R] device (Figure 10–4).

Administration of a drug by powder aerosol has two primary advantages: 1) proper breathing pattern is required to activate device, and therefore better deposition of aerosol is likely; and 2) no propellant gas (such as freon) is used. Although the amount of freon associated with the use of MDI devices may not seem significant, current recommendations suggest the elimination of gas-propelled MDIs within the next 5 years. It is likely that research will continue to develop powder-aerosol forms of currently used drugs to replace the widespread use of gas-propelled MDIs.

INSTILLED MEDICATIONS

Another route of administration frequently used by respiratory care practitioners is direct instillation of drugs through an endotracheal tube or intratracheal catheter. Instillation

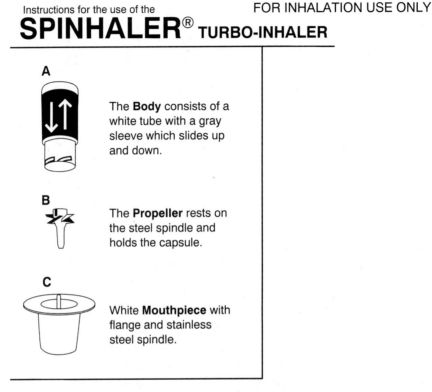

Instructions for the use of the   FOR INHALATION USE ONLY

SPINHALER® TURBO-INHALER

A

The **Body** consists of a white tube with a gray sleeve which slides up and down.

B

The **Propeller** rests on the steel spindle and holds the capsule.

C

White **Mouthpiece** with flange and stainless steel spindle.

FIGURE 10–3   Description of Spinhaler[R] Turbo-Inhaler. Courtesy of Fisons Corporation.

consists of injecting a bolus (3–5 mL) of a drug directly into the tracheobronchial tree via a tube or catheter. This route typically is used for the administration of wetting agents or mucolytics, surface-active agents (such as surfactant replacement), and advanced cardiac life support drugs during cardiac resuscitation.

Instillation of wetting agents (such as normal saline) usually is used as a part of the airway management protocol for intubated or tracheotomized patients when mucus plugging or retention of secretions has developed. Patients with indwelling transtracheal oxygen catheters also are taught to self-instill a bolus of saline to counteract the drying effect of gas delivered directly to the trachea.

Current surfactant replacement therapy requires direct instillation of the synthetic surfactant into an endotracheal tube and vigorous ventilation of the infant for distribution (these agents and specific dosage recommendations are discussed in Chapter 15).

Instillation of cardiac resuscitation drugs through the endotracheal tube long has been known to be a satisfactory route when cardiac output is reduced and/or intravenous routes have not been established. Drugs administered directly to the pulmonary mucosal surface may be effectively absorbed (similar to sublingual administration) in situations in which the cardiac output and perfusion are reduced.

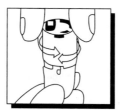 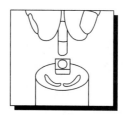 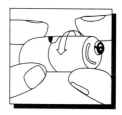

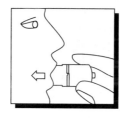 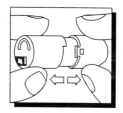

FIGURE 10–4 Description of Rotahaler^R. Courtesy of Fisons Corporation.

Disadvantages and Limitations of Drug Delivery by Instillation

The primary disadvantage of this method of drug delivery is its tendency to stimulate bronchospasm and a violent cough reflex. In patients with retained secretions, the cough is a necessary part of secretion removal, but special care must be taken to protect the artificial airway and/or the stoma site.

When this method of drug delivery is used during cardiac resuscitation, the dosage of drug retained cannot be determined absolutely because some may be suctioned from the airway. Coughing typically is not a consideration for the patient in full cardiac arrest.

Transient *hypoxemia* secondary to airway obstruction has been associated with the instillation of artificial surfactant. Monitoring of cardiac rhythms and pulse oximetry during such therapy is strongly recommended and is usually part of the treatment protocol.

POSTTEST: PRINCIPLES OF AEROSOLIZED AND INSTILLED MEDICATION ADMINISTRATION

For each of the following questions, try to select the *one* best answer from those choices given.

1. Which of the following is the recommended range of particle sizes for deposition in smaller airways and lung periphery?
   a. less than 1 micron

    b. 1–5 microns

    c. 5–10 microns

    d. 10–15 microns

    e. greater than 15 microns

2. Which of the following is the recommended breathing pattern for maximal deposition of medication by aerosol?

    a. normal breathing

    b. normal breathing with a 3-second pause at end-inspiration

    c. slow, deep breathing with a 3–5-second pause at end-inspiration

    d. rapid inspiration with a 3–5-second pause at end-inspiration

    e. none of the above is correct

3. Which of the following are advantages of drug administration by aerosol?

    I.   fewer systemic side effects than other routes

    II. rapid onset of therapeutic effects of drug

    III. precise amount of drug is given only to target organ

    IV. technique is cost-effective because patient effort is not required

    a. I and II only

    b. II and IV only

    c. I, II, and III only

    d. I and III only

    e. I, II, and IV only

4. Which of the following is the recommended flow rate to be used to power a SVN?

    a. 1–3 L per minute

    b. 3–4 L per minute

    c. 4–6 L per minute

    d. 7–10 L per minute

    e. none of the above

5. When taking a drug by MDI, a spacer is used to:

    a. concentrate the medication

    b. prolong the life of the MDI

    c. capture the patient's exhaled air

    d. provide a reservoir and improve drug delivery

    e. eliminate the need for the patient to inhale deeply

6. Approximately what percentage of medication is actually deposited on mucosal lung surfaces during a SVN treatment?

    a. less than 5 percent

    b. 5–10 percent

    c. 10–20 percent

    d. 20–30 percent

    e. more than 30 percent

7. A rapid breathing pattern (or rapid inspiratory flow rate) would most likely deposit an aerosol in:

    a. the oropharynx

    b. large airways (trachea and bronchi)

    c. medium airways (bronchi and segmental airways)

    d. small airways and lung periphery

    e. alveoli

8. The purpose of a brief breath-hold at end-inspiration during an aerosol treatment is to:

    a. improve treatment effectiveness and drug deposition

    b. guarantee drug deposition in the hilar region

    c. prevent hyperventilation during treatment

    d. assure proper drug mixing in nebulizer

    e. assure appropriate treatment length

9. Drugs are instilled into an artificial airway for which of the following reasons?

    I.   provide precise amount of desired drug

    II. stimulate a cough and aid in secretion removal

    III. utilize pulmonary mucosa for drug absorption in low cardiac output state (i.e., cardiac resuscitation)

    IV. minimize systemic effects of drugs

    V. assure drug is not swallowed

    a. I, IV, and V only

    b. I, II, and III only

    c. II, III, IV, and V only

    d. II and III only

    e. I, III, and IV only

10. When using a MDI the patient should be instructed to squeeze the cannister:

    a. at end-inspiration

    b. at end-exhalation

    c. during the middle of inspiration

    d. at the beginning of exhalation

    e. at the beginning of inspiration

11. If the cannister of a MDI floats on its side in a bowl of water, its contents are approximately:

    a. full

    b. 3/4 full

    c. half-full

    d. 1/4 full

    e. empty

12. When using MDI treatments for pediatric patients:

    a. a spacer is not recommended

    b. a spacer is recommended

    c. the breathing pattern is not important

    d. care should be taken to avoid coughing

    e. only patients 8 years or older should use MDI

REFERENCES/RECOMMENDED READING

Aerosol Consensus Statement, from the Consensus Conference on Aerosol Delivery, *Respir Care* 36:916–921, 1991.

Alvine GF, et al: Disposable jet nebulizers: How reliable are they? *Chest* 101:316, 1992.

Dolovich M: Clinical aspects of aerosol physics. *Respir Care* 36:931–938, 1991.

Gay PC, et al: Metered dose inhalers for bronchodilator delivery in intubated, mechanically ventilated patients. *Chest* 99:66, 1991.

Guidry GG, et al: Incorrect use of metered dose inhalers by medical personnel. *Chest* 101:31, 1992.

Kacmarek RM, Hess D: The interface between patient and aerosol generator. *Respir Care* 36:952–976, 1991.

Laube BL, Georgopoulos A, Adams GK: Preliminary study of the efficacy of insulin aerosol delivered by oral inhalation in diabetic patients. *JAMA* 269:2106, 1993.

Maguire GP, et al: Comparison of a hand-held nebulizer with a metered dose inhaler-spacer combination in acute obstructive pulmonary disease. *Chest* 100:1300, 1991.

Newman SP: Aerosol generators and delivery systems. *Respir Care* 36:939–951, 1991.

Pierson DJ: Toward international consensus on clinical aerosol administration. *Chest* 100:1100, 1991.

Rau, JL: Delivery of aerosolized drugs to neonatal and pediatric patients. *Respir Care* 36:514, 1991.

Scanlan CL: Humidity and aerosol therapy. In CL Scanlan, CB Spearman, RL Sheldon (eds), *Egan's Fundamentals of Respiratory Care*, 5th ed. CV Mosby Company, St. Louis, 1990, pp 557–581.

Sly RM: Aerosol therapy in children. *Respir Care* 36:994–1007, 1991.

Svedmyr N: Clinical advantages of the aerosol route of drug administration. *Respir Care* 36:922–930, 1991.

Tenholder MF, Bryson MJ, Whitlock WL: A model for conversion from small volume nebulizer to metered dose inhaler aerosol therapy. *Chest* 101:634, 1992.

Ziment I: *Respiratory Pharmacology and Therapeutics*. WB Saunders Co, Philadelphia, 1978.

CHAPTER 11

BRONCHODILATOR THERAPY

LEARNING OBJECTIVES

After completion of this chapter and its learning activities, the student will be able to:
1. Define bronchoconstriction.
2. Describe the pharmacological routes of bronchodilation (relief of mucosal edema and/or bronchospasm).
3. Describe the neurochemical physiology of the bronchial smooth muscle (what chemicals are present, what nerve endings are stimulated, and how dilation is achieved).
4. Define three categories of bronchodilators and describe the mode of action of bronchodilators in each category (sympathomimetic, anticholinergic, and xanthine).
5. Define the dosage ranges and concentrations of each bronchodilator.
6. Describe the contraindications, hazards, and side effects of each bronchodilator.
7. Given a patient case study, be able to suggest the most appropriate bronchodilator therapy, including the drug of choice, route of delivery, and recommended dosage.

INTRODUCTION

Bronchodilator therapy may be the most critical and challenging aspect of respiratory care pharmacology. Acute bronchoconstriction often is relieved most effectively by aerosol therapy, the respiratory care practitioner (RCP) may be the most knowledgeable individual regarding the *best drug for a specific patient under given circumstances*.

The RCP may be asked to recommend the most appropriate drug, its dosage (in either solution [cubic centimeters or milliliters] or by weight [milligrams]), and even its route of administration. Considering the wide range of patients seen by practitioners and the variety of such drugs available, it is critical for the RCP to possess a working knowledge of *how* each bronchodilator achieves its purpose, *how much* of each agent is appropriate, *how often* it is safe to administer, *how long* the effects will last, and what contraindications and side effects exist for each drug.

The art of respiratory care utilizes the skill and knowledge of the RCP to recommend or select the best drug for each situation. The challenge is to select the drug with the most beneficial effects, the least negative side effects, and the optimal duration. Because patients often develop a rapidly occurring tolerance (tachyphylaxis) to sympathomimetic drugs, the RCP may be in the best position to notice this phenomenon and recommend a course of therapy with an alternative drug. Combinations of drugs from several categories frequently are used in the management of chronic bronchospasm or severe acute symptoms (i.e. status asthmaticus). Knowledge of the mechanism by which each bronchodilator achieves its goal is a key factor in the safe, effective, and efficient care of patients with reactive airway disease.

BRONCHOCONSTRICTION

The term *bronchoconstriction* often is used incorrectly as a synonym for *bronchospasm*. Bronchospasm is one of the major factors of bronchoconstriction, but not the only one! Bronchoconstriction means a condition in which the diameter (lumen) of the airway is reduced or constricted. This condition may be due to bronchospasm, mucosal edema, or the presence of secretions (or often some combination of these). In the selection of the best bronchodilator for each patient, the RCP must have some knowledge of the pathophysiology of the disease or injury being treated.

Bronchodilators achieve relief of bronchoconstriction by acting on the cause, or mechanism, of the constriction. Asthmatics frequently exhibit all three aspects (bronchospasm, mucosal edema, and excessive secretions), whereas a croup patient may have only mucosal edema. The drug, or drugs, of choice in treating bronchoconstriction are determined by the mechanism of constriction, as well as factors such as patient history and sensitivity, other medications the patient is receiving, and the *acuity* (criticalness) of the situation.

METHODS OF BRONCHODILATION

Relief of Mucosal Edema

Drugs that reduce bronchoconstricion by relief of mucosal edema include both sympathomimetics with an α effect (α-adrenergic), which promotes vasoconstriction (*decongestant*), and corticosteroids, which have a general anti-inflammatory effect. The corticosteroids are covered in Chapter 14.

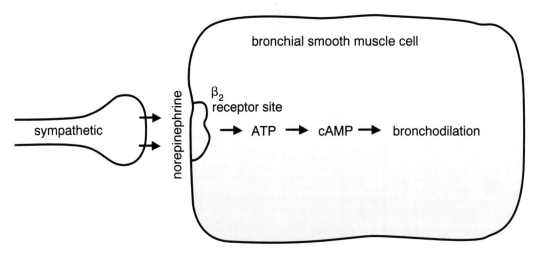

FIGURE 11–1   Effect of Sympathetic Stimulation in Bronchial Cells.

Relief of Bronchospasm

Bronchodilation is a complex process, and bronchodilators often are categorized according to the mechanism by which each achieves relief of bronchospasm. The three categories of bronchodilating drugs are sympathomimetics (β-adrenergics), anticholinergics (parasympatholytics), and xanthines. Respiratory care practitioners administer both sympathomimetic and anticholinergic drugs by aerosol or instillation, and must be aware of the effects of xanthines and their role in the relief of bronchospasm.

Bronchodilation through relief of bronchospasm is achieved in the pulmonary smooth muscle by either *directly stimulating bronchodilation* (sympathomimetics) or *blocking*

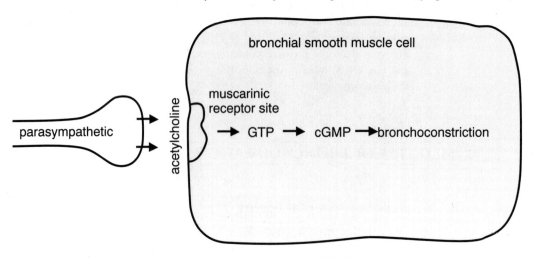

FIGURE 11–2   Effect of Parasympathetic Stimulation in Bronchial Cells.

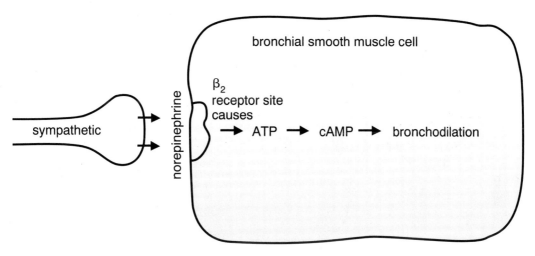

FIGURE 11–3 Sympathomimetic Drugs: Stimulate cAMP.

bronchospasm (anticholinergics or xanthines). When the sympathetic nervous system is stimulated, its effects in the pulmonary system include bronchodilation and vasoconstriction. Bronchodilators in this category thus are referred to as *sympathomimetic*, meaning they mimic or imitate the sympathetic nervous system, or as *adrenergic*, meaning they utilize neurotransmitters similar to adrenalin (epinephrine). When the parasympathetic nervous system is stimulated, its effects in the pulmonary system include bronchoconstriction. Bronchodilators in this category thus are referred to as *anticholinergic*, meaning they block the bronchoconstricting effects of the parasympathetic system, or as *parasympatholytic*, meaning the drug lyses or dissolves the effect of the parasympathetic system.

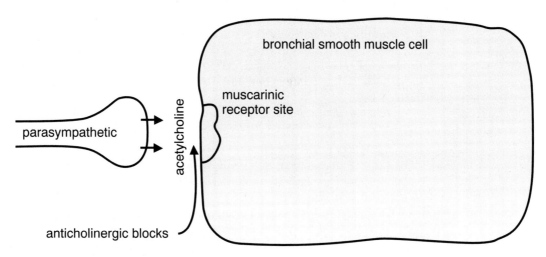

FIGURE 11–4 Anticholinergic Drugs: Block Parasympathetic Stimulation.

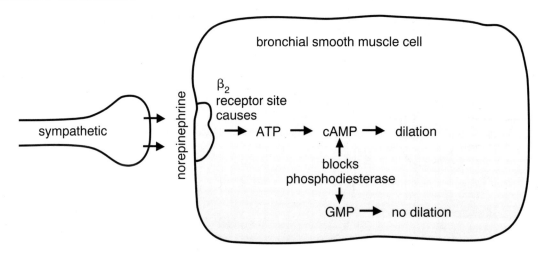

FIGURE 11–5   Xanthines: Inhibit Phosphodiesterase.

Neurochemical Mediators in Bronchodilation

Research has shown that when nerve endings in the autonomic nervous system are stimulated, they release *transmitters* (chemicals) that bind to receptor sites on the adjoining nerve ending (or neuroeffector site) to cause an effect. As described in Chapter 2, the neurotransmitter that stimulates bronchodilation is norepinephrine, which binds with a β_2 receptor and stimulates intracellular production of *cyclic 3'5'-adenosine monophosphate* (cAMP). When a sympathetic nerve in the bronchial tree is stimulated, it promotes the conversion of adenosine triphosphate (ATP) to cAMP, which leads to relaxation of smooth muscle (Figure 11–1). This mediator (cAMP) constantly is broken down into an inactive form (AMP) by the presence of the enzyme *phosphodiesterase*. When AMP is present in large quantities, it interferes with stimulation of bronchodilation.

When a parasympathetic nerve in the bronchial tree is stimulated, it promotes the conversion of guanosine triphosphate (GTP) to *cyclic 3'5'-guanosine monophosphate* (cGMP). Intracellular levels of cGMP in bronchial smooth muscle cells promote bronchoconstriction (Figure 11–2).

Thus we can categorize bronchodilators by three modes of action:

1. Stimulation of production of cAMP (*sympathomimetic*) (Figure 11–3)
2. Blockage of production of cGMP (*anticholinergic*) (Figure 11–4)
3. Inhibition of phosphodiesterase (*xanthines*) (Figure 11–5)

The primary goal of bronchodilator therapy is to increase levels of cAMP or decrease levels of cGMP in the smooth muscle cells in the pulmonary tree. Often a combination of drugs from these categories is needed in the management of acute or chronic bronchospasm (e.g., asthma).

SYMPATHOMIMETIC BRONCHODILATORS

Bronchodilators in this category historically have been referred to as sympathomimetic *amines*. This term refers to the chemical composition of the drug (its *catecholamine* properties) and can no longer be used to refer to all drugs in this category. Many of the newer agents in this category have higher specificity (they promote bronchodilation with fewer side effects) and are noncatecholamine. It is preferable to refer to these drugs as simply sympathomimetic because this term is sufficient to describe the mechanism of action.

When sympathomimetic drugs are used, there are three potential effects on the cardiovascular system:

1. alpha (α) effects (vasoconstriction)
2. beta-1 (β_1) effects (increase heart rate)
3. beta-2 (β_2) effects (reverse bronchospasm)

Ideal bronchodilators in this category are β_2-specific, meaning they promote bronchodilation while minimizing side effects. A few drugs in this category have both α and β effects. Table 11–1 summarizes the α, β_1, and β_2 characteristics of each bronchodilator now in use in the United States and Canada.

Calculating Drug Dosages (Weight vs. Solution Strength)

Although bronchodilators most frequently are ordered in volume measurements (milliliters [mL] or cubic centimeters [cc]), it is important to know how much of the drug actually is being administered. To determine the *weight* of the drug (in milligrams [mg]), the solution percentage must be converted to a weight/volume. For example:

> **Albuterol** is marketed in a 0.5% solution (**Proventil**[R], **Ventolin**[R], [C] **Salbutamol** [Canadian]). If the physician orders 0.5 mL Proventil[R] in 3 mL normal saline (NS), how much of the drug is the patient receiving?

Answer:

> A 0.5% solution means there is 0.5 g of the drug dissolved in 100 mL of diluent, or 0.5 g/100 mL. So, if 0.5 g = 500 mg, then 500 mg/100 mL = 5 mg/1 mL. If 0.5 mL is given, the patient receives 2.5 mg of drug.

Therapeutic Indications

The primary indication for the use of bronchodilators is the relief of acute bronchoconstriction that is caused by bronchospasm. Recent research has suggested that some of the newer sympathomimetic agents also may have some beneficial effect in the prevention of bronchospasm (such as that associated with exercise, or *exercise-induced asthma*). This action

TABLE 11–1   Sympathomimetic Bronchodilators

	α (VASOCONSTRICTION)	β₁ (HEART RATE)	β₂ (BRONCHODILATION)	DURATION (hr)	OTHER SIDE EFFECTS (NAUSEA, HEADACHES, TREMORS)
Albuterol (Proventil^R, Ventolin^R, [C] Salbutamol)	None	Mild	Strong	3–6	Few
Isoetharine (Bronkosol^R)	None	Moderate	Good	1.5–2	Few
Isoproterenol (Isuprel^R)	None	Strong	Strongest	0.5–1	Frequent and severe
Metaproterenol (Alupent^R, Metaprel^R)	None	Mild	Strong	3–4	Tremors
Racemic epinephrine (Micronefrin^R, Vaponefrin^R, Racepinephrine^R)	Strong	Moderate	Mild	0.5–1	Mild
Terbutaline (Brethine^R, Bricanyl^R)	None	Mild	Strong	2–6	Few
Bitolterol (Tornalate^R) (MDI)	None	Mild	Strong	5–8	Few
Pirbuterol (Maxair^R) (MDI)	None	Mild	Strong	3–5	Few

seems to be related to the increased intracellular levels of cAMP that are stimulated by sympathomimetic drugs.

SYMPATHOMIMETIC AND ANTICHOLINERGIC BRONCHODILATOR DRUGS

This section describes the specific sympathomimetic and anticholinergic bronchodilating drugs currently in use in the United States and Canada, including the brand names, drug action, contraindications, side effects, dosage, duration of action, and special considerations. Although there are other drugs available with bronchodilating effects (i.e., aminophylline), this section concentrates primarily on those drugs that are administered by the RCP in the acute or long-term care setting.

Sympathomimetic Bronchodilators

Albuterol (Proventil^R, Ventolin^R, [C] Salbutamol).

Actions: sympathomimetic; stimulates production of cAMP. Strong β_2 and minimal β_1 effects, no α effects.

Duration: rapid onset, effective for 4–6 hours.

Contraindications: tachycardia and hypersensitivity.

Side effects: (occasional) tachycardia, tremors, nervousness, hypertension, nausea, and headache.

Dosage: approved for adults and children over 12 years old. Give 0.20 to 0.50 mL of 0.5% solution with 2.5 mL diluent, administerd by aerosol every 3–4 hours (0.50 mL of 0.5% solution = 2.5 mg albuterol).

Epinephrine (Primatene Mist^R MDI, [C] Bronkaid, [C] Mistometer).

Actions: sympathomimetic; stimulates production of cAMP. Strong α, β_1, and β_2 effects.

Duration: rapid onset, relatively short duration (60 minutes).

Contraindications: use with extreme caution in patients with preexisting cardiovascular disease.

Side effects: profound cardiovascular side effects, including tachycardia, palpitations, hypertension, headache, and nausea.

Dosage: give 0.25–0.50 mL epinephrine 1:100 (1%) with 1.50 mL diluent, administered by aerosol every 2–4 hours; patient should be monitored very closely for adverse reactions.

Special considerations: use of aerosolized epinephrine should be restricted to a few selected critical care situations, such as *status asthmaticus*, and should be administered only in the acute care setting where cardiac and hemodynamic monitoring is available.

Isoetharine Hydrochloride (Bronkosol^R).

Actions: sympathomimetic; stimulates production of cAMP. Mild β_1 with moderate β_2 effects; no α effects.

Duration: rapid onset, but effective duration is only 90–120 minutes.

Contraindications: hypertension, tachycardia, and hypersensitivity.

Side effects: (occasional) tachycardia, nervousness, nausea, and hypertension.

Dosage: give 0.25–0.50 mL of 1% solution with 3.0 mL diluent, administered via aerosol every 3–4 hours (0.50 mL of 1% solution = 5.0 mg isoetharine).

Isoproterenol Hydrochloride (Isuprel[R], Vapo-N-Iso[R], Medihaler-Iso[R]).

Actions: sympathomimetic amine; stimulates production of cAMP. Strong β_1 and β_2 effects, no α effects; promotes pulmonary vasodilation with rapid systemic absorption.

Duration: rapid onset but short duration; therapeutic effectiveness 30–60 minutes.

Contraindications: tachycardia, hypertension, cardiovascular disease, hypersensitivity [allergy], and acute myocardial infarction.

Side effects: tachycardia, palpitation, flushing of skin, nausea, vomiting, nervousness, hypertension, hypotension, headache, and *increased myocardial oxygen consumption.*

Dosage: give 0.25–0.50 mL of 1:200 solution with 2.5–3.0 mL diluent (NS or distilled water [DW]), administered by aerosol every 3–4 hours (0.50 mL of 1:200 solution = 2.5 mg of isoproterenol).

Special considerations: a 1:200 solution means there is 1 g of the drug dissolved in 200 mL of diluent, or 1000 mg/200 mL. Thus, the patient receives 5 mg/1 mL when using the 1:200 (0.50%) solution. A 1:100 solution = 1% (1 g/100 mL); Thus, the patient receives 10 mg/1 mL when using 1:100 solution. Because of its systemic absorption, Isuprel[R] has strong but relatively short-duration bronchodilating effects. Because of its catecholamine properties, it is less effective in the presence of acidosis and the patient is likely to develop tachyphylaxis. In *acute status asthmaticus,* it may be administered as an aerosol bolus of 2.5 mg (0.50 mL of 1:200 solution) diluted 1:1 and followed by aerosolized saline; the patient must be *closely monitored.*

Metaproterenol Sulfate (Alupent[R], Metaprel[R]).

Actions: sympathomimetic; stimulates production of cAMP. Strong β_2 effects, minimal β_1 stimulation, and no α effects.

Duration: rapid onset, effective for 3–4 hours.

Contraindications: tachycardia and hypersensitivity.

Side effects: (occasional) tachycardia, tremors, nervousness, hypertension, nausea, and headache.

Dosage: approved for adults and children over 12 years old. Give 0.20–0.30 mL of 5% solution with 2.50 mL diluent, administered by aerosol every 3–4 hours.

Special Considerations: tremors associated with the use of metaproterenol typically diminish with successive treatments. Patients should be instructed to monitor this side effect and discontinue use of the drug if tremors persist.

Racemic Epinephrine (Micronefrin[R], Vaponefrin[R], Racepinephrine[R]).

Actions: sympathomimetic; stimulates production of cAMP. Moderate β_1, mild β_2, and strong α effects.

Duration: rapid onset; effective for 30–60 minutes.

Contraindication: sensitivity.

Side effects: tachycardia, hypertension, and headache.

Dosage: give 0.25–0.50 mL of 2.25% solution in 3.0 mL diluent, administered by aerosol every 1–2 hours (0.50 mL of 2.25% solution = 11.25 mg racemic epinephrine).

Special considerations: drug of choice in the treatment of bronchoconstriction associated with *mucosal edema* (e.g., croup, post-extubation laryngeal edema, inhalation injuries). It is rapidly metabolized, and can be given safely as frequently as every hour with close monitoring. The primary drug action is α; therefore, it is not useful in patients with severe bronchospasm.

Terbutaline Sulfate (Brethine[R], Bricanyl[R]).

Actions: sympathomimetic; stimulates production of cAMP. Strong β_2 specificity, minimal β_1 and no α effects.

Duration: slower onset than other sympathomimetic drugs but has effective bronchodilating effects for 2–6 hours.

Contraindication: sensitivity.

Side effects: (occasional) tremors, palpitations, tachycardia, and gastrointestinal distress.

Dosage: give 0.75–2.5 mg in 3 mL diluent, administered by aerosol every 4–6 hours. Ampules contain 0.1% solution (1 mg/1 mL).

Special considerations: neither multiple-dose nor unit-dose vials of terbutaline are available for aerosol administration. Ampules for subcutaneous injection currently are used for aerosolization. *This method of administration is not currently approved by the Food and Drug Administration.*

Bitolterol Mesylate (Tornalate^R) and Pirbuterol Acetate (Maxair^R). These are two potent β_2-specific bronchodilators in use the United States that currently are available only in metered-dose inhalers (MDIs). Because this method of administration now is commonly utilized in the inpatient care setting, it is important to note them by generic and brand names. The administration and dosage guidelines are comparable for each.

Actions: sympathomimetic; stimulate production of cAMP. Strong β_2 specificity, minimal β_1 and no α effects.

Duration: Tornalate^R, 5–8 hours; Maxair^R, up to 5 hours.

Dosage: Tornalate^R, 2 puffs every 4–6 hours; Maxair^R, 1–2 puffs every 4–6 hours.

General Sympathomimetic Special Considerations. It should be noted as a special consideration for *all* β-*adrenergic* bronchodilators that their effectiveness will be significantly reduced in patients who are on β-blocking drugs (e.g., **Inderal^R**) for control of hypertension.

The diluent of choice for most bronchodilators should be normal saline, unless specifically contraindicated. Recent studies have found that bronchodilators diluted with NS show greater efficacy than those diluted with sterile distilled water for aerosolization.

Research has demonstrated that any drug therapy that increases cAMP also increases *clotting time* by inhibiting platelet aggregation. This has particular significance for RCPs because many patients receiving bronchodilator therapy also have arterial punctures for blood gas analysis. Special attention to the arterial puncture site, including digital pressure and/or the use of a temporary pressure bandage, should be considered.

Anticholinergic Bronchodilators

Bronchodilators in this category also are referred to as *parasympatholytics*. Anticholinergic bronchodilators achieve bronchodilation through *decreased* levels of cGMP, which promotes bronchospasm when its formation is stimulated by the parasympathetic system. Anticholinergic bronchodilators *block* the effects of the parasympathetic system.

Stimulation of the parasympathetic nervous system causes several effects in the tracheobronchial tree:

1. Increased secretions
2. Slowing of the heart rate
3. Bronchoconstriction (by stimulating cGMP)

Bronchoconstriction occurs secondary to the formation of cGMP in the smooth muscle cell. When acetylcholine reaches a parasympathetic smooth muscle receptor, it stimulates the conversion of GMP to cGMP and smooth muscle constriction occurs. Use of anticholinergic (parasympatholytic) drugs to block the effects of the parasympathetic system therefore will lead to:

1. Drying of pulmonary secretions
2. Increasing heart rate
3. Bronchodilation (refer to Figure 11–4)

Atropine Sulfate (atropine [generic]).

Action: parasympatholytic; blocks production of cGMP.

Duration: onset within 15 minutes, reaching peak effectiveness within 1–2 hours; duration is dose dependent, usually 3–6 hours.

Contraindications: sensitivity, glaucoma, prostatic hypertrophy, tachycardia, and myocardial ischemia. Use with caution in patients with unstable cardiac status associated with acute hemorrhage.

Side effects: tachycardia, bradycardia, palpitations, angina, headache, nervousness, drowsiness, dizziness, insomnia, fever, confusion, agitation, nausea, vomiting, dysphagia, heartburn, *thickening of secretions*, and *mucus plugging*.

Dosage: give 0.3–0.5 mg in 3 mL NS, no more frequently than 4 times/day by aerosol. Use in *geriatric* and *pediatric* patients is limited because *side-effects* are more *pronounced* and dosage is difficult to titrate.

Special considerations: Refer to the *Physicians' Desk Reference* (PDR) for specific dosage recommendations for adults and children at varying body weights. Side effects are dose dependent. The recommended dosage above is the safe and effective range for the average adult. A short course of therapy alternating with sympathomimetic drugs may be the best therapeutic approach because useful additive effects have been noted. Special attention to *adequate hydration* should be observed in patients receiving aerosolized atropine (because of the potential drying of secretions and mucus plugging).

Ipratropium Bromide (Atrovent^R, [C] Atrovent [Solution]).

Actions: parasympatholytic; blocks production of cGMP.

Duration: onset within 15 minutes, reaching peak effectiveness within 1–2 hours and maintaining therapeutic effect for 4–6 hours.

Contraindication: sensitivity.

Side effects: very mild; occasional dryness of mouth may occur.

Dosage: *Available in the United States in MDI only.* Approved for use by adults and children over 12 years old; 1–2 inhalations (18 μg/inhalation) 4 times/day. *Available in Canada in 0.025% solution.* ADULTS: 250–500 μg (1–2 mL) every 4–6 hours. CHILDREN (5–12 years): 125–250 μg (0.50–1.0 mL) every 4–6 hours.

Special considerations: Ipratropium is not well absorbed systemically and therefore has almost none of the side effects seen with atropine. Mucus plugging and thickening of secretions is not seen within prescribed dosage ranges. Ipratropium is very helpful in the management of chronic bronchospasm (e.g., asthma) because of its duration of effectiveness and limited side effects. It often is administered in conjunction with albuterol for optimal bronchodilating effects.

XANTHINES

Although there are no bronchodilators in the xanthine category that are administered by aerosol, it is important for the RCP to be familiar with these drugs. Xanthines frequently are used in the management of acute and chronic bronchoconstriction associated with asthma and chronic obstructive pulmonary disease (COPD). The RCP must be aware of the actions, side effects, and drug interactions associated with xanthines so that optimal patient care can be achieved safely.

Xanthines are administered by oral or intravenous (IV) routes and have numerous effects in addition to bronchodilation. They promote pulmonary vasodilation, coronary vasodilation, cardiac stimulation (both rate and contractility are increased), skeletal muscle stimulation (including enhanced diaphragmatic contractility), central nervous system stimulation (medullary), and diuresis. Caffeine, theobromine, and theophylline constitute the xanthine group, but only theophylline and its derivatives are used therapeutically.

Mechanism of Bronchodilation

Xanthines are known to inhibit the action of phosphodiesterase and therefore have been thought to achieve bronchodilation by *indirectly* increasing the available levels of cAMP (refer to Figure 11–5). Although this is true, it is now known that this effect alone cannot explain their bronchodilating effects, and further research is being done to determine the specific pathways by which xanthines promote bronchodilation. For simplicity, xanthines still are classified as phosphodiesterase inhibitors.

Therapeutic Use of Xanthines

Xanthines commonly are prescribed for the long-term management of bronchospasm in asthmatic and COPD patients. Xanthines have a slow onset but long duration of effectiveness and are reasonably well tolerated by many patients. They also are used in the

TABLE 11–2 Aminophylline Brand Names		
TABLETS	**LIQUID**	**SUPPOSITORY**
Amoline[R] Phyllocontin[R]	Somophyllin[R]	Truphylline[R]

treatment of neonatal apnea and bradycardia because of their central nervous system stimulation. Because of their vasodilating effects, xanthines are sometimes used in the management of acute pulmonary edema.

Side Effects of Xanthines

Patients receiving xanthines must be closely monitored through measurement of serum levels of the drug because the therapeutic range is very narrow and quite close to toxicity.

TABLE 11–3 Theophylline Brand Names	
CAPSULES/TABLETS	**LIQUID/SUSPENSION**
Aerolate[R]	Accurbron[R]
Bronkodyl[R]	Aerolate[R]
Duraphyl[R]	Aquaphyllin[R]
Elixophyllin[R]	Asmalix[R]
LaBID[R]	Elixomin[R]
Lodrane[R]	Elixophyllin[R]
Quibron[R]	Lanophyllin[R]
Respid[R]	Lixolin[R]
Slo-Bid[R]	Slo-Phyllin[R]
Slo-Phyllin[R]	Theoclear[R]
Somephyllin[R]	Theolair[R]
Sustaire[R]	Theon[R]
Theobid[R]	Theostat[R]
Theochron[R]	
Theoclear[R]	
TheoDur[R]	
Theolair[R]	
Theophyl[R]	
Theospan[R]	
Theo-Time[R]	
Theovent[R]	
Uniphyl[R]	

Side effects primarily are manifested in the central nervous system, cardiovascular system, or gastrointestinal system, and include:

1. Dizziness, convulsions, or seizures
2. Headache, insomnia, restlessness, irritability, depression, and abnormal speech or behavior
3. Palpitations, tachycardia, arrhythmias, or hypotension
4. Nausea, vomiting, diarrhea, epigastric pain, anorexia, and hematemesis.

Because of the wide range of side effects and the delicacy of maintaining therapeutic levels without toxicity, the use of xanthines as a preventive measure is under review. Many pulmonologists are managing asthmatic patients with **cromolyn sodium** and reducing or eliminating the dosage of xanthines where possible. **Cromolyn sodium** and **nedocromil sodium** are described and discussed in Chapter 14.

Description of Xanthines

Theophylline and its salt, aminophylline, are the primary xanthines used therapeutically. These drugs are marketed for oral and IV use in several forms and under many brand names (see Tables 11–2 and 11–3). **Dosage:** ranges for xanthines vary widely based on type of drug and patient weight and tolerance. Refer to specific drug information in PDR or product inserts for dosage administration guidelines. **Special considerations:** Special care must be taken when administering chest physiotherapy or drawing an arterial blood gas on a patient with an IV infusion of aminophylline. Disruption or infiltration of the IV site may lead to localized irritation and tissue necrosis.

POSTTEST: BRONCHODILATOR THERAPY

For each of the following questions, try to select the *one* best answer from those choices given.

1. Which of the following terms is synonymous with β-*adrenergic*?
   a. parasympatholytic
   b. sympathomimetic
   c. α-adrenergic
   d. anticholinergic
   e. xanthinergic
2. Which of the following drugs is a sympathomimetic bronchodilator?
   I. terbutaline
   II. albuterol
   III. theophylline
   IV. isoproterenol
   V. ipratropium bromide
   a. I, II, and IV only

b. I, III, IV, and V only

c. I and IV only

d. II and V only

e. III and V only

3. Which of the following drugs stimulate production of cAMP?

    a. metaproterenol

    b. isoproterenol

    c. isoetharine

    d. albuterol

    e. all of the above

4. Which of the following is a brand name of isoetharine?

    a. Methine[R]

    b. Brethine[R]

    c. Bronkosol[R]

    d. Alupent[R]

    e. Both *b* and *c*

5. What is the primary goal of drugs that promote bronchodilation?

    a. increase levels of cGMP

    b. increase levels of cAMP

    c. decrease levels of cAMP

    d. block production of ATP

    e. increase levels of phosphodiesterase

6. Which of the following sympathomimetic drugs has an alpha effect?

    a. ipratropium bromide

    b. isoetharine

    c. metaproterenol

    d. racemic epinephrine

    e. albuterol

7. Which of the following drugs are xanthines?

    I.   theophylline

    II. aminophylline

    III. caffeine

    IV. bromide

    V. atropine

    a. I, II, and III only

    b. II only

    c. I, II, and IV only

    d. I, II, III, and IV only

    e. I and II only

8. What is the enzyme that breaks down cAMP?

    a. atropinase

    b. diabinase

    c. phosphodiesterase

d. theophyllase

e. Pepto-Bismol

9. What are three categories of bronchodilators?

a. sympatholytics, anticholinergics, and xanthines

b. parasympathomimetics, cholinergics, and xanthines

c. parasympatholytics, cholinergics, and xanthines

d. sympathomimetics, xanthinergics, and β-adrenergics

e. sympathomimetics, anticholinergics, and xanthines

10. Drying of secretions and mucus plugging may occur as a side effect from the use of which bronchodilator?

a. atropine

b. albuterol

c. aminophylline

d. racemic epinephrine

e. metaproterenol

11. Which of the following is an appropriate dosage for one treatment of aerosolized Ventolin[R]?

a. 0.2–0.3 mL in 2.5 mL diluent

b. 2.5 mL in 2.5 mL diluent

c. 0.2–0.5 mL in 1.5 mL diluent

d. 2.0 mg in 2.5 mL diluent

e. both *a* and *d*

12. Which of the following side effects may occur with the use of metaproterenol?

a. β blockade

b. tremors

c. hematemesis

d. seizures

e. bradycardia

13. Which of the following sympathomimetic bronchodilators has a pulmonary vasodilating effect?

a. racemic epinephrine

b. isproetharine

c. isoproterenol

d. aminophylline

e. atropine

14. Which of the following are brand names of metaproterenol?

a. Alupent[R]

b. Metaprel[R]

c. Albuterol[R]

d. Atrovent[R]

e. Both *a* and *b*

15. Which of the following bronchodilators is the drug of choice in the presence of mucosal edema?

   a. atropine
   b. Atrovent[R]
   c. albuterol
   d. racemic epinephrine
   e. aminophylline

REFERENCES/RECOMMENDED READING

Fanta H: Emergency management of acute, severe asthma. *Respir Care* 37:551, 1992.

Howder L: *Cardiopulmonary Pharmacology*. Williams & Wilkins, Baltimore, 1992.

Hutchison D: Platelet function, disorders and testing. In *Coagulation Education*. American Hospital Supply Corporation, Miami, 1983, pp 77–96.

Kornberg AE, et al: Effect of injected long-acting epinephrine in addition to aerosolized albuterol in the treatment of acute asthma in children. *Pediatr Emerg Care* 7:1, 1991.

Measen FPV, et al: The effect of maximal doses of Formoterol and Salbutamol from a metered dose inhaler on pulse rates, ECG, and serum potassium concentrations. *Chest* 99:1367, 1991.

Orlowski L, et al: Effect of Salbutamol on specific airway resistance in infants with a history of wheezing. *Pediatr Pulmonol* 10:191, 1991.

Rau JL: *Respiratory Care Pharmacology*, 3rd ed. Year Book Medical Publishers, Inc, Chicago, 1989.

Spitzer WO, et al: The use of beta-agonists and the risk of death and near death from asthma. *N Engl J Med* 326:501, 1992.

Tashkin DP: Dosing strategies for bronchodilator delivery. *Respir Care* 36:977, 1991.

van Lunteren E, Coreno A: Inhaled albuterol powder for pulmonary function testing. *Chest* 101:985, 1992.

Ziment I: *Respiratory Pharmacology and Therapeutics*. WB Saunders Co, Philadelphia, 1978.

CHAPTER **12**

WETTING AGENTS AND MUCOLYTICS

LEARNING OBJECTIVES:

After completion of this chapter and its learning activities, the student will be able to:

1. Define the terms *bland aerosol*, *mucolysis*, *mucolytic*, *hygroscopic*, *expectorant*, and *bronchorrhea*.
2. Discuss the therapeutic indications for the use of bland aerosols and mucolytic agents in airway maintenance.
3. Compare and contrast the three major types of mucolytic aerosols.
4. Define the dosage ranges and concentrations of each mucolytic agent.
5. Describe the contraindications and hazards of each mucolytic agent.
6. Describe the nonrespiratory applications of acetylcysteine.
7. Given a patient case study, be able to suggest the most appropriate mucolytic therapy, including the drug of choice, route of delivery, and recommended dosage.

INTRODUCTION

Bland aerosols and mucolytic agents are used in respiratory care to humidify the respiratory tract and help loosen, thin, and remove pulmonary secretions. These secretions are normally thin and watery, much like the consistency of saliva, but in many diseases or medical conditions (such as the patient who is intubated), secretions may be excessive and may become thick and concentrated. One of the important roles of the respiratory care practitioner (RCP) is recognizing when a patient may need an aerosol, and knowing which agent is the most effective to recommend to the physician. The therapist also must be knowledgeable about the dosage and concentration of the drug he or she recommends. It also is critical that the RCP understands and recognizes the potential side effects or consequences of using such drugs.

BLAND AEROSOLS

Bland aerosols are those that do not have a direct effect on the mucus molecule and usually do not cause any significant side effects. These agents include:

- Normal saline (0.9% sodium chloride [NaCl]
- Hypotonic saline (less than 0.9% NaCl, most commonly 0.45% NaCl, or *half-normal saline*
- Hypertonic saline (greater than 0.9% NaCl, most commonly 5% or 10% NaCl solutions)
- Sterile distilled water

Therapeutic Indications

Bland aerosols may be given on a continuous basis through a large-volume nebulizer such as a jet nebulizer, Babington nebulizer, or ultrasonic nebulizer. They also may be given by small-volume (hand-held) nebulizer, but this use generally is limited to acting as a diluent for other potent drugs, such as bronchodilators or mucolytics. Bland aerosols are appropriate for the patient who requires humidification of the respiratory tract, such as the intubated or tracheotomized patient. They also may be helpful as a thinning agent when administered by heated nebulizer prior to postural drainage and chest percussion. Another use of bland aerosols is for *sputum induction*, a procedure used to promote coughing and expectoration of a sputum sample for laboratory analysis.

Normal Saline

Normal saline (NS) refers to a saline solution that has the same *osmotic pressure* as body fluids; therefore, it is physiologically normal. It is the most common agent used to dilute bronchodilator drugs. Because NS is similar to body fluids, it is unlikely to cause bronchospasm. However, in the treatment of cardiac patients who may be on a strict low-sodium diet, the amount of sodium in NS should be taken into account if the patient receives frequent treatments throughout the day. For example:

$$0.9\% \ NaCl = 0.9 \ g \ NaCl/100 \ mL \ water$$
$$= 900 \ mg \ NaCl/100 \ mL \ solution$$
$$= 9 \ mg \ NaCl/mL \ solution$$

Thus, if a patient receives small-volume nebulizer treatments every four hours with a bronchodilator and 3 mL NS, this would contribute 162 mg NaCl/day!

$$(24 \ hr/4 \ hr)(9 \ mg/mL)(3 \ mL) = (6)(27 \ mg) = 162 \ mg$$

Although only part of the aerosol actually is absorbed (because much is lost during exhalation), if the patient's diet should be restricted to 500 mg sodium/day, the treatments could contribute up to one fifth of this. If the patient has an artificial airway in place that is instilled with saline prior to suctioning, the amount of saline administered through the day may contribute to the overall sodium intake. The therapist always should be aware of any significant patient orders, even those that do not directly affect respiratory care. In a case such as this, sterile distilled water may be suggested as a diluent for the bronchodilator therapy instead of normal saline.

Hypotonic Saline

Hypotonic saline refers to a solution that has an osmotic pressure *less* than that of body fluids. The most commonly used hypotonic solution is 0.45% NaCl, or *half-normal* saline. Indications for the use of hypotonic saline include use in large-volume nebulizers when the patient cannot tolerate sterile distilled water, or as a diluent in the case of severe salt restriction (as in the above example).

Hypertonic Saline

Hypertonic saline refers to a solution that has an osmotic pressure greater than that of body fluids. The most commonly used hypertonic solutions are 5% NaCl and 10% NaCl. These solutions are used only for sputum induction because they both irritate the airway and are *hygroscopic* in nature. Hygroscopic means that the aerosol droplets tend to attract humidity as they travel in suspension and therefore they become larger in size. The combined effect of the nature of hypertonic saline is that the patient produces more mucus to dilute the higher salt concentration and is stimulated to cough.

This procedure, the administration of a hypertonic saline solution by aerosol, is referred to as *sputum induction*. It often is used when a patient has a dry, nonproductive cough but the physician needs a sputum sample for microbiological culture and sensitivity. Care should be taken whenever administering hypertonic saline to a patient who has reactive airway disease and may develop bronchospasm. It is recommended that a bronchodilator be available (metered dose inhaler is the most common method) when performing an induced sputum procedure.

When hypertonic saline is used for sputum induction, the recommended *dosage* should not exceed 1500 mg/day. This is equivalent to 10 mL of 15% NaCl, 15 mL of 10% NaCl, or 30 mL of 5% NaCl.

Sterile Distilled Water

Sterile distilled water is the most commonly used agent in large-volume nebulizers for the humidification of the respiratory tract. It also is used as a diluent for small-volume nebulizer treatments with bronchodilators or other potent drugs. Occasionally a patient with reactive airway disease (i.e., asthma) may experience bronchospasm from aerosolized sterile water. In such cases, half-normal saline may be a better agent for general humidification.

MUCOLYTICS

Mucolytics are agents that disrupt the mucus molecule so that secretions may be removed more effectively by a natural cough or by suctioning the airway. Mucolytics cause *mucolysis*, or the breaking apart (lysis) of the mucus molecule itself. In contrast to wetting agents, which tend to add water to secretions and make them less viscous by thinning, mucolytics actually affect the composition of pulmonary secretions. Thus, although they are more potent in treating patients with exceptionally thick or copious secretions, they also should be used with more caution and may have side effects that are not seen with the use of wetting agents.

There are three major categories of mucolytics, based on the method of mucolysis. To understand how a mucolytic works, and therefore select the best agent for a specific patient's needs, it is necessary to have a general understanding of the composition of the mucus molecule itself.

Properties of the Mucus Molecule and Mucolysis

The normal mucus molecule is a *mucopolysaccharide* chain. This means that the molecule is composed of strands of alternating amino sugars and amino acids that are connected by disulfide bonds (Figure 12–1). The two commonly used mucolytics break apart this molecule by different mechanisms. One works on the disulfide bonds and the other affects the stability of the amino acid chains. **N-acetylcysteine (Mucomyst**[R]**, Mucosil**[R]**)** works by disrupting the disulfide bonds (shown in Figure 12–2). Sodium bicarbonate works by disrupting the stability of the mucopolysaccharide strands (Figure 12–3).

A third potential mucolytic process involves disruption of mucus proteins and/or proteinacious secretions such as those seen in cystic fibrosis or bronchiectasis. This category of mucolytics is referred to as *proteolytic*, meaning that they break apart proteins that make

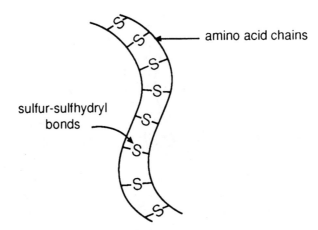

FIGURE 12–1 Structure of Mucus Molecule.

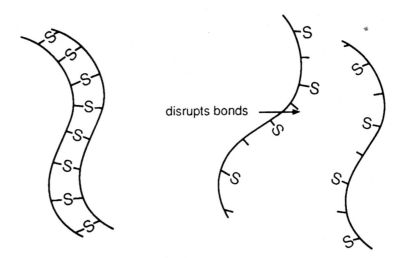

FIGURE 12–2   Mucolytic Action of *N*-acetylcysteine.

up the secretions. There are no commercially available agents in this category at present, although the drug **pancreatic dornase (Dornavac^R)** had been in use until the mid-1980s. Clinical studies currently are being conducted using *recombinant human deoxyribonuclease* (**rhDNase**) to reduce the viscosity of pulmonary secretions in cystic fibrosis patients. The drug shows promise as a mucolytic in these patients, but further study is needed.

It should be noted that intervention with mucolytics and other methods of airway maintenance always should be a secondary treatment. Primary treatment should be assuring adequate hydration and fluid intake through other mechanisms such as oral and

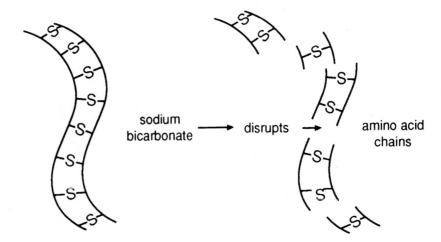

FIGURE 12–3   Mucolytic Action of Sodium Bicarbonate.

intravenous fluids. Mucolytic therapy often may be avoided, even in patients with chronic excessive secretions, by adequate fluid intake and the consistent use of coughing and other pulmonary hygiene techniques.

Indications for Mucolytics

Mucolytics may be administered by aerosol or by direct instillation into the airway. The method of administration is related to the goals of therapy and the ability of the patient to promote a spontaneous cough. If a patient has generalized thickened and inspissated secretions and is able to cooperate and generate a deep breath for good aerosol deposition, aerosolized mucolytic therapy is indicated. If the patient has an artificial airway in place (e.g., endotracheal or tracheostomy tube), mucolytic therapy may be administered by aerosolization in-line with a ventilator or by manual resuscitator bag, or by direct instillation into the tracheal tube. Occasionally a patient may require placement of a transtracheal catheter (i.e. intracath) and instillation of a mucolytic for cough stimulation and mobilization of secretions.

The decision to use N-acetylcysteine or sodium bicarbonate may be based upon several factors. N-acetylcysteine has been proven to be a more effective mucolytic than sodium bicarbonate, but this characteristic also increases its side effects and potential hazards. Either agent may be helpful in mobilizing pulmonary secretions in the patient who has excessive secretions, or purulent secretions, or thickened and inspissated secretions.

Contraindications and Hazards of Mucolytics

Sodium Bicarbonate.   Sodium bicarbonate is a somewhat benign mucolytic, but there are some contraindications to its use. If a patient is on a severely sodium-restricted diet, sodium bicarbonate may be contraindicated. Similarly, sodium bicarbonate should not be used if the patient has a severe preexisting metabolic alkalosis.

There are few side effects or hazards when using a 4.2% solution of sodium bicarbonate as a mucolytic. Suction equipment always should be available when administering a mucolytic agent, because the sudden mucolysis may cause airway obstruction.

N-Acetylcysteine.   N-acetylcysteine (**Mucomyst**[R], **Mucosil**[R]) is a potent mucolytic that should be used with caution in patients who have an inadequate cough or an artificial airway in place. Suction equipment should be readily available for such patients, the therapist should remain with the patient for 10–15 minutes after aerosolized or instilled administration of N-acetylcysteine, and nursing or other support staff should be alerted to monitor for signs of sudden airway obstruction due to mucus plugging.

N-acetylcysteine also has been reported to stimulate bronchospasm, even in those patients without primary pulmonary disease. It is recommended that aerosolized N-acetylcysteine be administered in conjunction with a bronchodilator, and the drug is compatible with most β-adrenergic (sympathomimetic) bronchodilators.

N-acetylcysteine may have a corrosive effect on metal parts and may irritate the mucosal membranes of the oropharynx. If a reusable nebulizer (such as the Puritan-Bennett twin-jet nebulizer) is used to nebulize the drug, care should be taken to rinse all metal surfaces thoroughly after the treatment. Patients also should be instructed to rinse their mouths vigorously following the treatment.

Although N-acetylcysteine has a distinctive, and somewhat offensive, odor (associated with its sulfhydryl groups), it is actually tasteless. If a patient does not smell the drug prior to administration, it is unlikely that this odor should create cause for concern or the use of an alternative agent.

Dosage and Concentrations of Mucolytics

Sodium Bicarbonate.   As mentioned, sodium bicarbonate often is administered as a 4.2% solution, although concentrations of 2% also have been used. Dosages of 3–5 mL of 4.2% sodium bicarbonate may be administered as frequently as necessary to promote mucolysis. Unit-dose vials of sodium bicarbonate are available in 4.2% solution. 30-mL vials and 50-mL syringes of 4.2% solution also are available. Multiple-dose vials should be refrigerated after opening and discarded after 24 hours.

If a bronchodilator is used in conjunction with sodium bicarbonate, it should be mixed only at the bedside immediately prior to administration. When bicarbonate is mixed with a sympathomimetic drug (e.g., **isoetharine, metaproterenol, albuterol**), the stability of the solution will be altered and discoloration may occur, typically causing the solution to turn pink. There is evidence that the alkaline solution reduces the potency of catecholamine-type bronchodilators such as **isoproterenol**; the effect is less pronounced when used with the newer β-adrenergic bronchodilators such as metaproterenol and albuterol.

N-Acetylcysteine.   N-acetylcysteine is commercially available in two concentrations, 10% and 20%. Unit-dose vials of both concentrations are available, as are 10-mL and 20-mL multiple-dose vials. N-acetylcysteine is an effective and potent mucolytic, the 10% solution usually is adequate and tends to cause fewer adverse reactions such as bronchospasm. If the only available concentration is 20% and the physician has ordered 10%, the 20% solution should be diluted in a 1:1 ratio with sterile distilled water or NS.

If multiple-dose vials are used, the unused portion of the drug must be refrigerated after opening. Vials should be dated when opened and discarded after 4 days (96 hours), because the potency of the drug diminishes after exposure to air. N-acetylcysteine should be administered in dosages of 3–5 mL per aerosolized treatment and should not be used more frequently than every 4 hours (primarily because of the necessity of using a bronchodilator when administering N-acetylcysteine).

Nonrespiratory Use of N-Acetylcysteine

N-acetylcysteine has been found to be an effective antidote for **acetaminophen** (e.g., **Tylenol**[R]) overdose when administered orally or by nasogastric tube. The metabolites associated with acetaminophen normally are broken down (detoxified) in the liver by glutathione, but this agent cannot be administered to combine with the excess metabolites freed by an acetaminophen overdose. N-acetylcysteine is similar in chemical structure to glutathione and can be effectively administered (orally) to protect the liver from toxicity associated with acetaminophen overdose.

When *N*-acetylcysteine is requested by the physician for this use, the order may be routed to the RCP because that department may have the primary in-hospital supply of the drug. Although the RCP does not administer the drug, he or she must be aware of this use and be able to respond to the physician's request. A typical order for a patient who has ingested an acetaminophen overdose may be 20–50 mL of 20% *N*-acetylcysteine, often mixed with a cola beverage and drunk by the patient. It also may be instilled directly into a nasogastric tube. The dosage of *N*-acetylcysteine for this use is determined by the physician based upon the amount of acetaminophen ingested, the patient's age and weight, and the time since ingestion occurred. The physician should refer to the *Physicians' Desk Reference* or other medical reference for such dosage information.

EXPECTORANTS AND BRONCHORRHEIC AGENTS

Bronchorrhea refers to the condition associated with excess thin and watery pulmonary secretions. It is similar to the rhinorrhea process in the nose, which usually is seen in the common cold and is often referred to as having a *runny nose*. Bronchorrhea can be induced by the use of drugs such as expectorants, one of which (hypertonic saline) already has been discussed.

Expectorants increase the amount of fluid in the respiratory tract and thus stimulate a cough. Expectorants are available in a wide variety of over-the-counter cough and cold remedies and are not routinely administered by RCPs. The use of hypertonic saline for sputum induction is the primary clinical application of bronchorrheic agents in respiratory care.

The use of saturated solution of potassium iodide (SSKI) as an expectorant in the treatment of asthma and chronic bronchitis has been reported since 1939. SSKI typically is not administered by the aerosol route, but rather by ingestion (mixed with water and drunk) or orally (as sodium iodide) in tablet form.

POSTTEST: WETTING AGENTS AND MUCOLYTICS

For each of the following questions, try to select the *one* best answer from those choices given.

1. Which of the following is a bland aerosol?
   a. normal saline
   b. half-normal saline
   c. sterile distilled water
   d. 0.9% NaCl
   e. all of the above

2. Which of the following agents are hypertonic?
   a. 0.9% NaCl
   b. 5% NaCl
   c. 10% NaCl
   d. all of the above
   e. *b* and *c* only

3. Which of the following may be considered expectorants?
   a. normal saline
   b. hypotonic saline
   c. hypertonic saline
   d. SSKI
   e. both *c* and *d*

4. Which of the following agents are hygroscopic?
   I.   normal saline
   II. half-normal saline
   III. hypertonic saline
   IV. 5% NaCl
   V.   sterile distilled water
   a. I, II, and V only
   b. III, IV, and V only
   c. I, II, III, IV, and V
   d. III and IV only
   e. IV only

5. Sodium bicarbonate may be administered by aerosol in which of the following concentrations?
   a. 5% and 10%
   b. 0.9% only
   c. 2% and 4.2%
   d. 10% and 20%
   e. 5% only

6. Mucomyst[R] is the brand name of:
   a. sulfur hydroxide
   b. *N*-acetylcysteine
   c. pancreatic dornase
   d. none of the above
   e. *a* and *b* only

7. *N*-acetylcysteine may be administered orally for which of the following conditions?
   I.   acetylsalicylic acid overdose
   II. acetaminophen overdose
   III. diabetic coma
   IV. Tylenol[R] overdose
   V.   barbiturate overdose

    a. I, II, and IV

    b. II and IV only

    c. III only

    d. I, II, III, and IV

    e. I and V only

8. The solution of choice for most large-volume nebulizer therapy is:

    a. normal saline

    b. sterile distilled water

    c. half-normal saline

    d. hypertonic saline

    e. hypotonic saline

9. The most effective method of mucolysis is:

    a. aerosolized mucolytics

    b. aerosolized wetting agents

    c. vigorous nasotracheal suctioning

    d. adequate hydration and fluid intake

    e. postural drainage

10. Side effects of aerosolized N-acetylcysteine may include:

    a. bronchospasm, acute airway obstruction, and oropharyngeal irritation

    b. bronchodilation, oropharyngeal irritation, and acute airway obstruction

    c. bronchospasm and acute airway obstruction

    d. fluid overload, bronchospasm, and oropharyngeal irritation

    e. liver damage, bronchospasm, and corrosion of metal parts of dental work

11. Which of the following are contraindications for the use of N-acetylcysteine as an aerosol?

    I. Tylenol[R] overdose

    II. administration without a bronchodilator

    III. administration to a semicomatose patient without suction equipment and monitoring

    IV. administration in concentrations over 10%

    V. administration with a bronchodilator

    a. I only

    b. I, II, and IV

    c. II, III, and IV

    d. II and III

    e. I, IV, and V

12. In which of the following patients should the RCP consider diluting the bronchodilator with sterile distilled water rather than normal saline for a small-volume nebulizer treatment given every 3 hours?

    I. post–acute myocardial infarction

    II. severe salt restriction

    III. diabetic coma

    IV. acute hypertensive episode

V. acetaminophen overdose
   a. I, II, and IV
   b. II only
   c. III only
   d. I, II, and V
   e. I, III, and V

13. What is the mechanism of action of *N*-acetylcysteine in promoting mucolysis?
    a. disruption of plasma proteins
    b. lysis of proteins in mucus
    c. increasing alkalinity of mucus
    d. hygroscopic properties
    e. disrupting disulfide bonds

14. What is the mechanism of action of sodium bicarbonate as a mucolytic?
    a. disruption of disulfide bonds
    b. lysis of proteins in mucus
    c. altering pH and disrupting amino acid chains
    d. airway irritation and cough stimulation
    e. stimulation of bronchorrhea

15. Which of the following statements are true regarding the use of bronchodilators with sodium bicarbonate in aerosol therapy?
    I.   sympathomimetic amines are incompatible with sodium bicarbonate.
    II. noncatecholamine sympathomimetic amines are compatible with sodium bicarbonate.
    III. sympathomimetic amines should be mixed with sodium bicarbonate at least 30 minutes before administration
    IV. metaproterenol and albuterol are compatible with sodium bicarbonate.
    a. I only
    b. II only
    c. II and III only
    d. II and IV only
    e. II, II, and IV

REFERENCES/RECOMMENDED READINGS

Aitken ML, et al: Recombinant human DNase inhalation in normal subjects and patients with cystic fibrosis. *JAMA* 267:9147, 1992.

Hubbard X, et al: A peliminary study of aerosolized recombinant human deoxyribonuclease I in the treatment of cystic fibrosis. *N Engl J Med* 326:812, 1992.

Rau JL: *Respiratory Care Pharmacology.* Year Book Medical Publishers, Inc, Chicago, 1989.

Scanlan CL, Spearman CB, Sheldon, RL, (eds): *Egan's Fundamentals of Respiratory Care,* 5th ed. CV Mosby Co, St. Louis, 1990.

Ziment I: *Respiratory Pharmacology and Therapeutics.* WB Saunders, Co, Philadelphia, 1978.

CHAPTER **13**

AEROSOL ANTIMICROBIAL THERAPY

LEARNING OBJECTIVES

After completion of this chapter and its learning activities, the student will be able to:

1. Define six specific indications for the use of antimicrobial agents by the aerosol route.
2. List eight disadvantages or limitations of aerosol administration of antimicrobial drugs.
3. List several pulmonary infectious processes that may be appropriately treated by aerosolized antimicrobial agents.
4. List four major categories of antimicrobial drugs that are administered by aerosol.
5. Given a drug category (e.g., antiviral), list drug(s) that may be administered by the aerosol route, including generic name, brand name, and dosage.
6. Describe contraindications and side effects of each drug that may be administered by aerosol as an antimicrobial agent.
7. Describe any special equipment required for aerosol administration of antimicrobial agents.
8. Given a patient case study, be able to suggest the most appropriate antimicrobial therapy, including the drug of choice, route of delivery, and recommended dosage.

INTRODUCTION

Although systemic administration of antimicrobial agents is still the best first-line approach in most cases, certain therapies are more effectively accomplished by the aerosol route. Aerosolized **pentamidine** for the treatment of acquired immunodeficiency syndrome (AIDS)-associated *Pneumocystis carinii* pneumonia now is considered the most effective route of administration. In other cases, the basic rationale for the delivery of aerosolized medications (i.e., reduced systemic side effects and direct deposition) are attractive for the delivery of antimicrobial drugs by aerosol. Pulmonary infections that have not responded well to systemic administration of antibiotics sometimes are resolved successfully with the addition of aerosol drugs. This chapter describes the general indications and rationale for the aerosol or instilled route of delivery for antimicrobial agents. Specific drugs that have been used successfully by these routes also are presented.

INDICATIONS FOR AEROSOLIZED ANTIMICROBIAL DRUGS

Chapter 10 discussed general reasons for aerosol delivery of medications to the pulmonary tract, including 1) deposition of drug at a specific site of action, and 2) reduced systemic side-effects of the drug. These reasons also provide the primary rationale for the use of anti-infective (antimicrobial) agents by the aerosol route. Aerosol administration of antimicrobials is limited and somewhat controversial. The currently accepted indications for administering antimicrobial drugs by aerosol are:

1. As an adjunct to systemic antimicrobial therapy when this has been unsuccessful
2. For direct topical deposition of an antimicrobial that is not appropriate for systemic administration (e.g., **nystatin**)
3. For topical deposition within a pulmonary infectious process in which perfusion is limited and systemic therapy has failed (e.g., aspergillosis)
4. For topical deposition of an antimicrobial that is more effective by this route (e.g., **pentamidine**)
5. To eliminate an organism that is colonizing the respiratory tract (e.g., infected sputum in cystic fibrosis or bronchiectasis)
6. To reduce the severity of systemic side effects (when an antimicrobial is selected that is poorly absorbed through the lung)

These indications and the rationale for aerosolizing antibiotics are illustrated in Figure 13–1.

DISADVANTAGES AND LIMITATIONS OF AEROSOLIZED ANTIMICROBIALS

There remain many limitations and disadvantages of aerosol administration of antimicrobials. Most aerosol therapy is somewhat patient dependent (except those treatments provided in-line for the mechanically ventilated patient). Because the effectiveness of an aerosol treatment requires patient effort and cooperation, there is no absolute assurance

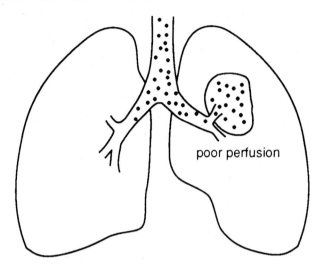

FIGURE 13–1   Aerosol Deposition of Antimicrobials.

that an inhaled antimicrobial will reach the site of infection. Bronchospasm is a frequent adverse reaction to inhaled antimicrobials, and the drug may be inactivated by combining with DNA strands in the infected sputum. There is little consensus regarding the optimal nebulization technique or dosages that are appropriate for this route of delivery. The aerosolized drug also enters the ambient air, so that practitioners or other patients may be exposed; this phenomenon actually may lead to increased nosocomial infections (by allowing resistant organisms to proliferate) or to the development of sensitivity to the drug by those exposed. In summary, the limitations and disadvantages of aerosolized antimicrobials are:

1. Bronchospasm is a common adverse reaction.
2. Systemic side effects *may* occur.
3. Drug may be inactivated by sputum proteins.
4. Drug may not be deposited at desired (infected) site.
5. Dosages of aerosolized antimicrobials have not been established.
6. Optimal delivery and equipment techniques have not been determined.
7. Ambient air may be contaminated by drug (exposing other personnel and visitors to the antimicrobial).
8. Hospital microbial population may develop a tolerance (subsequent to #7) and nosocomial infections may increase.

Many anti-infective agents are not approved by the Food and Drug Administration for administration by inhalation. The practice of medicine is an evolving art, in which the clinical experiences of both physician and practitioner will be used for decision making. If there is a significant question regarding the appropriateness of aerosol delivery of an anti-infective agent, experimental protocols should be developed. Patients should be informed of the experimental nature of this route of administration and a written informed consent should be developed and utilized. All available resources for such decisions should be used, including the hospital formulary and clinical pharmacist, attending physician, consulting medical staff (including the respiratory care medical director), and an institutional review board.

PULMONARY INFECTIOUS PROCESSES

Certain pulmonary diseases may be treated effectively by aerosol delivery of anti-infectives. Diseases characterized by reduced perfusion to a specific area (such as *cavitating* processes like tuberculosis, pulmonary aspergilloma, and coccidioidomycosis) may respond favorably to aerosol delivery of drugs to the pulmonary tree. In these cases, systemic (oral or parenteral) administration of antibiotics may fail because the cavity itself cannot achieve sufficiently high concentrations of the drug to eliminate the infecting organism. This phenomenon sometimes also is seen in patients with severe bronchiectasis and those with pulmonary abscess.

Patients who are susceptible to gram-negative pulmonary infections, such as those with cystic fibrosis, may tolerate aerosolized agents that are not effective orally. Thus, they may be able to avoid intravenous antibiotic therapy and maintain outpatient therapy or their home-care regimen.

Recent extensive experience in treating *Pneumocystis carinii* pneumonia also has demonstrated superior effectiveness when the antiprotozoal drug **pentamidine** is given by aerosol. Clearance of the pneumonia is much more dramatic when treated by aerosol than when treated by the oral or parenteral routes.

CATEGORIES OF ANTIMICROBIAL DRUGS ADMINISTERED BY AEROSOL

Although the entire group of antimicrobial drugs is large (as described in Chapter 8), relatively few have been used successfully by aerosol. These include drugs in four major categories: antibacterials (antibiotics), antifungals, antivirals, and antiprotozoals. The following sections describe the pulmonary pathology that may be treated successfully by drugs in each category. Specific drugs, including dosages, side effects, and contraindications, also are discussed.

ANTIBACTERIAL (ANTIBIOTIC) DRUGS

Antibiotics that have been administered successfully by aerosol include **amoxicillin, carbenicillin, colistin, gentamicin, kanamycin, neomycin, polymixin B,** and **sisomicin.** The most common use of antibiotics by aerosol is probably for cystic fibrosis. These patients often colonize *Pseudomonas aeruginosa* in the lower respiratory tract. The rationales for providing aerosolized antibiotics for these patients are:

1. It provides direct deposition of drug at the site of infection and reduces systemic effects.
2. There are no effective oral antibiotics for the treatment of *P. aeruginosa* infections.
3. Some antibiotics (e.g., aminoglycosides) may not achieve sufficient therapeutic levels in the lung even when given systemically.

The following descriptions of antimicrobial drugs cover only those drugs that have been shown to be safe and effective when given by aerosol. For each drug, the relative spectrum of effectiveness is noted, but specific susceptibility of an organism to the antimicrobial always should be determined by laboratory analysis (i.e., sputum culture and sensitivity).

Amoxicillin (Amoxil^R, Larotid^R, Polymox^R, Trimox^R)

Actions: aminopenicillin; interferes with bacterial cell wall synthesis.

Indications: broad spectrum; effective against gram-positive (including staphylococci and streptococci) and gram-negative (e.g., *Escherichia coli*, *Haemophilus influenzae*, and *Proteus*) organisms. *Has been used successfully in the treatment of purulent bronchiectasis.*

Contraindication: hypersensitivity to penicillin. Use with caution in asthmatics (hypersensitivity and bronchospasm are likely to occur) and in neonates (because of renal clearance).

Side effects/adverse reactions: hypersensitivy and anaphylaxis may develop. Skin rashes, ecchymoses, erythema, hives, fever, wheezing, laryngospasm, dyspnea, hypotension, and vascular collapse may occur. Gastrointestinal (GI) symptoms include nausea, abdominal cramps, vomiting, diarrhea, and increased thirst. May cause hematuria, pyuria, oliguria, and albuminuria.

Dosage: give 500 mg/treatment, nebulized with normal saline to provide at least 3 mL of solution; recommended twice/day.

Special considerations: initial treatment should be monitored closely for adverse reactions such as bronchospasm. Bronchodilator administration prior to antibiotic is recommended.

Carbenicillin (Geopen^R)

Actions: extended-spectrum penicillin; interferes with bacterial cell wall synthesis.

Indications: broad spectrum; effective against a wide range of both gram-positive and gram-negative organisms. *Has been used successfully in treating colonized Pseudomonas in cystic fibrosis; compatible with gentamycin, with which it has been used in combination for this purpose.*

Contraindication: same as for amoxicillin.

Adverse reactions/side effects: same as those with amoxicillin.

Dosage: give 125–1000 mg/treatment, not to exceed 2800 mg/day. Dilute with sufficient saline to provide 3 mL solution; nebulize 2–4 times/day.

Special considerations: same as with amoxicillin.

Colistin (Coly-Mycin S^R)

Actions: polypeptide; increases bacterial cell wall permeability.

Indications: bactericidal against gram-negative bacilli, *except Proteus. Has been used successfully in treating colonized P. aeruginosa in cystic fibrosis patients.*

Contraindication: sensitivity to colistin or polymixin B. Use with caution in patients with renal or neuromuscular disease.

Adverse reactions/side effects: neuromuscular symptoms and renal insufficiency are the most common side effects. Paresthesias, numbness or tingling of extremities or the tongue, and generalized itching or urticaria have been reported. May cause GI upset, vertigo, and slurring of speech.

Dosage: give 2–300 mg/treatment, nebulized 2–4 times/day (100 mg/treatment is usual adult dosage). A 150-mg vial is reconstituted with 2 mL sterile water; a 100-mg dose would require about 1.3 mL. Additional sterile water should be added to provide at least 3 mL of total solution for nebulization.

Special considerations: less likely to cause bronchospasm than other aerosolized antibiotics, particularly polymixin.

Gentamicin (Garamycin^R)

Actions: aminoglycoside; inhibits protein synthesis and cellular reproduction.

Indications: broad spectrum; effective against gram-negative infections (i.e., *Pseudomonas, E. coli, Proteus, Klebsiella, Serratia, Providencia, Acinebacter,* and *Enterobacter*), as well as gram-positive organisms (*Staphylococcus aureus* and *Streptococcus faecalis*). *Has been used successfully by instillation or aerosol in treating Pseudomonas-infected sputum.*

Contraindication: hypersensitivity. Use with caution in patients with neuromuscular disorders (may increase muscle weakness) and in neonates or patients with impaired renal function (drug is excreted through glomerular filtration).

Side effects/adverse reactions: may cause an array of symptoms in various organs/systems:

- Nervous system: numbness, tingling, tremor, muscle twitching or weakness, confusion, disorientation, depression, lethargy, headache, fever, respiratory depression, nystagmus, and visual disturbances
- GI tract: nausea, vomiting, anorexia, stomatitis
- Ear, nose, and throat: tinnitus, vertigo, dizziness
- Renal: proteinuria, hematuria, azotemia, oliguria, elevated blood urea nitrogen, and granular casts
- Cardiovascular: myocarditis, palpitations, hypotension, hypertension, hyperkalemia
- Pulmonary: bronchospasm, pulmonary fibrosis

Dosage: give 250 mg/treatment, administered in 2–3 mL saline, 3–4 times/day for 3–4 days.

Special considerations: because the aerosol may induce bronchopasm, a bronchodilator may be given prior to or mixed with the antibiotic. The patient should rinse his or her mouth thoroughly after treatment to minimize mucosal irritation (stomatitis).

Kanamycin (Kantrex[R], Klebcil[R])

Actions: aminoglycoside; inhibits protein synthesis and cellular reproduction.

Indications: broad spectrum; effective against many gram-negative organisms and staphylococci but is *not effective against Pseudomonas or Bacteroides. Has been used successfully in treating susceptible gram-negative infections in cystic fibrosis.*

Contraindication: same as for gentamicin.

Adverse reactions/side effects: same as those with gentamicin.

Dosage: give 250 mg/treatment diluted in saline to provide 3 mL of solution, nebulized 3–4 times/day for 3–4 days (maximum recommended course of therapy is 8 days).

Special considerations: has beneficial *mucokinetic* effect and generally is well tolerated with few adverse reactions. A bronchodilator should be given before or in combination with the antibiotic aerosol; kanamycin is compatible with all sympathomimetic dilators.

Polymyxin B (Aerosporin[R] [Sterile Powder])

Actions: polypeptide; increases bacterial cell wall permeability.

Indications: bactericidal against most gram-negative bacilli *except Proteus. Has been used successfully in treating colonized Pseudomonas in cystic fibrosis patients and by instillation in treating Pseudomonas-infected sputum.*

Contraindication: same as for colistin. Use with extreme caution in asthmatics because severe bronchospasm may occur.

Adverse reactions/side effects: same as those with colistin.

Dosage: give 5–50 mg/treatment (usual adult dosage is 50 mg/treatment), 2–4 times/day.

Special considerations: because of likelihood of bronchospasm, a bronchodilator should be given prior to or in combination with the antibiotic aerosol.

ANTIFUNGAL DRUGS

There are two antifungal drugs that have been given successfully by aerosol for the treatment of pulmonary mycoses and occasionally for opportunistic oral and tracheobronchial colonization by fungi. Both **amphotericin B** and **nystatin** have been nebulized with significant clinical improvement and few adverse reactions. Instillation of these drugs directly through an endotracheal tube or endobronchial catheter (e.g., during bronchoscopy) also has been effective.

Amphotericin B (Fungizone^R)

Actions: antimycotic polyene antimicrobial; alters fungal cellular permeability and reproduction. Has no effect on bacteria or viruses.

Indications: fungicidal, *has been used successfully in the treatment of pulmonary fungal infections such as aspergillosis, coccidioidomycosis, and candidiasis.*

Contraindication: hypersensitivity. Use with caution in asthmatics and patients with renal disease.

Adverse reactions/side effects: fever, headache, anorexia, nausea, vomiting, diarrhea, malaise, and muscle and joint pain are common side effects. Renal insufficiency may occur, and rare pulmonary complications include acute dyspnea, bronchospasm, and hypoxia.

Dosage: give 1–20 mg/treatment (usual adult dosage is 5–10 mg/treatment), nebulized 2–4 times/day. A 50-mg vial is reconstituted with 10 mL sterile water *without a bacteriostatic agent.* After reconstitution, the vial should be refrigerated and protected from exposure to light; discard after 24 hours.

Special considerations: amphotericin does not penetrate tissue barriers well and therefore is not likely to leave the pulmonary system after aerosol administration (thus fewer systemic side effects [i.e., renal dysfunction] are seen). May cause bronchospasm in asthmatics, use of a bronchodilator is recommended.

Nystatin (Nystatin, USP [generic], Mycostatin^R)

Actions: antimycotic polyene antimicrobial; alters fungal cellular permeability and reproduction. Has no effect on bacteria or viruses.

Indications: fungicidal, *has been used successfully in treating pulmonary aspergillosis and Candida albicans.*

Contraindication: hypersensitivity.

Adverse reactions/side effects: occasional nausea, vomiting, and diarrhea.

Dosage: give 25,000 units/treatment, nebulized 2–4 times per day or instilled directly into the endotracheal tube.

Special considerations: *Candida albicans* may colonize the tracheobronchial tree of patients receiving large doses of antibiotics. Nebulized or instilled nystatin has been helpful in clearing these opportunistic fungal infections.

ANTIVIRAL DRUGS

The only antiviral agent administered by aerosol is **ribavirin**. This agent is indicated only for use in the severely ill infant or child who has a known respiratory tract infection caused by *respiratory syncytial virus* (RSV). The drug has serious adverse effects even when administered by aerosol and should not be considered unless the diagnosis of RSV has been confirmed by laboratory analysis (ELISA: enzyme-linked immunosorbent assay test) and the child is seriously ill.

Ribavirin must be aerosolized only by a *small particle aerosol generator* (SPAG) nebulizer and usually is given via some enclosure, such as an oxygen hood or tent. Treatments may be administered by mask, but continuous nebulization for 12–18 hours per day make this method much less desireable. Ribavirin has been shown to be teratogenic (may cause birth defects), so pregnant women (i.e., parent, visitors, nursing or other staff) should avoid any exposure to the drug or its aerosol.

Ribavirin (Virazole^R)

Actions: mechanism of action is unknown; may inhibit protein synthesis and cellular reproduction.

Indications: antiviral; selectively inhibits RSV, influenza, and herpes simplex virus. *Recommended by aerosol **only** for infants or children with severe respiratory tract infection that is **known** to be caused by RSV.*

Contraindications: should be used cautiously in patients who are receiving continuous assisted ventilation. The drug may precipitate, causing inadvertent positive end-expiratory pressure, airway plugging, malfunction of exhalation valve, and interference with safe and effective ventilation. Use with caution in premature infants or patients with preexisting cardiopulmonary disease.

Adverse reactions/side effects: deterioration of respiratory function, bacterial pneumonia, pneumothorax, apnea, and ventilator dependence have been reported. Cardiac arrest, hypotension, and digitalis toxicity also have occurred. Less severe side effects include rash and conjunctivitis. Teratogenicity of the drug has been shown.

Dosage: give 300 mL of a 2% solution, nebulized by SPAG for 12–18 hours/day (via tent, hood, or face mask) for 3–7 days. A 100-mL vial (containing 6 g of drug) is reconstituted with sterile water *without a bacteriostatic agent*. The final concentration of drug is 20 mg/mL: 6 g = 6000 mg, and 6000 mg/300 mL = 60 mg/3 mL = 20 mg/mL; A 2% solution = 2 g/100 mL = 2000 mg/100 mL = 20 mg/mL.

Special considerations: scavenger systems should be considered to reduce exposure of visitors and personnel. Recent trials using particle filters and one-way valves have allowed successful use of the drug in-line with ventilated patients (as demonstrated by reduced period of assisted ventilation, improved oxygenation, and reduced hospital length of stay).

ANTIPROTOZOAL DRUGS

The only antiprotozoal drug administered by aerosol is **pentamidine**. This agent is indicated only for treatment of *Pneumocystis carinii* pneumonia, a pneumonia seen in immunosuppressed and AIDS patients. Recent studies have demonstrated the effectiveness of aerosolized pentamidine as both a prophylactic and therapeutic agent in the treatment of AIDS-associated *P. carinii* pneumonia.

Studies also have shown, however, that factors such as breathing pattern and pulmonary function (which are considered of primary importance in many aerosol therapies), are less important than the quality of aerosol provided in the nebulization of pentamidine. The major factor influencing pentamidine deposition in the lung is aerosol delivery, with the AeroTech[R] nebulizer delivering between 2.5 and 5 times as much drug as other nebulizers studied.

Another characteristic of aerosolized pentamidine is the airway irritation and fatigue experienced by patients receiving therapy. Studies are underway to determine the most appropriate form (salt) of pentamidine for aerosol administration.

Pentamidine Isoethionate (Pentam^R, [C] Pentacarinat, [C] Pneumopent)

Actions: mechanism of action is not fully understood, but inhibition of RNA, DNA, and protein synthesis is likely.

Indications: antiprotozoal; indicated for the prophylaxis and treatment of *P. carinii* pneumonia.

Contraindications: there are no contraindications for the use of pentamidine once the diagnosis of *P. carinii* pneumonia has been confirmed. Use with caution in patients with renal or hepatic disease, hypertension, hypotension, hyperglycemia, hypoglycemia, anemia, thrombocytopenia, or leukopenia.

Adverse reactions/side effects: bronchospasm, fatigue, severe cough, burning sensation in back of throat, and mild hypoglycemia have been reported following aerosol administration. Serious systemic side effects have not been noted with aerosol administration of the drug.

Dosage: give 600 mg dissolved in 6 mL of sterile water and nebulized for 20–30 minutes, once per day. The drug should be nebulized in a specialized micronebulizer approved for administration of pentamidine.

Special considerations: administration of a bronchodilator prior to treatment is indicated if the patient has a history of smoking or asthma (or has previously reacted to pentamidine). Scavenger systems and *strict isolation* should be used with all aerosolized pentamidine treatments. Pentamidine may degrade in a heated environment; therefore, nebulization via ultrasonic or heated nebulizer is not recommended. Patient fatigue is a common side effect of treatment.

GENERAL CONCLUSIONS AND CONSIDERATIONS REGARDING AEROSOLIZED ANTIMICROBIALS

Although there are many factors that limit the effectiveness and use of antimicrobial aerosols, certain clinical conditions respond favorably to aerosol administration of specific drugs. It is critical for the respiratory care practitioner to be well educated in the use of appropriate antimicrobial drugs by aerosol or instillation. In most cases, aerosol administration of these drugs should be used as an adjunct rather than as the primary method of administration.

Risks to visitors or health care providers should be minimized by the use of scavenger systems whenever possible. Exhaled aerosols or the exhaust of aerosolized antimicrobials may contribute to the development of resistant microorganisms and contribute to nosocomial infections in the hospital environment.

The respiratory care department and its medical director should develop protocols for the aerosol administration of these drugs. Drugs that are not approved by the Food and Drug Administration for aerosol administration should be subject to experimental protocols, and informed consent should be utilized.

POSTTEST: AEROSOL ANTIMICROBIAL THERAPY

For each of the following questions, try to select the *one* best answer from those choices given.

1. Which of the following drugs would be *contraindicated* for a patient with known sensitivity to penicillin?
   a. pentamidine
   b. amoxicillin
   c. kanamycin
   d. amphotericin B
   e. gentamicin

2. Which of the following drugs is an antifungal agent?
   a. amphotericin B
   b. amoxicillin
   c. colistin
   d. ribavirin
   e. carbenicillin

3. Which of the following drugs is indicated for aspergillosis?
   a. amoxicillin
   b. kanamycin
   c. pentamidine
   d. isoetharine
   e. nystatin

4. Which of the following side effects may be associated with aerosolized antibiotics?
   a. hypoglycemia
   b. bronchospasm
   c. bulemia
   d. fatigue
   e. euphoria

5. Which of the following drugs may be useful in treating colonized *Pseudomonas* in the cystic fibrosis patient?
   I. kanamycin
   II. carbenicillin
   III. amphotericin B
   IV. polymixin
   a. I and II only
   b. II and IV only

    c. I, II, and IV only

    d. II, III, and IV only

    e. I, II, III, and IV

6. Which of the following drugs requires a SPAG nebulizer?

    a. pentamidine

    b. nystatin

    c. colistin

    d. kanamycin

    e. ribavirin

7. Which of the following is *not* an appropriate clinical indication for the use of an aerosolized antimicrobial?

    a. to deliver the antimicrobial directly to the respiratory tract (e.g., infected/colonized sputum)

    b. to reduce the severity of systemic side effects

    c. as an adjunct (additional) therapy when systemic administration of antimicrobials has been unsuccessful

    d. to avoid the development of drug sensitivity

    e. when alternative routes are not available

8. Which of the following drugs is appropriately aerosolized in treating *Pneumocystis carinii* pneumonia?

    a. pentamidine

    b. Virazole[R]

    c. carbenicillin

    d. nystatin

    e. polymixin B

9. Which of the following antimicrobials also has a beneficial mucokinetic effect?

    a. gentamicin

    b. kanamycin

    c. colistin

    d. ribavirin

    e. polymixin B

10. Which of the following are *true* statements about the use of aerosolized antimicrobials?

    I. the primary use of antibiotics is in the treatment of cystic fibrosis patients with colonized/infected sputum.

    II. the primary use of antiviral drugs is in the treatment of pneumonia caused by RSV.

    III. the only clinical indication for the use of pentamidine is the presence of pneumonia caused by RSV.

    IV. the aerosol dosages are well established.

    V. ambient air may become contaminated by the drug.

    a. I, II, and IV only

    b. II, III, IV, and V only

    c. I, II, III, and V only

d. I, II, and V only

e. I and II only

11. Which of the following drugs is fungicidal?

    a. amoxicillin

    b. colistin

    c. amphotericin B

    d. ribavirin

    e. kanamycin

REFERENCES/RECOMMENDED READING

Castellano AR, Nettleman MD: Cost and benefit of secondary prophylaxis for *Pneumocystis carinii* pneumonia. *JAMA* 266:820, 1991.

Debs R, et al: Biodistribution, tissue reaction, and lung retention of pentamidine aerosolized as three different salts. *Am Rev Respir Dis* 142:1164, 1990.

Herzog KD, et al: Impact of treatment guidelines on use of ribavirin. *Am J Dis Child* 144:1001, 1990.

Jensen T, et al: Colistin inhalation therapy in cystic fibrosis patients with chronic *Pseudomonas aeruginosa* lung infection. *J Antimicrob Chemother* 19:831, 1987.

Leoung GS, et al: Aerosolized pentamidine for prophylaxis against *Pneumocystis carinii* pneumonia. *N Engl J Med* 323:769, 1990.

Physicians' Desk Reference, 46th ed. Medical Economics Co, Inc, Montvale, NJ, 1992.

Smaldone GC, et al: Deposition of aerosolized pentamidine and failure of *Pneumocystis* prophylaxis. *Chest* 101:82, 1992.

Smaldone GC, et al: Factors determining pulmonary deposition of aerosolized pentamidine in patients with human immunodeficiency virus infection. *Am Rev Respir Dis* 143:727, 1991.

Smith DW, et al: A controlled trial of aerosolized ribavirin in infants receiving mechanical ventilation for severe respiratory syncytial virus infection. *N Engl J Med* 325:24, 1991.

Waskin H: Toxicology of antimicrobial aerosols: A review of aerosolized ribavirin and pentamidine. *Respir Care* 36:1026, 1991.

Ziment I: *Respiratory Pharmacology and Therapeutics*. WB Saunders Co, Philadelphia, 1978.

CHAPTER 14

ANTI-INFLAMMATORY AND ANTIASTHMATIC DRUGS

LEARNING OBJECTIVES

After completion of this chapter and its learning activities, the student will be able to:

1. Describe mucosal edema as it relates to difficulty breathing or respiratory distress.
2. List clinical conditions or diseases that may lead to bronchoconstriction caused by mucosal edema.
3. Describe the mechanism of action of α-adrenergic agents.
4. List the primary α-adrenergic drugs used by respiratory care practitioners, including brand names.
5. List the dosage range, concentration, side effects, contraindications, and any special considerations for the use of racemic epinephrine.
6. Describe the mechanism of action of corticosteroids used in the treatment of airway inflammation.
7. List the primary corticosteroids used in the treatment of airway inflammation, including brand names.
8. List the dosage range, side effects, contraindications, and any special considerations for the use of corticosteroids in the treatment of airway inflammation.
9. Describe the mechanism of action of cromolyn sodium.
10. List the brand names, dosage ranges, side effects, contraindications, and any special considerations for the use of cromolyn sodium.
11. Describe the mechanism of action of nedocromil sodium.
12. List the brand name, dosage ranges, side effects, contraindications, and any special considerations for the use of nedocromil sodium.
13. Given a patient case study, be able to suggest the most appropriate drug therapy, including the drug(s) of choice, route of delivery, and recommended dosage(s).

INTRODUCTION

Drugs that reduce inflammation and swelling in the airway often are aerosolized for the management of acute inhalational injuries (e.g., poisonous fumes, steam), laryngeal trauma (e.g., intubation/extubation) or infection (croup), severe allergic reactions (e.g., anaphylaxis) and in both acute and chronic asthma. Two of these drugs were briefly mentioned in Chapter 11, but there are other agents that also have the primary result of increasing the airway lumen by reducing mucosal swelling and edema. Drugs in this category are primarily α stimulants (which reduce mucosal edema by vasoconstriction) or corticosteroids (which have a nonspecific anti-inflammatory action). Mucosal edema within the airway may be a life-threatening situation that requires immediate treatment. Providing an aerosolized drug directly to the airway may improve ventilation and reduce hypoxemia rapidly, and enhance the effectiveness of systemic drugs.

Current research regarding asthma and its clinical management suggests that treating the *inflammation* associated with asthma may be more important than treating its bronchospasm (even though we have primarily treated the bronchospasm for decades). The most recent studies of asthma conclude that treatment of the inflammation and mucosal edema is the most important aspect of control of symptoms.

A front-line antiasthmatic drug is **cromolyn sodium**. This drug has neither bronchodilating nor anti-inflammatory actions, but rather is *preventive* in nature. Its actions, when properly used, prevent the histamine release that triggers the asthmatic reaction in extrinsic asthmatics. **Nedocromil sodium** (presently available only Canada) displays both anti-inflammatory properties and inhibition of the release of inflammatory mediators. Use of corticosteroids, cromolyn sodium, and nedocromil sodium may become more important than the traditional use of xanthines and β adrenergic bronchodilators.

Respiratory care practitioners (RCPs) are often among the first health care providers to treat patients who present with difficulty breathing. It is vitally important that RCPs understand the pathology behind a patient who is wheezing, and that we are able to suggest and deliver the most appropriate drug to improve the situation. In many cases, a combination of drugs may be appropriate; in other cases the administration of a bronchodilator for a patient who is suffering from mucosal edema may be inappropriate and may waste precious time. It is equally important that we understand which drugs have immediate effect in the relief of symptoms, in contrast to those agents that are preventive or that require more time to take effect.

BRONCHOCONSTRICTION AND MUCOSAL EDEMA

Mucosal edema refers to the accumulation of fluid within the mucosal membrane. When this process occurs within the airway, this membrane must invade the airway lumen, because all structures in the airway are bound by cartilaginous support (Figure 14–1). In the nose, when someone inhales an antigen, the response is a sneeze, followed by a "stuffy

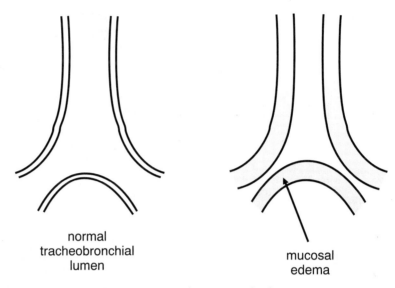

normal
tracheobronchial
lumen

mucosal
edema

FIGURE 14-1   Bronchoconstriction by Mucosal Edema.

and runny nose." The same response in the lung results in a cough, followed by bron-choconstriction and increased mucus production. The response in the lung, however, may become life-threatening if the mucosal edema causes enough airway restriction to limit ventilation. This scenario could lead to hypercarbia and hypoxia, which may contribute to cardiac arrhythmias and sudden death.

There are several pulmonary injuries, infectious processes, and diseases or conditions that may cause mucosal edema (Table 14–1). The degree of severity of each disorder is difficult to predict, but clinical signs and symptoms usually determine the appropriate treatment decisions. When it can be determined that a patient who is experiencing dif-ficulty breathing, tachypnea, tachycardia, and wheezing may have been exposed to one of the causes listed in Table 14–1, an α-adrenergic drug probably is indicated. In severe and life-threatening situations, the drug should be given systemically (intravenously [IV] or intramuscularly [IM]). If an IV line cannot be established or perfusion is poor, the drug may be instilled directly through an endotracheal tube or a transtracheal catheter. In less severe situations, aerosolized administration of the drug provides rapid therapeutic response with few systemic side effects.

α-ADRENERGIC SYMPATHOMIMETIC DRUGS

There are several α-adrenergic drugs available, but only one is commonly used by RCPs for the reversal or reduction of mucosal edema. **Racemic epinephrine**, a modified form of epinephrine, typically is administered by small-volume nebulizer, or in-line for me-chanically ventilated patients. **Epinephrine** is not frequently given as an aerosol by small

TABLE 14–1 Causes of Pulmonary Mucosal Edema
Infectious processes
Croup (tracheolargynobronchitis)
Epiglottitis
Bronchiolitis
Trauma
Intubation/extubation
Laryngeal injury
Smoke inhalation
Poisonous fumes inhalation
Superheated air or steam inhalation
Diseases
Bronchitis
Asthma
Conditions
Severe allergic reactions
Anaphylaxis

volume nebulizer because of its profound side effects (although it is a component of many metered dose inhalers [MDIs]). **Phenylephrine** is a potent α-adrenergic but is used primarily by inhalation via *atomizer* directly into the nasal passages, and is not currently used for nebulization and inhalation into the lung. **Phenylephrine (Neo-Synephrine[R])** is likely to cause *rebound* when its use is suddenly discontinued; this characteristic makes it undesireable. The original formulation of **Bronkosol[R]** included **isoetharine** and **phenylephrine** (combining both α and β effects), but the Food and Drug Administration (FDA) has gradually discouraged or eliminated these combination drugs. (Refer to Chapter 11 for the current drug components and actions of Bronkosol[R]).

This section describes the specific sympathomimetic α-adrenergic drugs currently in use, including brand names, drug action, contraindications, side effects, dosage, duration of effectiveness, and special considerations.

Epinephrine (1:100 Epinephrine Hydrochloride [Solution for Nebulization]; Contained in MDIs: Asthmahaler[R], Bronitin Mist[R], Bronkaid Mist[R], Medihaler-Epi[R], Primatene Mist[R]

Actions: sympathomimetic amine, stimulates production of cAMP. Strong α, β_1, and β_2 effects.

Duration: rapid onset by inhalation (3–5 minutes) but short duration (less than 60 minutes).

Contraindications: cardiovascular disease (particularly hypertension or cardiac arrhythmias), hypersensitivity, and concurrent digitalis therapy.

Side effects: tachycardia, arrhythmias, palpitations, hypertension.

Dosage: give 0.25–0.50 mL of 1% solution with 2.5 mL diluent, administered by small volume nebulizer. Also may be administered by hand-bulb nebulizer using 8–15 drops (0.5–1.0 ml) of 1% solution, self-administer *only 2–3 puffs*. May take another 2–3 inhalations after 5 minutes, then cannot receive another dosage for 4 hours. MDI dosage: 1–2 puffs, no more frequently than 6 times daily.

Special Considerations: epinephrine is the drug of choice for acute allergic reactions (i.e., anaphylaxis) and severe acute asthma, but it is usually administered IM in these cases. Although it is a potent bronchodilator and vasoconstrictor, its use as an aerosol is infrequent because of its serious side effects. Epinephrine sometimes is used in the early management of acute status asthmaticus, but safer drugs (β_2-specific bronchodilators or racemic epinephrine) are preferred for routine use by the aerosol route.

Racemic Epinephrine (Micronefrin[R], Vaponefrin[R], Racepinephrine[R])

Actions: sympathomimetic amine; stimulates production of cAMP. Strong α, mild β_2, and moderate β_1 effects.

Duration: rapid onset, effective for 30–60 minutes.

Contraindication: hypersensitivity.

Side effects: tachycardia, hypertension, and headache.

Dosage: give 0.25–0.50 mL of 2.25% solution in 3 mL of diluent, administered by aerosol every 1–2 hours (0.50 mL of 2.25% solution = 11.25 mg racemic epinephrine).

Special considerations: drug of choice in the treatment of bronchoconstriction associated with mucosal edema (e.g., croup, postextubation laryngeal edema, inhalation injuries). It is rapidly metabolized, and can be given safely as frequently as every hour with close monitoring. The primary drug action by aerosol is α (vasoconstriction).

CORTICOSTEROID ANTI-INFLAMMATORY DRUGS

Glucocorticosteroids (referred to for simplicity as *corticosteroids* in this chapter) are used in the management of acute and chronic asthma, and were introduced in Chapter 7. These drugs have many medical uses because of their nonspecific anti-inflammatory action, but they also have serious systemic side effects. Use of corticosteroids by aerosol has been adopted wherever practical in the management of asthma because of the reduction of systemic effects. However, in contrast to other drugs that have rapid onset when administered by aerosol, corticosteroids given systemically (IV) are more effective than those given by aerosol in the acute or emergency setting. Thus, administering **hydrocortisone** by aerosol to a croup or status asthmaticus patient is not as effective as IV administration, often in combination with aerosol administration of sympathomimetic drugs.

There are four FDA-approved aerosol corticosteroids currently in use in the United States, and a fifth in the investigational and clinical trial stage. The advantages and disadvantages of this route, indications for use, contraindications, side effects, and adverse reactions are comparable among these drugs.

Advantages and Disadvantages of Aerosolized Corticosteroids

Advantages of aerosolized corticosteroids in comparison with oral administration are related primarily to the reduction of serious systemic side effects. With optimal doses of aerosol steroids, neither Cushing syndrome (the *moon-faced* appearance associated with fluid retention) nor adrenal suppression occurs, and there is a very low risk of steroid dependency. These advantages, when considered in light of the excellent localized (i.e., pulmonary) anti-inflammatory action, have led many pulmonary physicians to utilize steroids by aerosol.

Disadvantages to this route of administration include:

1. Aerosol steroids are more expensive than oral dosage.
2. Aerosol steroids are not helpful in status asthmaticus.
3. Risk of superinfection is higher with aerosol steroids than with oral dosage.
4. Airway side effects (hoarseness, coughing, dry throat) are experienced only when aerosolized corticosteroids are given; this side effect is not associated with oral dosage.
5. Patient effort and *understanding* are required for effective aerosol corticosteroid therapy. Patients must be able to take a satisfactory MDI treatment and must reliably follow their prescribed regimen. Improper use of aerosol corticosteroids (i.e., as a bronchodilator) is a hazard.

Indications for Aerosolized Corticosteroids

Aerosolized corticosteroid therapy should be considered for any patient who requires long-term steroidal therapy for control of airway inflammation. It should be considered an adjunct to asthma management in patients who demonstrate little responsiveness to sympathomimetic drugs (e.g., bronchodilators). Use of corticosteroids by aerosol provides good clinical improvement with few side effects, but systemic effects cannot be eliminated. Therefore, when steroids are used in the management of *chronic asthma*, they should be tried in the following order:

1. Aerosolized corticosteroids
2. Oral steroid therapy on alternating days
3. Daily oral corticosteroids

In *status asthmaticus*, the therapy regimen is very different:

1. IV or IM corticosteroids as *first-line drugs*
2. taper with oral steroids
3. manage with aerosol drugs

An interesting and important beneficial effect of corticosteroids is their ability to *potentiate* the effectiveness of β-adrenergic drugs. One of the actions of corticosteroids is to increase the affinity of the receptors on the cell surfaces to β agonists (sympathomimetics). When an asthmatic is given corticosteroids, particularly as a bolus in the early stage of status asthmaticus, the response to β-adrenergic drugs is improved and more invasive critical care (e.g., intubation and mechanical ventilation) may be avoided.

Contraindications/Precautions for Aerosolized Corticosteroids

As with all medical decisions involving the use of drugs, the costs and benefits of each type of therapy must be weighed. Use of inhaled corticosteroids may allow the patient to reduce the dosage of sympathomimetic drugs (and avoid their side effects), or enhance the action of sympathomimetics, but the corticosteroids also have associated risks.

Hypersensitivity to any drug is an absolute contraindication to its use, and benefits must clearly outweigh fetal risks if the drug is used during pregnancy. Presence of a systemic fungal infection, renal failure, or severe diabetes mellitus contraindicates the use of steroids.

Patient education and understanding of the drug regimen is critical, particularly when drugs such as corticosteroids and cromolyn sodium are used in asthma management. Steroids have *no bronchodilating effects* and should not be used during an acute attack. Frequent use or overuse of corticosteroid MDIs not only may delay necessary treatment, it also may lead to fungal infections of the mouth and pharynx (because of the immunosuppressant actions). Patients who successfully use MDI corticosteroids must be cooperative, willing and able to follow dosage directions, and able to take an effective aerosol inhalation from the MDI (see Chapter 10). Another important patient education issue is *compliance*. The patient should not adjust the prescribed dosage and should never discontinue use of the drug unless under a physician's care. Corticosteroid use, even by aerosol, should be tapered gradually until finally discontinued. Transferring a patient from oral to aerosolized steroids also should be done through a weaning process, to allow gradual recovery of full adrenal function.

Side Effects/Adverse Reactions of Aerosolized Corticosteroids

Systemic side effects of corticosteroids (i.e., Cushing syndrome, immunosuppression, and diabetes) are not seen in the dosages used by aerosol administration (less than 1000 μg/day). Throat irritation, hoarseness, coughing, and dry mouth are the most frequent side effects of aerosolized corticosteroids. These effects can be prevented almost completely by having the patient thoroughly rinse the mouth and gargle after each MDI treatment.

Occasionally a patient will develop oral candidiasis or aspergillosis (fungal super-infections) following aerosolized corticosteroid therapy. This also is avoidable by having the patient thoroughly rinse the mouth and gargle after a treatment, preferably with an alcohol-based mouthwash such as **Cepacol**[R]. If discontinuation or interruption of aerosol therapy is contraindicated, or rapid clearance of the fungal infection is desired, the patient may be given **nystatin** lozenges.

Aerosolized corticosteroids should be used cautiously in patients with bronchiectasis, or those who are susceptible to pneumonias or purulent bronchitis. Studies have shown that inhaled steroids seem to predispose some patients to pulmonary infections.

Aerosol Corticosteroid Drugs

All of the following aerosol corticosteroids are administered by MDI. Please refer to Chapter 10 for special considerations and techniques for optimal drug deposition by MDI inhalation. Dosages are provided in *micrograms* (μg).

Beclomethasone (Beclovent[R], Vanceril[R]).

Duration: rapidly absorbed and relatively long acting.

Dosage: MDI provides 42 μg/inhalation (puff). ADULTS: 2 inhalations 3–4 times/day, *not to exceed 20 inhalations/day.* CHILDREN (6–12 years old): 1–2 inhalations 3–4 times/day, *not to exceed 10 puffs/day.*

Special Considerations: beclomethasone sometimes is used as an alternative drug for patients who do not tolerate cromolyn sodium.

Dexamethasone (Decadron Respihaler[R]).

Duration: rapidly absorbed.

Dosage: MDI provides 84 μg/inhalation. ADULTS: 2–3 inhalations, 3–4 times/day, *not to exceed 12 inhalations/day.* CHILDREN: (6–12 years old): 2 inhalations 3–4 times/day, *not to exceed 2 puffs/treatment or 8 puffs/day.*

Flunisolide (AeroBid[R]).

Duration: rapidly absorbed but has a short plasma half-life; thus, several days of therapy may be required before maximal clinical improvement is seen.

Dosage: MDI provides 250 μg/inhalation. ADULTS and CHILDREN (6–15 years old): 2 inhalations/treatment, 2 times/day (one treatment in morning, one in evening), *not to exceed 4 inhalations/day.*

Special considerations: AeroBid^R dosage is the most concentrated of the currently used aerosolized corticosteroids. Special care must be taken in patient instructions to avoid overuse, particularly if the patient has had previous experience with a different cortico-steroid MDI.

Triamcinolone (Azmacort^R).

Duration: Intermediate acting; because of very short plasma half-life, full therapeutic effects may require 5–10 days. Onset of clinical improvement within 1–3 days.

Dosage: MDI provides 100 μg/inhalation. ADULTS: 2 inhalations 3–4 times/day, *not to exceed 16 inhalations/day.* CHILDREN (6–12 years old): 1–2 inhalations 3–4 times/day, *not to exceed 12 inhalations/day.*

Budesonide (Investigational).

Duration: rapidly absorbed, onset of anti-inflammatory action is comparable to that of dexamethasone (but not as rapid as beclomethasone).

Dosage: MDI provides 50 μg/inhalation. ADULTS: 400–1600 μg/day, in 2–4 treatments. CHILDREN (6–12 years old): 200–400 μg/day in 2–4 doses. *Maximal daily dosages have not been established.*

Special considerations: this drug shows promise as an initial intervention in newly diagnosed asthma and may be preferable to β agonists in some patients.

ANTI-ASTHMATIC (MAST CELL STABILIZER) DRUGS

As discussed in Chapter 7, when histamine is released following an antigen–antibody reaction, the classic allergic reaction occurs. This reaction includes increased capillary permeability, increased mucus production, mucosal inflammation and edema, and bronchospasm. Histamine is stored within *mast cells*; when the antigen–antibody reaction occurs these cells *degranulate* (rupture) and histamine is released (Figure 14–2).

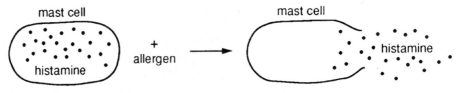

FIGURE 14–2 Allergic Response: Ruptured Mast Cell Releases Histamine.

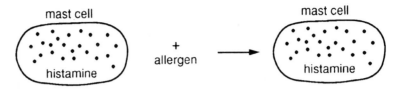

FIGURE 14–3 Cromolyn Sodium: Stabilizes Mast Cell to Prevent Histamine Release.

Antihistamines have limited value as preventive drugs because they antagonize the effects of histamine once it has been released. **Cromolyn sodium** was developed as a true *preventive* drug because it does not allow the mast cell to degranulate when the patient is exposed to an antigen; therefore, the allergic reaction itself is prevented (Figure 14–3).

Cromolyn Sodium

Cromolyn sodium, when properly used, has revolutionized the management of chronic asthma. Success also has been reported for the use of cromolyn sodium in severe inhalation allergies that are not associated with asthma (i.e., hay fever). Cromolyn sodium has been marketed in the United States since the mid-1970s, but its initial form of administration (powder aerosol) was irritating to many asthmatics and the drug was prohibitively expensive. Patient compliance also was a problem (asthmatics tend to independently reduce their drug dosage when not symptomatic). Cromolyn sodium is now available in solution as well as the original Spinhaler[R] capsules, and competitive pricing and emphasis on patient education have made the drug an invaluable part of the long-term management of chronic asthma.

Mechanism of Action. Cromolyn sodium is referred to as a *mast cell stabilizer*, because it prevents the cell from degranulating. When the mast cell is exposed to an allergen, calcium ions enter the cell and cause its rupture. Cromolyn sodium prevents the influx of calcium ions and therefore prevents the rupture. It is only when mast cells rupture that the allergic reaction occurs (after the release of mediators that have been stored within the cell).

Indications for Use. Cromolyn sodium is indicated for the management of chronic extrinsic asthma and also is effective as a prophylactic in patients who have *intrinsic* asthma. Although these patients do not have the allergic asthma associated with exposure to an antigen, when an attack is stimulated by some *endogenous* stimulus, the mast cells degranulate and the inflammatory response follows. Intrinsic asthmatics are subject to nonallergic asthma attacks, which may be triggered by infection, cold air, stress, exercise, emotional stimuli, or even unknown etiology.

Limitations and Concerns. Cromolyn sodium is not recommended for the occasional asthmatic attack or the seasonal asthmatic. It is effective only when administered by aerosol (liquid or powder), and its prophylactic effects require 2–4 weeks to reach maximal levels. In many ways, cromolyn sodium should be considered similar to anti-hypertensive drugs when conducting patient education. Initial dosages may be reduced gradually once the therapeutic serum level has been reached, but the drug should be used continually once therapy has been initiated.

Careful physician supervision is required through the initial stages, and the patient must understand that this drug is to be used regardless of the presence of symptoms. If the patient regards cromolyn sodium in the same manner as other asthma drugs (i.e., bronchodilators or steroids) that are safely reduced when symptoms are absent, the drug will fail. It is also imperative that the patient understands what cromolyn sodium cannot do:

1. It *should not be used in an acute attack*.
2. It has *no bronchodilator* effects.
3. It has *no anti-inflammatory* effects.
4. It has *no antihistamine* effects.

Cromolyn Sodium (Intal^R, Nasalcrom^R [Nasal Solution]).

Actions: mast cell stabilizer.

Contraindication: sensitivity to cromolyn sodium. The drug should be used cautiously in patients with renal or hepatic disease, during pregnancy, and by children under 5 or in patients who may not be able to comply with the treatment regimen.

Adverse reactions/side effects: bronchospasm, wheezing, and cough may occur. Dizziness, headache,and nausea have been reported. Occasionally allergic reactions such as rash, urticaria, sneezing, epistaxis, and joint swelling may occur.

Duration: onset is rapid, but prophylactic effects do not occur until 2–4 weeks after beginning therapy.

Dosage: drug is available in two forms (2-mL liquid ampule and powder capsule); both provide the same dosage per treatment (20 mg). It also is available in MDI (800 μg/ inhalation). Adult and child dosages are the same. Initial dosage is 20 mg/treatment, 4 times/day (at regular intervals). MDI dosage is 2 inhalations, 4 times/day (not to exceed 8 MDI doses/day). *For prevention of exercise-induced bronchospasm*: give 20 mg (ampule or capsule) inhaled (or 2 MDI inhalations) no more than 60 minutes prior to exercise.

Special considerations: bronchospasm is not infrequent; use of a bronchodilator prior to cromolyn sodium is recommended if bronchospasm occurs. Use of powder capsule by Spinhaler^R is not recommended for children under age 5. (Spinhaler^R procedure is described in Figure 14–4, p. 234.)

Nedocromil Sodium

Mechanism of Action. Nedocromil sodium is a new antiasthmatic drug that is available in Canada under the brand name (C) **Tilade**. This drug exhibits both mast-cell stabilization (comparable to that of cromolyn sodium) and specific anti-inflammatory properties. Its usage is comparable to that of cromolyn sodium in the management of chronic bronchitis and chronic asthma, and is particularly useful in extrinisic (*allergic*) disease.

Indications for Use.   Nedocromil sodium is indicated as part of the treatment regimen for the management of chronic allergic bronchitis and asthma. It has been shown to be useful on an occasional basis in the prevention of bronchospasm induced by such external factors as pollutants, cold air, or exercise. It is intended for *daily* use as a maintenance drug and should not be used during an acute asthmatic attack.

Limitations and Concerns.   As for cromolyn sodium, nedocromil sodium is not recommended for the occasional asthmatic attack or the seasonal asthmatic. It is only effective when administered by aerosol, it is available only in MDI, and its therapeutic benefits usually require 1 or more weeks to reach maximal levels. Initial dosages may be reduced gradually once the therapeutic serum level has been reached, but the drug should be used continually once therapy has been initiated.

Careful physician supervision is required through the initial stages, and the patient must understand that this drug is to be used regardless of the presence of symptoms. Patients should be instructed carefully about the proper use and dosage of nedocromil sodium and should be cautioned not to change dosage without physician supervision. As with cromolyn sodium, it is also imperative that the patient understands what nedocromil sodium cannot do:

1. It *should not be used in an acute attack*.
2. It has *no bronchodilator* effects.
3. It has *no antihistamine* effects.

Nedocromil Sodium ([C] Tilade).

Actions: mast cell stabilizer, anti-inflammatory.

Contraindication: sensitivity to nedocromil sodium. The drug should be used cautiously by nursing mothers or during pregnancy, and by patients who may not be able to comply with the treatment regimen.

Adverse reactions/side effects: few side effects have been noted, but headaches, nausea, and vomiting have been reported. The most common side effect is an unpleasant taste.

Duration: onset is rapid and the drug may be effective within a few minutes when using prior to exposure to an irritant (cold air, exercise). Prophylactic therapeutic effects usually are apparent within 1 week of initiating daily usage.

Dosage: Drug is available in MDI only (2.0 mg/inhalation). Adults and children over 12 years old: initial dosage is 4.0 mg/treatment (2 inhalations), 4 times/day (at regular intervals). *For prevention of stimulant-provoked bronchospasm:* give 4.0 mg (or 2 MDI inhalations) inhaled no more than 60 minutes prior to exposure.

FOR INHALATION USE ONLY

1

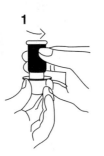

Make sure your hands
are clean and dry.

Loading the SPINHALER

Hold SPINHALER vertical
with white mouthpiece held
downwards. Unscrew body
of inhaler counter-clockwise.

2

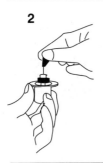

Keep mouthpiece down-
wards and propeller on
spindle. Insert **colored**
end of capsule **firmly**
into propeller cup. Ex-
cessive handling of the
capsule causes it to
soften.

3

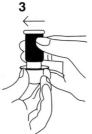

Screw body back into
mouthpiece, making
certain it is securely
fastened.

4a

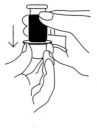

Keep SPINHALER vertical
and mouthpiece down-
wards...slide the gray
sleeve down firmly
until it stops (to pierce
the capsule)...then
slide the gray sleeve up
as far as it will go.

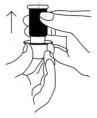

**Do this only once.
Do not repeat.**

4b

5

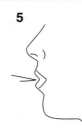

**Use of SPINHALER
Check again to make
sure that the mouth-
piece is securely
attached to the body.**
Holding SPINHALER
well away from mouth
breathe out fully
emptying air from lungs
as much as possible.

FIGURE 14–4 Procedure for Using Spinhaler[R] Turbo-Inhaler. Courtesy of
Fisons Pharmaceutical Corporation.

6

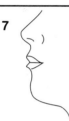

With head tilted back-
wards and teeth apart,
close lips and teeth
around the mouthpiece.

Inhale a deep and
rapid breath.
DO NOT BREATHE
OUT THROUGH
SPINHALER®

7

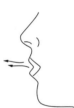

Remove SPINHALER
from your mouth and
hold your breath for a
few seconds.

8

Holding SPINHALER well
away from mouth
breathe out completely.

Repeat steps 5, 6, 7, and
8 several times until
the powder is inhaled.

A light dusting of
powder remaining
behind in the capsule
is normal and is not
an indication that
the SPINHALER or
capsule is faulty.

9

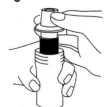

Discard empty capsule,
return SPINHALER to
container and screw
lid on securely.

10

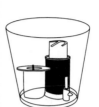

Cleaning SPINHALER
At least once a week,
dismantle parts A, B,
and C and wash them
in clean, warm water.
Pay particular attention to
washing the inside of the
propeller shaft, by moving
the propeller on and off
the steel spindle under
water. Shake out excess
water and allow all parts
to dry before re-assembly.

How to care for the capsules

1. Do not remove capsules
from foil except for immediate use.

2. Do not handle capsules
excessively. Moisture
from hands may make
capsules soft.

3. Protect from extremes
of temperature.

Note: In case of difficulty,
consult your physician
or pharmacist.

With care the SPINHALER should
provide useful service for up to 6
months. The SPINHALER should
be replaced after 6 months.

FIGURE 14–4 *Continued*

POSTTEST: ANTI-INFLAMMATORY AND ANTIASTHMATIC DRUGS

For each of the following questions, try to select the *one* best answer from those choices given.

1. Which of the following drugs has an α-adrenergic effect?
   - I.   epinephrine
   - II. cromolyn sodium
   - III. beclomethasone
   - IV. racemic epinephrine
   - V.   flunisolide
   - a. I and IV only
   - b. I, II, and IV only
   - c. II only
   - d. III and V only
   - e. I, II, and V only

2. A pediatric patient in the emergency room has a harsh, barking cough, inspiratory stridor, tachypnea, and tachycardia. Wheezing is not heard, and the parents report some improvement since the child has been sitting up and during the ride in the cold night air to the hospital. Which of the following drugs should the RCP recommend by aerosol?
   - a. epinephrine
   - b. Vanceril^R
   - c. Vaponefrin^R
   - d. Intal^R
   - e. Ventolin^R

3. What is the appropriate dosage of the drug recommended in question 2?
   - a. 0.30 mL of 1% solution in 3.0 mL of diluent
   - b. 0.50 mL of 2.25% solution in 3.0 mL of diluent
   - c. 0.25 mL of 1:100 solution in 3.0 mL of diluent
   - d. 0.20 mL of .5% solution in 2.5 mL of diluent
   - e. 20 mg of nebulized solution

4. How frequently can the drug recommended in question 2 be safely given (in the dosage suggested in Question 3)?
   - a. every hour
   - b. every 4 hours
   - c. 4 times per day
   - d. every 6 hours
   - e. none of the above

5. Which of the following drugs stabilizes the mast cell?
   - a. Intal^R
   - b. Vanceril^R
   - c. Nasalcrom^R
   - d. Azmacort^R
   - e. both *a* and *c*

6. Which of the following drugs has a general anti-inflammatory effect?
    I. Vanceril^R
    II. cromolyn sodium
    III. Azmacort^R
    IV. Decadron^R
    V. Nasalcrom^R
  a. II and V only
  b. III only
  c. I, II, and IV only
  d. I, III, and IV only
  e. III and V only

7. A patient is brought to the emergency room after experiencing shortness of breath, a "tight" feeling in his chest, and tachycardia while swimming at a local pool. The maintenance crew had added chlorine to the pool by tossing a bucket of solution over the surface just before the patient's symptoms began. Which of the following drugs should the RCP suggest by aerosol?
  a. Ventolin^R
  b. Vanceril^R
  c. epinephrine
  d. Micronefrin^R
  e. aminophylline

8. Which of the following drugs may be used to control the bronchospasm associated with an acute asthmatic attack?
    I. Intal^R
    II. Ventolin^R
    III. Vanceril^R
    IV. Alupent^R
    V. Alonefrin^R
  a. I and IV only
  b. III, IV, and V only
  c. II and IV only
  d. II, IV, and V only
  e. III only

9. The advantages of administering corticosteroids by aerosol include:
  a. rapid absorption at site of action with reduced systemic side effects
  b. prolonged duration with reduced side effects
  c. rapid absorption with reduced dosage
  d. rapid serum levels with reduced dosages
  e. immediate relief of bronchospasm

10. Which of the following drugs should *not* be recommended for the treatment of status asthmaticus?
  a. Intal^R
  b. Nasalcrom^R

    c. beclomethasone

    d. Vanceril[R]

    e. all of the above

11. Which of the following drugs often are used to control the inflammation associated with chronic asthma?

    I.   beclomethasone

    II. racemic epinephrine

    III. epinephrine

    IV. Decadron Respihaler[R]

    V. Vanceril[R]

    a. II and III only

    b. I, II, and IV only

    c. I, IV, and V only

    d. IV and V only

    e. I and V only

12. Which of the following considerations should be stressed when instructing a new patient in the use of aerosolized steroids?

    a. the patient should use the MDI steroids only when symptoms (e.g., wheezing) are severe.

    b. the use of steroids by MDI should be tapered gradually and under a physician's supervision.

    c. the patient should be able to adjust the dosage and frequency according to "feel" because steroids are very safe by MDI.

    d. the MDI steroids should be used on alternate days with other antiasthmatic drugs.

    e. MDI steroids are safe for use during pregnancy because they are deposited in the lung and do not reach fetal circulation.

13. With regard to β agonists, aerosolized steroids have which of the following effects

    a. they block the effects of bronchodilators.

    b. they have no effect on bronchodilating.

    c. they reduce systemic side effects of dilators.

    d. they potentiate (increase) bronchodilating effects.

    e. there are no data regarding this interaction.

14. Which of the following phrases best describes the action of cromolyn sodium?

    a. prevents degranulation of mast cell

    b. anti-inflammatory

    c. antihistaminic

    d. bronchodilator

    e. breaks down histamine inside of mast cell

15. The Spinhaler[R] is used specifically for the administration of:

    a. Vanceril[R]

    b. Intal[R]

    c. Beclovent[R]

    d. Azmacort[R]

    e. Atrovent[R]

REFERENCES/RECOMMENDED READING

Bergmann KC et al: A placebo-controlled, blind comparison of nedocromil sodium and beclomethasone dipropionate in bronchial asthma. *Curr Med Res Opin*, 11:533, 1989.

Carlsen K-H, et al: Allergic alveolitis in a 12–year old boy: Treatment with budesonide nebulizing solution. *Pediatr Pulmonol*, 12:257, 1992.

Cherniak RM, et al: A double blind group-comparative study of the efficacy and safety of nedocromil sodium in the management of asthma. *Chest* 97:1299, 1990.

Fanta CH: Emergency management of acute severe asthma. *Respir Care*, 37:551, 1992.

Haahtela T, et al: Comparison of a β-agonist, terbutaline, with an inhaled corticosteroid, budesonide, in newly detected asthma. *New Engl J Med* 325:388, 1991.

Haponik EF: Smoke inhalation injury: Some priorities for respiratory care professionals. *Respir Care*, 37:609, 1992.

Howder CL: *Cardiopulmonary Pharmacology*. Williams & Wilkins, Baltimore, 1992.

Thompson JE, Farrell E, McManus M: Neonatal and pediatric airway emergencies. *Respir Care*, 37:582, 1992.

CHAPTER 15

SURFACE ACTIVE AGENTS

LEARNING OBJECTIVES

After the completion of this chapter and its learning activities, the student will be able to:

1. Define surface tension.
2. Describe the clinical importance of surface tension as it relates to the work of breathing.
3. Define surfactant, specifically pulmonary surfactant.
4. Describe clinical indications (or protocol) for the use of surfactant replacement drugs.
5. List two surfactant replacement drugs currently in use in the United States, including:
   a. brand names
   b. indications
   c. contraindications
   d. side effects/adverse reactions
   e. dosage and route of administration
6. Define fulminant pulmonary edema, and alveolar pulmonary edema. Contrast these terms with interstitial pulmonary edema.
7. Describe clinical signs and symptoms of fulminant alveolar pulmonary edema.
8. List several causes of or predisposing factors for fulminant alveolar pulmonary edema.
9. List one surface-active drug indicated for the treatment of fulminant alveolar pulmonary edema, including:
   a. indications
   b. contraindications
   c. side effects/adverse reactions
   d. dosage and route of administration

INTRODUCTION

Surface tension is the physical property that creates tension at a fluid–air interface, similar to that of soap bubble. The physical property of surface tension is extremely important in respiratory care. Surface tension is a necessary component of passive exhalation (the tendency of the lung to return to its resting state). In the newborn, the first few breaths of life are the most difficult because the physiological detergent surfactant has not yet been distributed evenly throughout the lungs. In premature newborns, surfactant production may be inadequate, leading to poor distribution of ventilation and extreme work of breathing. Surfactant replacement therapy is now an integral part of resuscitation and management of premature newborns.

The use of surface-active agents in respiratory care is limited to the critical care setting. Surfactant replacement drugs have greatly improved the survival and reduced the morbidity of premature newborns, but this therapy should be given only by the most highly skilled practitioners in a critical care environment.

Another critical situation in which a surface-active agent may be indicated is *fulminant pulmonary edema*. For the patient who exhibits evidence of fulminant alveolar pulmonary edema, including diffuse patchy infiltrates on chest radiographs and frothy, foamy, pinkish sputum, administration of aerosolized ethyl alcohol to raise the surface tension of the edema froth has been shown to be life-saving because it improves oxygenation rapidly. The use of ethanol as a drying agent for the treatment of severe hypoxia associated with alveolar pulmonary edema often is a life-saving procedure and typically is performed in the emergency room or intensive care unit.

Although a practitioner may see only a few patients a year who may benefit from these therapies, it is imperative that we retain a working knowledge of the drugs and their applications.

SURFACE TENSION

Surface tension is the result of the attraction (cohesion) of like molecules at the surface of a liquid. Molecules on the surface are attracted inward; thus, surface tension makes the liquid contract to minimize its surface area. It is this property that makes a drop of water form a bead, or assume a semicircular shape instead of a formless puddle. When surface-active agents, such as detergents, are added to such a liquid, the drop actually dissolves into a puddle because the *cohesion* between the molecules on its surface has been broken.

A *detergent* is a substance that reduces surface tension; this is the basis on which laundry detergents work. When cleaning products are used, they reduce surface tension to allow the dirt or stain to be removed from the clothing. In the lung, detergents are used to reduce surface tension to reduce the work of breathing and improve distribution of ventilation.

SURFACTANT

Pulmonary surfactant is the naturally occurring (*endogenous*) detergent that reduces alveolar surface tension and allows lung inflation with normal breathing effort (Figure 15–1). Surfactant is a *phospholipid* (dipalmitoyl lecithin) that is produced by alveolar type II cells. Without surfactant, the surface tension of pulmonary secretions has a strong cohesive force that contributes to alveolar collapse and opposes inflation.

Surfactant has a relatively short half-life (hours), and is constantly produced and replenished when the alveolar type II cells are stimulated. Atelectasis sometimes occurs from the lack of stimulation of these cells by deep breathing, in this case, alveolar collapse occurs when the surface tension is not balanced by surfactant. Atelectasis also may persist in the premature newborn when insufficient surfactant is present at birth.

Under normal physiological conditions, an inspiratory effort of -5 to -10 cm H_2O pressure will generate enough force to provide a sufficient tidal volume. An infant's first breath may require -60 to -100 cm H_2O pressure, but the presence of surfactant makes subsequent breaths easier. Within moments of birth, the newborn's work of breathing is minimal (as it should be), because the surfactant is present and distributed throughout the lungs.

In the premature newborn, particularly if the infant is born at less than 28 weeks' gestation, surfactant may be absent or present in only small quantities. These infants quickly develop difficulty breathing as a result of the effort required to overcome surface tension on each breath (Figure 15–2).

The concept of surface tension is applied in two very different clinical situations: infant respiratory distress syndrome (IRDS) and fulminant alveolar pulmonary edema. Although the pathology of these two conditions is entirely unrelated, and different drugs are used in the treatments, it is the concept of using a *detergent* to reduce surface tension that is applied in both situations.

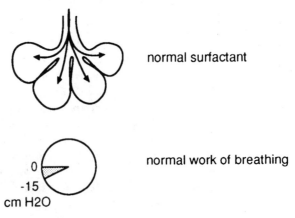

normal surfactant

normal work of breathing

0
-15
cm H2O

FIGURE 15–1   Normal Surfactant: Normal Work of Breathing.

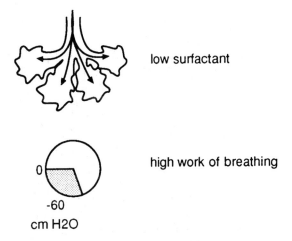

low surfactant

high work of breathing

FIGURE 15–2 Lack of Surfactant: Increased Work of Breathing.

INFANT (OR IDIOPATHIC) RESPIRATORY DISTRESS SYNDROME

Premature or low-birth-weight infants often develop IRDS. This syndrome is associated with difficulty breathing, poor ventilation and oxygenation, and excessive work of breathing, which often leads to fatigue, cardiac arrhythmias, and worsening blood gases. It has long been known that many of these infants are born with insufficient surfactant levels, and that it may require up to 72 hours after birth for adequate endogenous surfactant levels to be achieved. Over the past two decades, neonatology has greatly improved the survival of these infants, but use of traditional therapies (primarily mechanical ventilation, oxygen, and continuous positive airway pressure or positive end-expiratory pressure) also have contributed to long-term consequences such as bronchopulmonary dysplasia. There has been great scientific interest in developing a surfactant replacement that could be used for treatment of IRDS, but only recently has such research been successful.

Early attempts to provide surfactant replacement drugs concentrated on an aerosol drug that could be deposited in the lung by mechanical (assisted) ventilation or by patient effort. These drugs were not found to be effective. Current surfactant replacement therapy involves *instillation* of the surfactant replacement drug, followed by vigorous manual ventilation and position changes of the newborn to provide distribution of the drug.

Surfactant Replacement Drugs

There are currently two forms of surfactant replacement drugs approved by the Food and Drug Administration. Both are synthetic surface-active substances, rather than extracts from donors or other animal sources. These two drugs are similar in dosage and administration guidelines, as well as contraindications, side effects, and adverse reactions.

Both drugs describe *prophylactic* as well as *rescue* protocols. Studies have shown that low-birth-weight (less than 1250 g birth weight) infants may benefit from prophylactic treatment with a surfactant replacement drug, before the onset of respiratory failure associated with IRDS. The *rescue* protocol refers to infants who *develop* IRDS (often these are infants who did not meet the criteria for prophylactic use of surfactant replacement drugs, e.g., full-term gestation or a birth weight over 1250 g).

Beractant (Survanta[R] [Intratracheal Suspension]).

Actions: phospholipid, reduces alveolar surface tension to improve distribution of ventilation and reduce work of breathing.

Indications: *Prevention protocol*: Initial dose should be given within 15 minutes of birth for premature infants whose birth weight is less than 1250 g. *Rescue protocol*: Initial dose should be given within 8 hours of the onset of symptoms of IRDS (as manifest by radiographic findings and the need for mechanical ventilation).

Contraindications: none known.

Side effects/adverse reactions: bradycardia and oxygen desaturation occur in 10–12 percent of infants given Survanta[R]; if these occur, interrupt the drug administration and resuscitate. When the infant is stabilized, the dosage may be continued. Other less common adverse reactions include bronchospasm, pallor, vasoconstriction, hypertension, hypotension, hypocarbia, hypercarbia, and apnea.

Dosage: give 100 mg/kg, *instilled* directly via endotracheal tube and followed by vigorous manual ventilation and oxygenation. Maximum of four doses, given no more frequently than every 6 hours. Survanta[R] is supplied in single-dose 8-mL vials that contain 25 mg/mL (total of 200 mg of drug per vial).

Special Considerations: diffuse rales and acute partial airway obstruction occur with initiation of dosing procedure. Suctioning is *not recommended* unless bradycardia and arterial or transcutaneous oxygen desaturation persists. Survanta[R] should be given only in the tertiary newborn intensive care settings where appropriate personnel and equipment are available for resuscitation. Arterial or transcutaneous oxygen and carbon dioxide monitors should be utilized during dosing procedure and for patient monitoring following drug administration.

Colfosceril Palmitate, Cetyl Alcohol, Tyloxapol (Exosurf Neonatal[R]).

Actions: synthetic surfactant, reduces alveolar surface tension to improve distribution of ventilation and reduce work of breathing.

Indications: *Prevention protocol:* Initial dosage should be given as soon as possible after birth for infants whose birth weight is less than 1250 g or who have evidence of pulmonary immaturity (i.e., abnormal lecithin/sphingomyelin ratio). *Rescue protocol:* Initial dosage should be given as soon as possible after the diagnosis of IRDS has been confirmed.

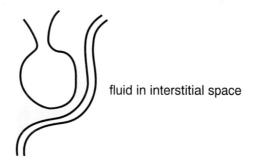

fluid in interstitial space

FIGURE 15–3   Interstitial Pulmonary Edema.

Contraindications: none known.

Side effects/adverse reactions: same as those for Survanta[R].

Dosage: *Prevention protocol:* Initial dosage of 5 mL/kg as soon as possible after birth; following doses (5 mL/kg) given every 12 hours (if the infant remains on mechanical ventilation). Drug is administered by *instillation* into endotracheal tube. Maximum of three dosages recommended. *Rescue protocol:* Initial dosage of 5 mL/kg given as soon as possible (by endotracheal instillation) after diagnosis of IRDS is confirmed. One additional dosage (5 mL/kg) is given 12 hours after first dose.

Special Considerations: all special considerations noted for Survanta[R] also apply to Exosurf Neonatal[R]. Dosing procedure for Exosurf Neonatal[R] requires administration of recommended dosages in *two half-doses*, changing the position of the infant for each dose to allow gravity to help disperse the drug. A videotape that demonstrates the dosing procedure is provided by the manufacturer and is strongly suggested as mandatory viewing for respiratory care practitioners and other health professionals prior to drug administration.

FULMINANT ALVEOLAR PULMONARY EDEMA

Pulmonary edema is the accumulation of fluid in the lung. This nonspecific term may mean *interstitial* or *alveolar* pulmonary edema, or a combination of both (Figures 15–3 and 15–4).

   Interstitial pulmonary edema is seen most often in patients with chronic or acute congestive heart failure in which the cardiac output is unable to keep up with circulatory needs and fluid "backs up" into the interstitial spaces. The earliest signs of congestive heart failure include pedal (foot) or ankle edema and some shortness of breath on exertion. This type of pulmonary edema is best treated with drugs that improve cardiac output (i.e., digitalis) and reduce excess fluids (i.e., diuretics).

   Fulminant alveolar pulmonary edema is a rapidly occurring accumulation of fluid within the alveolar sacs (fulminant means "coming in lightening-like flashes"). This type

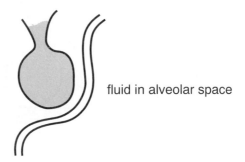

fluid in alveolar space

FIGURE 15–4 Alveolar Pulmonary Edema.

of edema may be associated with life-threatening acute congestive heart failure, or with traumatic causes such as head injuries (neurogenic pulmonary edema), acute mountain sickness, heroin overdose, burns, or acute inhalation injuries, such as poisonous fumes.

Clinical signs associated with alveolar pulmonary edema are much more dramatic than those seen in the chronic congestive heart failure patient. Alveolar pulmonary edema leads to profound hypoxia, which may render the patient unconscious within minutes. Cyanosis, diffuse bilateral rales, and the presence of frothy, foamy, pinkish pulmonary secretions are common. Chest radiographs will reveal diffuse bilateral patchy infiltrates, often described as having a *cotton-ball* appearance, throughout both lung fields. Medical treatment for alveolar pulmonary edema is similar to that for interstitial edema (digitalis, diuretics, rotating tourniquets), but the use of ethyl alcohol as a surface-active agent may provide enough immediate reduction of the edema froth to minimize end-organ hypoxic damage.

In contrast to the use of surfactant as a detergent to reduce surface tension and ease alveolar inflation, ethyl alcohol is sometimes referred to as a *drying agent*. The pathology of alveolar pulmonary edema leads to frothy, foamy secretions that create a barrier to gas (oxygen) diffusion. Ethyl alcohol raises the surface tension of the edema bubbles, causing them to "burst" and thereby reducing the physical barrier to gas diffusion and improving oxygen transport across the alveolar–capillary membrane (Figure 15–5). Administration of ethyl alcohol by aerosol, or by passing oxygen through a bubble diffuser filled with ethyl alcohol, has been shown to reduce the frothy secretions significantly and improve oxygenation.

Treatment of the underlying cause of the pulmonary edema always should be ongoing, whether or not ethyl alcohol is being used to treat the acute symptoms.

Drying Agents

Ethyl Alcohol/Ethanol.

Actions: drying agent; raises surface tension of frothy secretions associated with pulmonary edema.

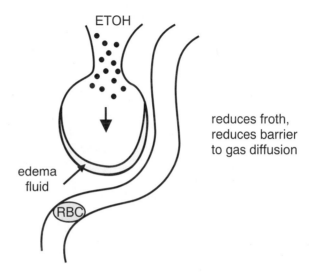

FIGURE 15–5   Use of Alcohol (ETOH) in Alveolar Pulmonary Edema. (RBC = red blood cell.)

Indications: as an *adjunct* in the treatment of acute alveolar pulmonary edema.

Contraindication: Antabuse[R] therapy (treatment for alcoholism).

Side effects: rarely causes any adverse reactions, but drying effect may irritate lung mucosa or cause bronchospasm. Mild intoxication may occur.

Dosage: give 5–15 mL of 30–50% ethyl alcohol administered by small-volume nebulizer or intermittent positive pressure breathing; gas source of oxygen is recommended. Short course of therapy (2–4 treatments) usually is sufficient; treatments may be given every 30 minutes.

Special Considerations: isopropyl or denatured alcohol are toxic when ingested and *must not be used* for this purpose. Use of aerosolized alcohol should be as an adjunct to traditional medical treatment of pulmonary edema. Noncardiac pulmonary edema (i.e., acute mountain sickness or neurogenic pulmonary edema) may be the most appropriate applications of this therapy.

POSTTEST: SURFACE ACTIVE AGENTS

For each of the following questions, try to select the *one* best answer from those choices given.

1. Surface tension:
   a. causes pulmonary edema
   b. is a cohesive force that creates tension at the surface of a liquid
   c. is an adhesive force that prevents alveolar collapse
   d. always opposes alveolar deflation
   e. is the force within a fluid that holds molecules together

2. Pulmonary surfactant:
   a. is a phospholipid
   b. is a detergent
   c. reduces surface tension
   d. is produced by alveolar type II cells
   e. all of the above

3. Surfactant replacement drugs are given:
   a. by aerosol
   b. by instillation
   c. by aerosol or instillation
   d. by aerosol or intravenous line
   e. none of the above

4. Which of the following are brand names of surfactant replacement drugs?
   a. Survanta^R and Exosurf Neonatal^R
   b. Surviva^R and Ethanol^R
   c. Tyloxapol^R and Exosurf^R
   d. Surfazox^R and Survanta^R
   e. Extrasurf^R and Surfazox^R

5. The *rescue* protocol for surfactant replacement drugs is used:
   a. for infants whose birth weight is less than 1250 g
   b. for infants whose birth weight is less than 1350 g
   c. for infants who are born at less than 28 weeks' gestation
   d. for infants who develop IRDS
   e. both *a* and *d*

6. Contraindications for the administration of surfactant replacement drugs include:
   a. persistent fetal circulation
   b. severe IRDS
   c. congenital heart disease
   d. Apgar score of less than 5 at birth
   e. none of the above

7. Adverse reactions of administration of surfactant replacement drugs include:
   I. tachycardia
   II. bradycardia

III. oxygen desaturation

IV. transient rales

V. tremors

    a. I, II, and III only

    b. II and III only

    c. II, III, and IV only

    d. I, II, III, and IV only

    e. I, II, III, IV, and V

8. *Fulminant* means:

    a. foaming

    b. frothy

    c. rapidly occurring

    d. alveolar

    e. all of the above

9. Which of the following signs and symptoms are seen in a patient with alveolar pulmonary edema?

    a. frothy, foamy secretions, cyanosis, patchy infiltrates (on chest radiograph), and bilateral diffuse rales

    b. hemoptysis, cyanosis, bilateral rales and rhonchi

    c. frothy secretions, pallor, patchy areas of consolidation on chest radiograph

    d. swollen ankles, difficulty breathing, history of smoking

    e. thick yellowish sputum, coarse rhonchi, barrel chest, and dyspnea on exertion

10. Which of the following circumstances may lead to alveolar pulmonary edema?

    I. congestive heart failure

    II. acetaminophen overdose

    III. heroin overdose

    IV. acute mountain sickness

    V. head injury

    a. I, IV, and V only

    b. II and III only

    c. III, IV, and V only

    d. I, III, IV, and V only

    e. I, II, III, IV, and V

11. Without adequate surfactant in the alveoli, how much negative pressure must be generated for alveolar inflation?

    a. -5 to -10 cm H_2O

    b. -10 to -20 cm H_2O

    c. -50 to -60 cm H_2O

    d. -60 to -100 cm H_2O

    e. none of the above

12. Surfactant production normally is stimulated by which of the following techniques?

    I. coughing

    II. stimulation of stretch receptors in the lung

   III. periodic sighs

   IV. instillation of synthetic surfactant

   V. administration of ethyl alcohol

   a. I, II, and III only

   b. II and III only

   c. IV only

   d. IV and V only

   e. II, III, and IV only

13. Respiratory failure secondary to surfactant deficiency in the newborn primarily is due to:

   a. ventilation–perfusion mismatching

   b. diffusion barrier

   c. fatigue, excessive work of breathing

   d. shunting

   e. persistent fetal circulation

14. Ethyl alcohol is a surface-active agent that is useful in the clinical management of:

   a. alveolar pulmonary edema

   b. congestive heart failure

   c. interstitial pulmonary edema

   d. pedal edema

   e. all of the above

15. Ethyl alcohol may be used as an aerosol in which of the following dosages?

   a. 3–5 mL of 2.25% solution

   b. 5–10 mL of 10% solution

   c. 5–15 mL of 30–50% solution

   d. 10–15 mL of 60–70% solution

   e. 5–15 mL of 80% solution

REFERENCES/RECOMMENDED READING

Barness LA: Pediatrics update. *JAMA*, 268:399, 1992.

Bhat R, et al: Effect of single dose surfactant on pulmonary function. *Crit Care Med*, 18: 590, 1990.

Kendig JW, et al: A comparison of surfactant as immediate prophylaxis and as rescue therapy in newborns of less than 30 weeks' gestation. *N Engl J Med*, 324:865, 1991.

Long W, et al: A controlled trial of synthetic surfactant in infants weighing 1,250 grams or more with respiratory distress syndrome. *N Engl J Med*, 325:1696, 1991.

Strandjord TP, Hodson WA: Neonatology. *JAMA*, 268:377, 1992.

Whitaker KC: *Neonatal and Pediatric Respiratory Care*. Delmar Publishing, Albany, NY, 1992.

Ziment I: *Respiratory Pharmacology and Therapeutics*. WB Saunders Co, Philadelphia, 1978.

SPECIAL APPLICATIONS

INTRODUCTION

There are several areas of respiratory care practice that involve medication administration but are not clearly related to preceding chapters of this text. These areas include infant/pediatric aerosol dosages, advanced cardiac life support (ACLS), and special procedures (such as bronchoscopy and pulmonary function diagnostics).

Respiratory care practitioners (RCPs) are involved in a wide variety of patient care and diagnostic settings. The patients range in age from premature newborns to geriatrics, and frequently have accompanying cardiac disease. The role of the RCP often is consultative in nature, assisting the physician and other health professionals in selecting the most appropriate drug or its dosage. Practitioners also assist in diagnostic procedures such as bronchoscopy and bronchial challenge testing. It is imperative that the RCP be knowledgeable about the full spectrum of drugs used in respiratory and cardiac care.

This chapter has been included to provide an overview of these topics, and refer the reader to appropriate references, resources, or agencies.

DOSAGE GUIDELINES FOR INFANTS AND CHILDREN

There are few authoritative definitions of *infant* or *child*. The American Heart Association defines an infant as *newborn to 1 year of age* and a child as *1 to 8 years of age*. These are arbitrary definitions, but are useful for the purpose of making initial treatment decisions. Because only 25 percent of all drugs approved by the Food and Drug Administration (FDA) are labeled as "safe and effective for children," considerable care must be taken when determining the appropriate dosage of a specific drug for use by the pediatric patient. In clinical practice, treatment decisions are based on the same criteria as for adults: What drug is the best drug for this patient under these circumstances? The *drug of choice* in all treatment decisions is that drug that produces the maximum benefit with the fewest adverse reactions and (where possible) at the least expense.

Dosage of drugs given by instillation or aerosol generally is determined by the patient response to an initial conservative dosage. In the infant or child, as a general rule, indications, contraindications, and hazards of specific drugs are comparable to these factors in the adult. Dosage is reduced in the pediatric patient, and careful monitoring during the initial administration provides a useful guide for future treatments. Although drug metabolism is a function of body weight, it also is affected by metabolic rate. Infants and children are given lower doses because of their smaller body weight, but side effects may be minimized by their accelerated metabolic rates. Thus there are few absolute rules for dosage guidelines in the infant/child patient.

Several rules have been suggested for initial drug dosages in infants and children. These rules should be used as *guidelines* only, with careful physiologic monitoring of the patient during and immediately following therapy.

- **Clark's Rule**

$$\text{Pediatric dosage} = \frac{\text{weight (pounds)}}{150} \times \text{adult dosage}$$

- **Cowling's Rule**

$$\text{Pediatric dosage} = \frac{\text{age next birthday}}{24} \times \text{adult dosage}$$

- **Fried's Rule**

$$\text{Pediatric dosage (children} <2 \text{ yr)} = \frac{\text{age (mo)}}{150} \times \text{adult dosage}$$

- **Young's Rule**

$$\text{Pediatric dosage (children 2-12 yr)} = \frac{\text{age (yr)}}{\text{age (yr)} + 12} \times \text{adult dosage}$$

Once an appropriate dosage range has been determined, the treatment should be given under close supervision and monitoring. Dosage adjustments may be made after the initial treatment, based on the child's therapeutic response and the severity of side effects.

Dosage *frequency* in infants and children also is adjusted according to therapeutic response and the presence and severity of side effects. In many cases, a drug that is given every 4 hours for an adult patient also can be given every 4 hours for a child. It is in this realm of medicine that the expertise and assessment skills of the practitioner are critical.

The American Academy of Pediatrics is working actively with the FDA for the provision of better drug dosage guidelines for infants and children. Research in many tertiary neonatal care units (Level 3 nurseries) may yield such guidelines in the future.

ASTHMA MANAGEMENT IN CHILDREN

The U.S. Department of Health and Human Services (DHHS) published an expert panel report in 1992 that provides some specific dosage recommendations for drugs used in asthma management. This document, the *Executive Summary: Guidelines for the Diagnosis*

TABLE 16-1 Recommended Dosages for Children (D-HHS)	
DRUG	**CHILD AEROSOL DOSAGE**
albuterol (5 mg/mL)	0.1–0.15 mg/kg in 2 cc saline every 4–6 hours; *maximum dosage of 5.0 mg*
metaproterenol (50 mg/mL)	0.25–0.50 mg/kg in 2 cc saline every 4–6 hours; *maximum dosage of 15.0 mg*
beclomethasone	2–4 MDI* puffs 2–4 times/day (42 µg/puff by MDI)
cromolyn sodium	20 mg nebulized 2–4 times/day (ampules) and capsules contain 20 mg) or 2 MDI puffs 2–4 times/day (1 mg/MDI puff)
*MDI = metered dose inhaler.	

and Management of Asthma, was the product of extensive research and clinical experience in the current treatment of asthma and was published as part of the National Asthma Education Program. The complete report may be obtained from the American Association of Respiratory Care (AARC) or from the DHHS, National Institutes of Health, Bethesda, MD 20892. The report provides dosage guidelines for children as listed in Table 16–1.

ADVANCED CARDIAC LIFE SUPPORT

Advanced cardiac life support is a specific combination of skills and knowledge that are utilized in cardiac resuscitation. Under the guidance of the American Heart Association, with the support of the National Academy of Sciences and the National Research Council, specific courses have been designed to train health professionals in ACLS. These courses include topics such as:

- Myocardial infarction (risks, signs/symptoms)
- Cardiac dysrhythmia recognition (electrocardiographic disturbances)
- Pharmacological agents and their administration routes in emergency cardiac care
- Airway management/ventilation
- Acid–base balance
- Defibrillation
- Invasive monitoring and therapeutic techniques
- Postresuscitation management
- Special resuscitation situations
- Neonatal, infant, and child resuscitation
- Medicolegal aspects of cardiac resuscitation

It is becoming increasingly common for RCPs to participate in such courses and function as key personnel on the resuscitation team. As resuscitation guidelines have

TABLE 16–2 Primary Advanced Cardiac Life Support Drugs

DRUG NAME	DRUG ACTION	LOCATION IN TEXT
Epinephrine	Increases myocardial contractility and rate	Chapter 2
Atropine	Increases myocardial contractility and rate	Chapter 4
Lidocaine	Reduces myocardial irritability	Chapter 5
Procainamide	Reduces myocardial irritability	Chapter 5
Bretylium	Antiarrhythmic	Chapter 5
Verapamil	Calcium channel blocker	Chapter 5
Morphine	Potent analgesic, reduces myocardial oxygen consumption	Chapter 4
Sodium bicarbonate*	Absorbs H^+ to correct metabolic acidosis	Chapter 5

*The use of sodium bicarbonate during cardiac resuscitation is controversial and currently under review. Use is very limited.

become more refined, specific courses have been developed for neonatal advanced life support (NALS) and pediatric advanced life support (PALS).

Although RCPs may not legally be allowed to administer drugs by the intravenous route, many ACLS drugs are safely and effectively administered by instillation during cardiac resuscitation. It is not within the scope or intent of this textbook to define current ACLS drugs or their dosages; however, it is recognized that the RCP must be knowledgeable about which drugs are included and should consider completion of an ACLS course when possible. Many drugs that are included in *ACLS cardiovascular pharmacology* have been described in this text.

The American Heart Association standards for cardiac resuscitation, as published and periodically updated in the *Journal of the American Medical Association*, have become the legal standard of care. The first such standards were published in 1975; they were revised in 1985 and most recently in 1992. Complete ACLS protocols, including drug dosage and administration guidelines, are published in the October 28, 1992 *JAMA* Supplement (Vol. 268, No. 16). The American Heart Association publishes learning materials for participants of ACLS courses, including the *Textbook of Advanced Cardiac Life Support*. The reader should refer to this textbook as the most current and authoritative description of accepted pharmacologic management of the cardiac patient.

Tables 16–2 and 16–3 list the current ACLS drugs, as described in *JAMA* (1992), with reference to the location of these drugs in this textbook. For specific drug dosage

TABLE 16–3 Secondary Advanced Cardiac Life Support Drugs		
DRUG NAME	**DRUG ACTION**	**LOCATION IN TEXT**
Norepinephrine	Increases myocardial contractility and vasoconstriction	Chapters 2 and 5
Dopamine	Vasopressor	Chapter 2
Dobutamine	Vasopressor	Chapter 2
Isoproterenol	Increases cardiac output and **myocardial oxygen consumption***	Chapter 2
Digitalis	Increases myocardial contractility	Chapter 5
Sodium nitroprusside	Coronary vasodilator	Chapter 5
Nitroglycerin	Coronary vasodilator	Chapter 5
Propranolol	β Blocker	Chapter 5
Furosemide	Diuretic	Chapters 2 and 5

*Isoproterenol rarely is used during resuscitation because it may worsen myocardial ischemia. It is used occasionally as a pharmacology "pacemaker" as an interim measure.

information and the clinical indications for the use of these drugs during cardiac resuscitation, please refer to the current *Textbook of Advanced Cardiac Life Support*, or revisions as published in *JAMA* supplements.

SPECIAL PROCEDURES: BRONCHOSCOPY AND BRONCHIAL CHALLENGE

Bronchoscopy

It is common for the RCP to assist a pulmonary physician in the performance of various pulmonary diagnostic procedures. *Bronchoscopy*, the direct visualization of the tracheobronchial tree by a rigid or flexible scope, may irritate the mucosal membranes during the procedure and lead to excessive coughing or bronchospasm. The insertion of the bronchoscope may be traumatic and may stimulate laryngospasm, bronchospasm, mucosal edema, and coughing. To avoid many of these side effects, a preprocedure small-volume nebulizer treatment may be given with an aerosolized local anesthetic. The most commonly used drug for this purpose is **lidocaine**.

Lidocaine is an effective and safe local anesthetic, typically used in 2% or 4% solutions, with or without **epinephrine**. Lidocaine also has an *antitussive* effect, helpfully suppressing the cough reflex during bronchoscopy. The combination of lidocaine with epinephrine commonly is used in dental procedures for the anesthetic effect as well as a favorable vasoconstricting (α) effect that limits bleeding during and after a procedure. This combination also is useful for bronchoscopy, particularly if a forceps biopsy is to be performed. If the patient has a known sensitivity (allergy) to epinephrine, however, this form of the drug should not be used.

Lidocaine Hydrochloride (Xylocaine[R]).

Actions: local anesthetic and antitussive; if used in combination with epinephrine, also will exhibit α (vasoconstricting) effects.

Duration: onset within 3 minutes; local anesthetic effects may persist up to 1 hour.

Contraindication: hypersensitivity to lidocaine (or epinephrine, if appropriate).

Side effects: light-headedness, dizziness, nervousness, apprehension, euphoria, confusion (all rare).

Dosage: give 4–7 mL of 2% **or** 4% solution.

Special considerations: bronchoscopy is a potentially hazardous procedure and requires careful patient monitoring. Continuous pulse oximetry and electrocardiographic monitoring is recommended; supplemental oxygen should be provided via Briggs adaptor (T-piece) during procedure for patients with known hypoxemia. If persistent coughing occurs during the procedure, additional lidocaine may be instilled directly into the trachea in a 0.5–1.0-mL bolus. (*Note:* **Procaine (Novocain[R])** is *not effective topically* and is *not* recommended for aerosol use.)

Bronchial Provocation or Bronchial Challenge Testing

Bronchial provocation is a procedure done in the pulmonary function laboratory to provide the physician with information regarding the *reactivity* of the patient's airways when exposed to an irritant. This is a sophisticated study and should be done only in a well-controlled laboratory that is equipped with scavenger devices to prevent the drug from contaminating the testing environment or adversely affecting personnel or visitors present during testing. Resuscitation equipment should be readily available and personnel should be certified in cardiopulmonary resuscitation and able to recognize and respond appropriately if severe or life-threatening reactions occur.

The two most common drugs used for this *challenge* testing are **methacholine** and **histamine**. Methacholine is a *parasympathomimetic* drug, meaning that it mimics or imitates the effects of the parasympathetic nervous system. When used as an aerosol agent, the primary effect is the stimulation of bronchoconstriction and increased bronchial gland secretion. Some patients who do not respond to a methacholine challenge will respond to histamine, a major mediator of inflammatory reactions. The general clinical indication for such testing is to diagnose reactive airway disease in patients who do not have clinically apparent asthma.

Pulmonary function laboratories typically maintain specific protocols for the performance of such provocation testing and describe the procedure in detail. Histamine is sometimes used for this provocation, but usually only after a methacholine challenge. This text describes methacholine, as the more common agent, and suggests that the reader refer to specific laboratory manuals if histamine is required.

Methacholine Chloride (Provocholine^R).

Actions: parasympathomimetic; stimulates cyclic 3′,5′-guanosine monophosphate. Stimulates bronchoconstriction and increases secretions from bronchial glands.

Duration: peak onset within 2 minutes (may occur within 30 seconds of inhalation); pulmonary function normalizes within 30–45 minutes after study.

Contraindications: methacholine should not be administered to nursing mothers, patients who are receiving β-blocking drugs (e.g., **propranolol**), or those with a known hypersensitivity to this or other parasympathomimetic drugs. In women of childbearing potential, methacholine should be given only within 2 weeks of a negative pregnancy test.

Side effects: side effects are rare, but headache, throat irritation, light-headedness, and itching have been reported.

Dosage: methacholine is provided in a vial containing 100 mg of powder. The powder is reconstituted with saline, according to package insert instructions, into progressively more dilute concentrations. The patient receives **5 inhalations** of the most dilute solution, followed within 5 minutes by a forced vital capacity (FVC) measurement. The study continues, using progressively more concentrated solutions, until the patient's forced expiratory volume in 1 minute (FEV_1) is reduced by 20 percent or the patient has received the maximum dosage (188.9 units).

Special considerations: a breath-activated nebulizing device that is capable of delivering metered aerosol during inspiration only is required. Baseline spirometry must be performed prior to bronchial challenge testing. Special care must be taken when mixing the powder to prevent accidental inhalation, and personnel with asthma or hay fever should not perform this task. Bronchodilators should be immediately accessible during testing in the event of severe reactions, and often are given after testing to enhance return of normal pulmonary function.

POSTTEST: SPECIAL APPLICATIONS

For each of the following questions, try to select the *one* best answer from those choices given.

1. Which of the following statements is true about pediatric drug administration dosages?
   a. the American Heart Association has established guidelines that are followed by most pediatricians.
   b. the American Academy of Pediatrics has published dosages for all pediatric drug use.
   c. there are very few drugs with established guidelines specifically for pediatric dosages.
   d. initial pediatric dosage should be about one-half of the recommended adult dosage.
   e. the *Physicians' Desk Reference* (PDR) has specific conversion tables for determining the appropriate pediatric dosage for all FDA-approved drugs.

2. After determining an initial drug dosage using clinical experience or an available "rule," subsequent dosages should be determined by:
   a. drug insert information
   b. PDR tables
   c. the same rule used for initial dosage
   d. patient response to initial dosage
   e. the clinical pharmacist

3. The American Heart Association defines "infant" and "child":
   a. according to weight
   b. as infant is up to 18 months, child is over 18 months old
   c. for the purposes of teaching cardiopulmonary resuscitation only
   d. for the purposes of teaching ACLS only
   e. as infant is up to 12 months, child is 1–8 years old

4. Dosage recommendations for pediatric patients have been published by the DHHS specifically for drugs used in the treatment of:
   a. asthma
   b. croup
   c. bronchitis
   d. respiratory syncytial virus
   e. all of the above

5. ACLS is an acronym for:
   a. adult–child life support
   b. advanced cardiac life support
   c. advanced child life support
   d. advanced critical life support
   e. adult cardiac life support

6. ACLS courses include skills and knowledge about:
   a. defibrillation, invasive hemodynamic monitoring, and cardiac resuscitation drugs
   b. cardiac dysrhythmia recognition and treatment, airway management, and medicolegal aspects of resuscitation

    c. acid–base balance, ventilation, and intubation

    d. postresuscitation management and special resuscitation situations

    e. all of the above

7. Most of the drugs recommended for use during cardiac resuscitation should be administered:

    I. orally

    II. intramuscularly

    III. intravenously

    IV. by aerosol

    V. by instillation

    a. II or III only

    b. II, III, or V only

    c. III or V only

    d. III or IV only

    e. I, II, III, IV, and V

8. The most recent revisions of ACLS standards were published:

    a. in *JAMA*, in 1992

    b. in *JAMA*, in 1987

    c. in the *Annals of Internal Medicine*, in 1991

    d. in *Chest*, in 1990

    e. none of the above

9. Isoproterenol is sometimes used during cardiac resuscitation as a:

    a. bronchodilator and antiarrhythmic

    b. temporary pacemaker

    c. vasopressor

    d. cardiac oxidant

    e. β agonist

10. Three *primary* drugs used during cardiac resuscitation include:

    a. isoproterenol, bretylium, and calcium chloride

    b. epinephrine, lidocaine, and atropine

    c. morphine, epinephrine, and levophed

    d. adrenalin, norepinephrine, and nitroglycerin

    e. sodium bicarbonate, epinephrine, and calcium

11. Dopamine and dobutamine are used during cardiac resuscitation to:

    a. increase cardiac output

    b. lower venous resistance

    c. reduce myocardial irritability

    d. increase urine output

    e. increase blood pressure

12. Sodium bicarbonate may be useful during cardiac resuscitation when:

    a. blood gases show a pH of less than 7.25

    b. perfusion is poor

    c. blood gases show a pH of greater than 7.25

d. the patient has a preexisting metabolic acidosis

e. both *a* and *d*

13. Which of the following cardiac resuscitation drugs may be useful for a patient with frequent premature ventricular contractions or runs of ventricular tachycardia?

    a. lidocaine and bretylium

    b. atropine and procainamide

    c. morphine and adenosine

    d. digitalis and bretylium

    e. epinephrine and lidocaine

14. Which of the following drugs may be useful as a prebronchoscopy aerosol agent?

    I. Novocain[R]

    II. lidocaine

    III. Xylocaine[R]

    IV. Narcan[R]

    V. procainamide

    a. I and II only

    b. II and III only

    c. II only

    d. I and IV only

    e. II, III, and V only

15. Which of the following is an appropriate drug and dosage for use prior to bronchoscopy?

    a. 4–6 mL of 2% lidocaine

    b. 4–7 mL of 4% Xylocaine[R]

    c. 3 mL of 1% Novocain[R]

    d. 3–5 mL of 2% procainamide

    e. both *a* and *b*

16. During bronchoscopy, the patient experiences paroxysmal coughing and some desaturation as noted by pulse oximetry. Which of the following should the RCP recommend?

    a. discontinue the procedure and place the patient on oxygen to restore saturation.

    b. instill 0.5–1.0 mL of 2% lidocaine into the trachea and add supplemental oxygen if desaturation persists.

    c. interrupt procedure until coughing has subsided, then add supplemental oxygen and continue.

    d. instill 3–5 mL of 4% lidocaine into the trachea and monitor oxygen saturation.

    e. instill 0.5–1.0 mL of 2% procainamide into the trachea and monitor oxygen saturation.

17. Bronchial provocation testing is performed:

    a. to determine which allergens cause bronchospasm in a specific patient

    b. to determine the degree of bronchospasm caused by a specific allergen in a given patient

    c. to determine if an asthma attack can be provoked by external stimuli such as stress or cold air

    d. to diagnose reactive airway disease in patients who do not have clinically apparent asthma

    e. both *a* and *d*

18. Methacholine can be categorized as a:

    a. β agonist

    b. β antagonist

    c. parasympathomimetic

    d. sympathomimetic

    e. xanthine agonist

19. Which of the following statements are true about methacholine?

    a. it increases bronchial secretions.

    b. it stimulates production of cyclic $3',5'$-guanosine monophosphate.

    c. it should be administered only by a breath-activated nebulizing device.

    d. onset may occur within 30 seconds of administration.

    e. all of the above

20. What is the recommended dosage of methacholine used during bronchial provocation testing?

    a. 2–3 breaths of the *strongest* solution, followed by measurement of FVC

    b. 3–5 breaths of the *strongest* solution, followed by measurement of inspiratory capacity

    c. 5 breaths of each dilution, beginning with the *most dilute* solution, followed by measurement of FVC after each dilution until 20% reduction in FEV_1 occurs

    d. 2–3 mL of each solution, beginning with the *most dilute* solution, test ends when 20% reduction in FVC occurs

    e. none of the above

REFERENCES/RECOMMENDED READING

American Heart Association: *Textbook of Advanced Cardiac Life Support*. American Heart Association, Dallas, 1987.

Emergency Cardiac Care Committee and Subcommittees, American Heart Association. Guidelines for cardiopulmonary resuscitation and emergency cardiac care. CPR Issue. *JAMA* 268(suppl):2199–2241, 1992.

Executive Summary: Guidelines for the Diagnosis and Management of Asthma. Publication No. 91–3042A, National Asthma Education Program, Office of Prevention, Education, and Control. National Heart, Lung, and Blood Institute, National Institutes of Health, Bethesda, MD, 1991.

Green E, Grauer K, Rothenberg M: Charting the future of emergency drug protocols. *Nursing* 92 June, 1992, pp 55–57.

Howder CL: *Cardiopulmonary Pharmacology*, Williams & Wilkins, Baltimore, 1992.

Ruppel G: *Manual of Pulmonary Function Testing*, 5th ed. Mosby-Year Book, Inc, St. Louis, 1991.

Whitaker K: *Neonatal and Pediatric Respiratory Care*. Delmar Publishing, Inc, Albany, NY, 1992, chap 9.

Ziment I: *Respiratory Pharmacology and Therapeutics*. WB Saunders Co, Philadelphia, 1978.

APPENDIX **A**

ANSWERS TO POSTTEST

CHAPTER 1

1. c
2. e
3. d
4. d
5. True

6. a
7. b
8. b
9. b
10. b

CHAPTER 2

1. c
2. d
3. d
4. c
5. True

6. a
7. c
8. d
9. a
10. c

CHAPTER 3

1. e
2. True
3. c
4. True
5. c
6. c

7. True
8. False
9. b
10. c
11. e
12. a

CHAPTER 4

1. c
2. a
3. c
4. b

5. True
6. False
7. d
8. True

CHAPTER 5

1. a	7. c
2. True	8. c
3. d	9. e
4. b	10. a
5. c	11. True
6. a	12. True

CHAPTER 6

1. b	4. c
2. True	5. b
3. c	6. True

CHAPTER 7

1. True	6. d
2. False	7. b
3. b	8. True
4. c	9. d
5. a	10. False

CHAPTER 8

1. False	6. False
2. c	7. a
3. True	8. b
4. b	9. True
5. e	10. c

CHAPTER 9

1. d	4. a
2. b	5. c
3. True	

CHAPTER 10

1. b	7. b
2. c	8. a
3. a	9. d
4. c	10. e
5. d	11. e
6. c	12. b

CHAPTER 11

1. b	9. e
2. a	10. a
3. e	11. e
4. c	12. b
5. b	13. c
6. d	14. e
7. a	15. d
8. c	

CHAPTER 12

1. e	9. d
2. e	10. a
3. e	11. d
4. d	12. a
5. c	13. e
6. b	14. c
7. b	15. d
8. b	

CHAPTER 13

1. b	7. d
2. a	8. a
3. e	9. b
4. b	10. d
5. c	11. c
6. e	

CHAPTER 14

1. a	9. a
2. c	10. e
3. b	11. c
4. a	12. b
5. e	13. d
6. d	14. a
7. d	15. b
8. c	

CHAPTER 15

1. b	9. a
2. e	10. d
3. b	11. d
4. a	12. b
5. d	13. e
6. e	14. a
7. c	15. c
8. c	

CHAPTER 16

1. c	11. e
2. d	12. d
3. e	13. a
4. a	14. b
5. b	15. e
6. e	16. b
7. c	17. d
8. a	18. c
9. b	19. e
10. b	20. c

APPENDIX B

CASE STUDIES

This appendix presents the following case studies:

1. Aerosol Techniques
2. Chronic Obstructive Pulmonary Disease
3. Acute Severe Asthma
4. Home Care for COPD
5. Cystic Fibrosis (Mucoviscidosis)
6. Severe Respiratory Syncytial Virus Infection
7. Positive Human Immunodeficiency Virus Status
8. Aspergillosis
9. Acute Asthma
10. Postextubation Stridor
11. Bronchiolitis
12. Acute Mountain Sickness—Pulmonary Edema
13. Infant Respiratory Distress Syndrome
14. Diagnostic Bronchoscopy
15. Methacholine Challenge
16. Ventricular Tachycardia

The answers to all case study questions can be found at the end of the appendix.

CASE 1: AEROSOL TECHNIQUES (CHAPTER 10)

Martha G., a 33-year-old (66-kg, 5'4") female, had nausea and vomiting for 4 days. She was examined in the outpatient clinic and sent home on trimethoprim-sulfamethoxazole (Bactrim[R]). The day before hospital admission, she was seen in the emergency room for asthma. She was treated with albuterol by metered dose inhaler (MDI) 3 times. Patient refused arterial blood gases and chest radiograph. She was sent home with albuterol and ipratropium inhalers. The next day she became increasingly dyspneic and was being driven by a friend to the emergency room (ER) when she collapsed in the car. Her friend pulled into a nearby fire station, where cardiopulmonary resuscitation (CPR) was initiated. She was intubated by ambulance paramedics and found to be in pulseless electrical activity (PEA). CPR was continued after arrival at the ER, with recovery of a pulse. The patient was stabilized and moved to the Pulmonary Medicine intensive care unit (ICU), where she was placed on a mechanical ventilator. The electrocardiogram (ECG) showed a pulse rate of 140/minute with ST segment depression throughout.

History and Physical Exam

History. Patient has a history of asthma and has had an appendectomy. Tob 1 PPD ×
10 years. No history of alcohol use.
Vital Signs. Heart rate-118 beats/minute; blood pressure-151/100 mm Hg; tempera-
ture-35°C.
Neurologic. No response to pain, silent electroencephalogram, and pupils fixed and
dilated.
Respiratory. Bilateral inspiratory and expiratory wheezes, minimal air movement, and
moderate amount of cloudy secretions.

Laboratory Values

Chest Radiograph. Hyperaeration.

Diagnosis

1. Status asthmaticus
2. PEA
3. Post-code anoxic encephalopathy

Hospital Orders

Medications.

Vecuronium (Norcuron^R)   Co-trimoxazole (Bactrim^R)
Midazolam (Versed^R)   Ranitidine (Zantac^R)
Diazepam (Valium^R)   Methylprednisolone (Solu-Medrol^R)
Furosemide (Lasix^R)   Theophylline (Slo-Bid^R)
Gentamicin   Acetaminophen
Albuterol (Ventolin^R)

Questions

1. On the day before admission, the patient was seen in the ER for asthma. What test
   would have helped evaluate this patient's degree of airway obstruction? Can the severity
   of airway obstruction be assessed by observation alone?
2. When the patient was seen in the ER the day before admission, she was given albuterol
   MDI 3 times and sent home on albuterol and ipratropium inhalers. Given the situation,
   how appropriate was this course of action?
3. During this patient's resuscitation, what avenues for drug administration became
   available?

CASE 2: CHRONIC OBSTRUCTIVE PULMONARY DISEASE (CHAPTER 11)

A 57-year-old female was admitted for increasing shortness of breath (SOB). She has had recurrent exacerbations of her chronic obstructive pulmonary disease (COPD). Her chief complaints are worsening SOB, yellow sputum production, and general malaise.

History and Physical Exam

History.   The patient was diagnosed as having COPD 10 years ago. She has hypertension, cor pulmonale, and hyperthyroidism. Her $FEV_{1.0}$ 6 months ago = 0.9 L.
Vital Signs.   Heart rate = 160 beats/minute; respiratory rate = 27 breaths/minute; blood pressure = 150/90 mm Hg; temperature 38°F.
Clinical Appearance.   Cushingoid.
Neurologic.   Pupils equal and react to light and accommodation.
Cardiovascular.   No jugular venous distention.
Respiratory.   Expiratory wheezes and decreased breath sounds. Use of accessory muscles. $FEV_{1.0}$ = 0.67 L before bronchodilator and 0.74 L after bronchodilator.

Laboratory Values

Chest Radiograph.   Mild diffuse emphysema with parenchymal fibrosis. Right upper lung diffusely replaced by blebs and bullae. No congestive heart failure, pneumonia, or pleural effusion.
Arterial Blood Gases.   On 2 L/minute nasal cannula: pH = 7.41; pCO_2 = 50 torr; pO_2 = 99 torr.
Electrolytes. Na^+ = 139 mEq/L; K^+ = 4.6 mEq/L; Cl^- = 95 mEq/L; HCO_3^- = 34 mEq/L.
Hematology.   Hgb = 15.8 g/dL; WBC count = 12, 400/mm^3.

Hospital Course

Days 1–4.   Although the patient slept better initially after receiving oxygen and bronchodilator therapy, she still had trouble clearing her secretions, despite PD&V. Acetylcysteine was ordered with the bronchodilator treatments. A sputum sample was obtained. Gram stain revealed gram-positive cocci in chains. A sputum culture and sensitivity test was ordered.
Day 5.   Acetylcysteine was not well tolerated. Sputum sample revealed heavy growth of α-hemolytic streptococci. Gentamicin 40 mg was ordered via aerosol therapy.
Day 7.   Patient developed slight edema of the extremities. Lasix[R] 20 mg PO ordered.
Day 11.   The patient complained of worsening SOB. Arterial blood gases on oxygen 2 L/minute by nasal cannula: pH = 7.41; pCO_2 = 60 torr; pO_2 = 63 torr. Patient was transferred to the Pulmonary Medicine ICU.

Hospital Orders

Respiratory Care.
1. Oxygen 2 L/minute by nasal cannula
2. Albuterol 0.5 mL in NS
3. Atrovent[R] 2 puffs
4. Postural drainage and vibration (PD&V)

Medications.

Ceftazidime

Methylprednisolone

Guaifenesin

Verapamil

Phosphate mixture

Heparin SQ

Questions

1. Why was 0.5 mL of albuterol used?
2. Is there any problem giving Atrovent[R] to patients with retained secretions?
3. Are inhaled steroids indicated for this patient?

CASE 3: ACUTE SEVERE ASTHMA (CHAPTER 11)

Sally C. is a 32-year-old female with a history of asthma admitted to the ER in acute distress. She was hospitalized 6 weeks prior to this admission for an acute exacerbation of asthma with acute bronchitis. She has had a respiratory infection with nonpurulent sputum production for the past week.

History and Physical Exam

History. This patient has been hospitalized for severe exacerbation of asthma four times over the last 2 years. Intubation was required during one admission.

Family History. Father deceased. Respiratory failure from asthma. Mother has chronic bronchitis, brother has asthma.

Vital Signs. Heart rate = 170 beats/minute; blood pressure = 130/70 mm Hg; respiratory rate = 30 breaths/minute.

Cardiovascular. Tachycardia.

Respiratory. Patient is in severe respiratory distress. Breath sounds decreased throughout, with inspiratory and expiratory wheezes.

Laboratory Values

Chest Radiograph. Hyperinflation without infiltrates.

Arterial Blood Gases. On oxygen 6 L/minute: pH = 7.29; pCO_2 = 48 torr; pO_2 = 152 torr.

Blood Chemistry. Theophylline 13 μg/mL.

Electrolytes. $HCO_3^- = 21$ mEq/L.

Hematology.   Hgb = 11.8 g/dL; Hct = 42.2 percent; WBC count = $11,500/mm^3$.

Hospital Course

Day 1.   Patient was placed on oxygen 6 L/minute by nasal cannula. Her $FEV_{1.0}$ was 35 percent of the predicted value. Blood was drawn for arterial blood gases, theophylline level, and blood chemistry. Both systemic β_2 agonists and corticosteroids were given immediately. An aerosol treatment via SVN with 0.5 mL of albuterol in 3 mL of saline was given with little improvement. Two puffs of Atrovent[R] then were given. After 20 minutes another treatment was given; the patient improved slightly. Continuous aerosol therapy with albuterol was initiated after another 20 minutes. The patient continued to improve gradually over the next 4 hours. She then was transferred to the Pulmonary Medicine service and placed on albuterol 0.5 mL/3 mL saline and beclomethasone MDI q2h. Inspiratory and expiratory wheezes cleared after treatments.

Day 2.   The patient continued to improve. Aerosol treatments were decreasd to 3 times a day. Chest radiograph showed a decrease in hyperinflation without infiltrates. Sputum culture revealed *Streptococcus pneumoniae*. Patient was titrated to room air with a S_aO_2 of 94%. Peak expiratory flow rate (PEFR) was 175 L/minute.

Day 3.   Aerosol treatments changed to albuterol MDI 4 times a day and beclomethasone MDI 4 times a day. Breath sounds are now clear and slightly decreased. PEF-265 L/minute.

Day 4.   No change in the patient's condition. PEF-250 L/minute. The patient was reminded to use her spacer with both MDIs and discharged on her previous home medications of prednisone, albuterol MDI, and beclomethasone MDI.

Questions

1. Why was the theophylline blood level checked in the ER and was it within therapeutic range?
2. Was continuous aerosol administration indicated in this situation? What side effects could be expected with maximal doses of β_2 agonists? What was the alternative course of action?
3. Given this patient's $FEV_{1.0}$ in the ER, does the arterial pCO_2 coincide with the degree of airway obstruction?

CASE 4: HOME CARE FOR COPD (CHAPTER 12)

A 69-year-old female was referred to pulmonary services by her home-town physician. She has had a 5-day history of increasing shortness of breath, dyspnea on exertion, and $\frac{1}{2}$ cup of yellow sputum production per day. Patient denies a history of hemoptypsis, chest pain, palpitations, or ankle swelling. She admits to having fever without chills, orthopnea, and postnasal drip. She has never been treated for COPD and has no known history of asthma or tuberculosis. She is not currently on any medication.

History and Physical Exam

History.   Chronic bronchitis.
Social History.   Heavy tobacco use (2 packs/day $\times$ 50 years); still smokes. Alcohol use ($\frac{1}{2}$ case beer/day) in past but not for several years.
Vital Signs.   Heart rate = 130 beats/minute; blood pressure = 146/86 mm Hg; respiratory rate = 37 breaths/minute; temperature = 37°C.
Clinical Appearance.   Clubbing, arthritis, and no edema.
Respiratory.   Decreased breath sounds with expiratory wheezes.

Laboratory Values

Chest Radiograph.   Changes consistent with emphysema. Possible bleb areas in right upper and left upper lobes. Haziness of left lower lobe may represent pneumonitis.
Arterial Blood Gases.   On room air: pH = 7.53; pCO_2 = 35 torr; pO_2 = 41 torr. On oxygen 4 L/minute via nasal cannula: pH = 7.53; pCO_2 = 35 torr; pO_2 = 61 torr.
Blood Chemistry.   Glucose = 186 mg/dL.
Electrolytes.   Within normal limits.
Hematology.   WBC count = 19,900/mm^3.

Hospital Course

Day 1.   Patient received IV steroids and bronchodilators, inhaled bronchodilators, and oxygen via nasal cannula at 4 L/minute. Arterial blood gases, blood chemistry, and sputum culture were obtained. Patient was started on antibiotics. Bedside pulmonary function tests: FVC = 0.9 L; $FEV_{1.0}$ = 0.7 L (34% of predicted value). Sputum production was decreased and work of breathing was reduced on oxygen.
Days 2–5.   Pneumonia resolving. WBC = 9600/mm^3. Ausculation reveals crackles and expiratory wheezes.
Day 6.   Crackles and wheezes persist in the lower lobes. Arterial blood gases: pH = 7.46; pCO_2 = 39 torr; pO_2 = 64 torr.
Days 7 and 8.   Pneumonia has resolved. Pulmonary condition remains unchanged. Patient is started on prednisone. Instructions for home use of albuterol MDI with spacer and ipratropium MDI with spacer are prescribed. Arrangements for home oxygen use also are started. Patient discharged.

Medications.

Solu-Medrol^R Lasix^R
Aminophylline   Benadryl
Ampicillin   TheoDur^R
Gentamycin   Prednisone
Alupent^R

Questions

1. What MDI instructions are important when spacers are used?
2. What other instructions for MDI use should be given when a patient is discharged?
3. What additional information relative to her pulmonary disease may benefit this patient?

CASE 5: CYSTIC FIBROSIS (MUCOVISCIDOSIS) (CHAPTER 12)

Toby W., a 17-year-old, white, 150-lb male, was admitted to the adolescent unit with a chief complaint of exacerbation of his previously diagnosed cystic fibrosis (CF) and weight loss of 3 months' duration.

History and Physical Exam

History. The patient was diagnosed as having CF at age 3 months (sweat chloride test +4). He is currently on enzyme replacement therapy, postural drainage and coughing (PD&C) QID, aerosol treatment QID, and oxygen PRN at 2 L/minute via nasal cannula. Usual childhood inoculations and illness.

Family History. Toby is the third of three children; the other children are living and well with no signs of CF. Both parents are living and well, as are both maternal and one paternal grandparent. Toby is in a mainstream school but is 2 years behind his age group in school. Patient denies smoking, alcohol or recreational drug use. Patient recently has started dating.

Vital Signs. Pulse = 84, steady and bounding; blood pressure = 130/80 mm Hg; respiratory rate = 18 breaths/minute; temperature = 99.9°F (oral); SpO$_2$ = 89 percent.

Neurologic. Pupils equal and react to light and accommodation. Oriented $\times$ 3.

Psychiatric. Toby is becoming depressed and fatalistic. Typical statements include "What's the use? CFers die early," "I get stared at all the time because of my coughing," and "Why can't I be like normal kids?"

Cardiovascular. Heart sounds bounding and slightly distant. ECG shows changes consistent with left ventricular hypertrophy (LVH).

Respiratory. Decreased lower lobe sounds bilaterally; crackles and ronchi noted in bases during active inspiration and expiration. Cough loose, "sticky," and nonproductive. Expiratory wheezing noted on exertion.

Gastrointestinal. Patient has lost 20 lb in last 3 weeks. No complaints of pain or discomfort. Appetite decreased; states, "I don't want to use enzymes any more; I want to eat what regular people do."

Skin. Dry, nonresilient.

Genitourinary. Within normal limits.

Laboratory Values

Chest Radiograph.   Comparison with films of 3 months age reveals increased opacities in lower lobes bilaterally and presence of air bronchograms. Increased left ventricular size. *Note:* Films are consistent with advanced CF and increased mucus production and retention. LVH suggests increased pulmonary vascular resistance.

Arterial Blood Gases.   pH = 7.36; pCO_2 = 44 torr; pO_2 = 80 torr; F_IO_2 = 0.21.

Electrolytes. Na^+ = 150 mEq/L; K^+ = 4.0 mEq/L; Cl^- = 115 mEq/L; HCO_3^- = 30 mEq/L.

Hematology.   White blood cell (WBC) count = 30,000/mm^3; hemoglobin (Hgb) = 20 g/dL; hematocrit (HCT) = 54 percent.

Diagnosis

1. Exacerbation of CF.
2. Pulmonary tract infection ? pneumonia.
3. Malnutrition/dehydration.
4. Depression.

Hospital Orders

Respiratory Care.

1. Continuous high-humidity aerosol with 24% oxygen.
2. Aerosolized $NaHCO_3$ 3–5 mL q4h via small-volume nebulizer (SVN)
   alternate with
3. Aerosolized CF "cocktail" via SVN q4h + PRN:
   3.0 mL 20% Mucomyst Solution^R
   3.0 mL normal saline (NS)
   3 drops Bronkosol^R 1:100
4. Ventolin^R MDI × 2 puffs 10 seconds before all aerosol treatments.
5. PD&C q4h.
6. Proceed PD&C with 1 puff Ventolin^R MDI.

Diet.

1. High-protein, high-calorie, low carbohydrate supplements to keep caloric intake over 5,000 kCal/day.
2. Monitor $ETCO_2$ TID.

Questions

1. What is the purpose of administering a Ventolin MDI treatment prior to each aerosol treatment? What is the rationale for giving another MDI treatment before PD&C?
2. How can the cystic fibrosis "cocktail" be modified to reduce its nebulization time?
3. Why is $NaHCO_3$ being nebulized? How do the effects of $NaHCO_3$ differ from those of Mucomyst?

4. What particular hazards must be anticipated as a result of the use of wetting agents (heated high humidity), bronchodilators, mucolytics, and PD&C?

5. What other strategies should/could be considered, instead of or in addition to the use of mucolytics and PD&C, to treat Toby's problem of thick, tenacious secretions?

6. What suggestions do you have for the type of solutions or drugs to be administered in the continuous high-humidity device? Why?

CASE 6: SEVERE RESPIRATORY SYNCYTIAL VIRUS INFECTION (CHAPTER 13)

Emily R. is a 7-month-old (5-kg) female. She was taken by her parents to the pediatric outpatient clinic because of increasing respiratory distress. Her parents state that she had a runny nose, cough, and poor appetite for 2 days prior to being seen in the clinic. After examining the infant, the pediatrician diagnosed bronchiolitis and mild dehydration. Hospital admission was recommended because of the medical history of the infant and the severity of the respiratory distress.

History and Physical Exam

History. The patient was a premature birth (30 weeks' gestational age) and has bronchopulmonary dysplasia (on low-flow oxygen at home).
Vital Signs. Heart rate = 140 beats/minute; respiratory rate = 68 breaths/minute; temperature = 38.5°C.
Respiratory. Chest wall retractions, nasal flaring. Cyanosis of mucous membranes. Bilateral retractions. S_aO_2 90 percent.

Laboratory Values

Arterial Blood Gases. pH = 7.48; pCO_2 = 35 torr; pO_2 = 58 torr.
Electrolytes. HCO_3^- = 28 mEq/L.
Hematology. Hgb = 11.0 g/dL; WBC count = 9100/mm^3.

Hospital Orders

1. Hydration.
2. Oxygen hood.
3. Maintain S_aO_2 above 90 percent.
4. Aerosol treatments with albuterol 4 times daily.
5. Secretion specimen to laboratory to test for presence of respiratory syncytial virus (RSV) (ELISA test).

Several hours later the physician was notified by the laboratory that RSV had been identified in the specimen. Based on this confirming evidence, the physician contacted the respiratory care department to initiate ribavirin therapy.

Questions

1. What criteria are used to determine the need for ribavirin delivery?
2. What equipment is appropriate for delivery of ribavirin to this infant?
3. What are the equipment concerns with respect to ribavirin administration?
4. What precautions should be taken to minimize the risk of ribavirin contact for health care personnel and family members?

CASE 7: POSITIVE HUMAN IMMUNODEFICIENCY VIRUS STATUS (CHAPTER 13)

John R. is a 28-year old male who was confirmed as having positive human immunodeficiency virus (HIV) status 4 years ago. He has felt well until recently, when he began to experience increased fatigue and weight loss.

History and Physical Exam

History. The patient has had the usual childhood diseases and is allergic to penicillin and sulfonamide antibiotics.
Social History. Intravenous drug use during age period 20–24 years. Quit smoking 3 years ago.
Vital Signs. Heart rate = 80 beats/minute; respiratory rate = 20 breaths/minute; blood pressure = 110/80 mm Hg; temperature = $37.2°C$.
Respiratory. Breath sounds clear to auscultation. S_aO_2 = 94 percent.

Laboratory Values

Chest Radiograph. Normal appearance.
Blood Chemistry. Glucose, blood urea nitrogen, and creatinine within normal limits.
Electrolytes. Within normal limits.
Immunodiagnostic Studies. CD4+ lymphocytes = $160/mm^3$.

Questions

1. What are the indications for administering pentamidine aerosol to this patient?
2. What factors are important in selecting equipment for delivery of the drug by aerosol?
3. What precautions should be taken to minimize risk to the care provider?
4. What adverse effects may occur in a patient who is given pentamidine aerosol?

CASE 8: ASPERGILLOSIS (CHAPTER 13)

Mark M. is a 24-year-old male who came to the ER complaining of increasing shortness of breath, chest pain, fever, and cough productive of brood-streaked sputum. He has had five previous admissions to the hospital with pulmonary infections, including the diagnosis and treatment of tuberculosis 2 years prior to this admission. He is known to be a chronic user of intravenous heroin. On physical examination, he is noted to be tachypneic and using accessory muscles of respiration. He appears pale and malnourished.

History and Physical Exam

Vital Signs.   Blood pressure = 130/85 mm Hg; heart rate = 110 beats/minute; respiratory rate = 35 breaths/minute; temperature = 39.2°C.
Cardiovascular.   Sinus tachycardia.
Respiratory.   Tachypnea, rhonchi bilaterally, and scattered wheezes. S_aO_2 = 90 percent.

Laboratory Values

Chest Radiograph.   Bilateral cavitations in upper lobes with "crescent sign" (solid mass separated from cavity wall by a crescent of air) suggestive of aspergillomas.
Arterial Blood Gases.   On room air: pH = 7.49; pCO_2 = 34 torr; pO_2 = 60 torr.
Blood Chemistry.   Blood urea nitrogen and creatinine within normal limits.
Electrolytes.   Within normal limits.
Hematology.   WBC count = 5600/mm^3; Hgb = 8.4 g/dL; HCT = 30 percent.

Hospital Orders

1. Sputum Gram stain, culture and sensitivity.
2. Acid-fast test.
3. Serum precipitins.

The acid-fast test is negative; *Aspergillus fumigatus* is identified in sputum. Positive precipitin test.
Treatment.
1. Intravenous amphotericin B therapy.
2. Nutritional supplementation.

Questions

1. What rationale may exist for the addition of aerosolized amphotericin B to the patient's medication regimen?
2. What other aerosolized medication should be administered when amphotericin B is delivered by SVN?
3. What are the limiting factors when delivering this anti-infective medication by aerosol?
4. What precautions should be taken to protect the health care worker during administration of the drug.

CASE 9: ACUTE ASTHMA (CHAPTER 14)

Cornelia A., a 55-year-old black female with a history of asthma, came to the emergency room complaining of SOB. She became increasingly dyspneic over the last 2 days. The patient was taking the following medicines at home: Ventolin[R] (hourly just before admission), Vanceril[R], and prednisone (55 mg/day per physician order). Yesterday, she was started on ampicillin for a "cold" that produced yellow-green sinus drainage and chest congestion. This is a well-developed, well-nourished black female in obvious respiratory distress.

History and Physical Exam

History.   Steroid-dependent asthma since 1988. Episodes of pulmonary infections. Home medications: prednisone 10 mg/day, Vanceril[R] MDI 2 puffs QID; Ventolin[R] MDI 2 puffs QID.

Family History.   Brother with adult-onset asthma.

Vital Signs.   Blood pressure = 150/90 mm Hg; heart rate = 100 beats/minute; respiratory rate = 28 breaths/minute; afebrile.

Respiratory.   Diffuse inspiratory and expiratory wheezing without crackles.

Laboratory Values

Chest Radiograph.   Hyperinflation without infiltrates.

Arterial Blood Gases.   pH = 7.35; pCO_2 = 37 torr; pO_2 = 65 torr.

Electrolytes.   Within normal limits.

Hematology.   WBC count = 9400/mm^3; Hgb = 12.4 g/dL; HCT = 37 percent.

Pulmonary Function.

MEASURED	PATIENT BASELINE	PREDICTED
$FEV_{1.0}$ 0.7	1.2 L	2.69 L
FVC 1.4	2.2 L	3.65 L
PEFR 115 L/min		

The patient is admitted to the pulmonary service and started on 2 L/minute oxygen by nasal cannula. As the nurse is settling the patient in her room, you are asked by the physician to recommend the type of respiratory medications the patient should receive. Keeping this request in mind, please answer the following questions.

Questions

1. Should the patient receive IV *and* aerosol steroid therapy? Explain your answer.
2. What type of bronchodilator should the patient receive? What frequency would you recommend?
3. Should the patient be started on cromolyn sodium? Explain your answer.

4. What type of test would you administer to monitor the effectiveness of the therapy? Explain your answer.

CASE 10: POSTEXTUBATION STRIDOR (CHAPTER 14)

Tommy N., a 35-year-old white, obese (192 kg [422 lbs]) male, presented in the ER with a complaint of SOB. Shortly after admission, the patient went into ventilatory failure and was electively intubated. Arterial blood gases at that time were pH = 7.30, pCO_2 = 63 torr, and pO_2 = 47 torr on room air. The patient had been having difficulty breathing for a long time, with extreme loud snoring and daytime somnolence. The patient also had been experiencing inability to stay awake, with periods of apneic breathing during sleep. Over the past 4 days the patient's dyspnea worsened until he could not walk to the bathroom. He had been sleeping sitting up.

History and Physical Exam

History. Abdominal surgery (?).
Social History. Smokes 2 packs/day, does not use alcohol. Unemployed.
Vital Signs. Blood pressure = 166/106 mm Hg; temperature = 37°C; heart rate = 100 beats/minute.
Neurologic. Pupils equal and react to light and accommodation.
Cardiovascular. Heart beat distant but regular. No jugular venous distention.
Respiratory. Basilar fine crackles.
Gastrointestinal. Old healed abdominal scar, unable to palpate liver or spleen.
Extremities. 4+ Pedal edema.

Laboratory Values

Chest Radiograph. Cardiomegaly with bilateral, fluffy infiltrates and pulmonary edema.
Electrolytes. Within normal limits.
Hematology. Red blood cell (RBC) count 5.34 M/mm^3; Hgb = 16 g/dL; WBC count = 21,000/mm^3.

Hospital Course

Days 1–3. The patient's ventilator settings are A/C = 14, V_T = 800 mL, F_iO_2 = 0.5, S_aO_2 = 97 percent. He slept for 36 hours and was unresponsive when first aroused. Wheezes were heard throughout the lung and suctioning returned a large amount of yellow secretions from the endotracheal tube. On Day 2, he was reintubated because of a large cuff leak. *Medications:* Lasix^R, Captopril^R, MDI albuterol, cefazolin, acetaminophen, Reglan^R, morphine, IV fluids containing KCl and albumin.
Days 4–6. Pitting edema is improved. The patient has lost 17.5 kg since admission. On Day 4, the patient was started on a pressure support trial of 5 cm H_2O. Pressure

support trials were progressively lengthened until, on Day 6, the pulmonary function parameters indicated the patient could be extubated. Following extubation, the patient developed stridor. *Medications:* Lasix[R], Captopril[R], MDI albuterol, cefazolin, acetaminophen, Provera[R]

Questions

1. What could be causing this patient's respiratory difficulty?
2. What respiratory drug could you recommend to the physician that would help relieve the patient's stridor? Explain the rationale for your recommendation.
3. Could another drug (systemic or respiratory) be given to the patient to treat the cause of the stridor?

CASE 11: BRONCHIOLITIS (CHAPTER 14)

Jerry M., a 5-month-old, 7-kg white male, was admitted with a chief complaint of respiratory distress. The infant was in good health until 3 days ago, when he developed a fever, cough, and runny nose. He was treated by his doctor with PO erythromycin. The infant's cough worsened and he was taken to the hospital ER by his parents. On admission, the baby was actively wheezing and retracting. His S_aO_2 was 75 percent on oxygen at 5 L/minute by facemask. Patient appears to be a well-developed, well-nourished, white male infant in severe respiratory distress.

Physical Exam

Vital Signs. Temperature = 38.8°C; heart rate = 200 beats/minute; respiratory rate = 80–90 breaths/minute.
Cardiovascular. Tachycardia, normal rhythm.
Respiratory. Diffuse wheezes bilaterally, tachypnea, nasal flaring, subcostal retractions.

Laboratory Values

Chest Radiograph. Hyperinflation with right upper lobe infiltrates.
Arterial Blood Gases.

	pH	pCO$_2$ (TORR)	pO$_2$ (TORR)	OXYGEN
Day 1	7.41	33	54	10 L/min, facemask (ER)
	7.39	30	120	100%, hood
Day 2	7.42	34	65	60%, hood

Electrolytes. Within normal limits.
Hematology. Hgb = 10.2 g/dL; WBC count = 10,700/mm^3; RBC count = 3.81 M/mm^3.

Hospital Orders

Respiratory Care.
1. Continuous albuterol 2 mL/hour.
2. Oxygen hood on 100 percent, wean for S_aO_2's greater than 95 percent.
3. Continuous pulse oximetry and transcutaneous monitor.

Other Medications.
IV Solu-Medrol^R	Acetaminophen
Cefuroxine	IV fluids

Hospital Course

Day 1.   The patient was admitted to the Pediatric ICU in respiratory distress. He was put in a oxygen hood at 100 percent oxygen with continuous aerosolized albuterol therapy. A secretion sample was obtained for RSV culture.

Day 2.   After the arterial blood gases on F_iO_2 of 1.0, the F_iO_2 was decreased to 0.60 in early A.M. Continuous aerosolized albuterol will be changed to q2h when baby improves. The patient's respiratory rate and breathing effort have decreased.

Day 3.   The baby is improved. Continuous aerosol therapy is discontinued and the baby was started on q2h albuterol treatments. RSV culture was positive.

Questions

1. Why was continuous aerosolized albuterol therapy used in this baby's illness?
2. While the infant was receiving continuous aerosolized albuterol, what dose of albuterol was the infant receiving each minute?
3. When the baby's bronchodilator therapy was changed from continuous administration to every 2 hours, if you used *Fried's rule*, what dose of albuterol should the infant receive during each treatment?
4. What other respiratory-related medications could have been used in the treatment of this baby's bronchiolitis?
5. Are bronchodilators the primary medication used in the treatment of bronchiolitis? Why or why not?

CASE 12: ACUTE MOUNTAIN SICKNESS—PULMONARY EDEMA (CHAPTER 15)

Giles K-B. was an otherwise healthy 42-year-old white male college professor until the day of admission. On that day he flew from Tampa, Florida (elevation, sea level [0 feet]) to Salt Lake City, Utah (altitude, 4280 feet [1320 m]) and from there traveled by car to a ski resort about 2500 feet (667 m) above Park City, Utah. This trip resulted in a change of altitude of over 9800 feet (2,970 m) over a 6–8-hour period. Over the next several hours, Giles complained of SOB, headaches, general malaise, nausea, and aches and pains in his joints. He was noted to be increasingly disoriented, with progressive loss of sensorium. His colleagues called the local Emergency Medical Services (EMS) system, who responded immediately, bringing him to the local clinic.

On arrival and examination, a provisional diagnosis of acute mountain sickness (AMS) was made by the rescue squad and confirmed by the EMS physician controller based on symptoms described by telemetry. Orders to transport to Salt Lake City via helicopter were given. As the chopper took off, Giles became increasingly more disoriented and SOB. As the chopper rose, the flight paramedics (a registered nurse and a registered respiratory therapy/emergency medicine intensive care technician) immediately noted the onset of acute pulmonary edema and ordered the chopper to land, requesting land transport.

History and Physical Exam

History.   Past medical history noncontributory. The patient is an acutely distressed middle-aged white male. He is gasping for breath and complaining of exertional chest pain, headache, joint pains, and fatigue. He is diaphoretic and exhibits +3/+4 pedal edema. He is cyanotic, with reduced capillary refill time. Patient denies drug use; alcohol use, 1 beer today.

Vital Signs: Heart rate = 110 beats/minute; blood pressure = 140/100 mm Hg; respiratory rate = 35 breaths/minute; temperature = 37.9°C tymp

Cardiovascular.   Pulse is rapid and thready. Heart sounds full but masked by breath sounds.

Respiratory.   Auscultation revels wet, bubbling rales in all lung fields. Percussion nonspecific. Moist bubbling sound apparent on both inspiration and expiration without stethoscope. S_pO_2 = 85 percent on 100 percent oxygen.

Questions

1. Why did the helicopter crew decide to abort the flight and rely instead on ground transportation?
2. The physician controller ordered that the patient be given an IV dose of a glucocorticosteroid (prednisone). What rationale is there for this decision?
3. The physician also ordered administration of ethyl alcohol (ETOH) by intermittent positive pressure breathing (IPPB) with pressures of 25–30 cm H_2O and a prolonged expiratory time. He requested that oxygen be used as the power gas. Explain the logic behind these orders.
4. Should the physician consider drugs or procedures to decrease pulmonary wedge pressure in this patient? If so, what would you suggest that could be instituted on the scene? Why?

CASE 13: INFANT RESPIRATORY DISTRESS SYNDROME (CHAPTER 15)

(Prematurity, ? 2° to maternal cocaine use)

Baby Boy Chou is a 590-g Oriental male born at a gestational age of 27 weeks by Ballard score. His mother has a positive history of recreational drug use, including cocaine, marijuana, alcohol, and tobacco. The mother claims drugs were discontinued at 2–3 months' gestation. Maternal drug screen was negative. Prenatal care was episodic and poorly compliant. The baby was born of a precipitous labor in the ER of the 150-bed general hospital that does not have a Neonatal ICU service. Luckily, you have been through a Premature Infant Stabilization Course (PISC) given by the local Level III Neonatal ICU and are certified to implement the PISC protocol. A local obstetrician is called and arrives shortly after the delivery.

Physical Examination

Length = 30.0 cm; weight = 590 g (1.3 lbs); head circumference = 19.5 cm; color: blue; APGARs = 2, 2, and 4 at 1, 5, and 10 minutes.

Vital Signs.   Respiratory rate = 60 breaths/minute; heart rate = 159 beats/minute.

Neurologic.   Slow, weak reactions to pain and auditory stimulation.

Cardiovascular.   Regular rhythm and rate without murmurs.

Respiratory.   Weak, gasping, grunting respirations with bilateral rales.

Laboratory Values

Chest Radiograph.   Endotracheal tube in place. Hazy bilateral lung fields. *Impression:* Infant respiratory distress syndrome (IRDS) secondary to prematurity and maternal drug use.

Arterial Blood Gases.   pH = 7.27; pCO_2 = 47 torr; pO_2 = 42 torr; F_iO_2 = 100 percent; saturation = 84 percent.

Diagnosis

1. Respiratory distress syndrome
2. Prematurity

Hospital Orders

1. Oxygen to bring pO_2 to 65 torr.
2. Intubate.
3. Surfactant instillation per PISC protocol.
4. Monitor arterial blood gases.
5. Transport to Level III Neonatal ICU.

The physician asks that you direct the care of this baby as it is related to the PISC protocol. (*Note:* The PISC is the standard administration methodology for this drug.) As you are administering the drug, other interested caregivers watch and ask you the following questions regarding the drug and the procedures.

Questions

1. What are the sources of surfactant and how does the surfactant from each source differ?
2. I have heard surfactant called a detergent. Can you explain that to me? Is it like my laundry detergent?
3. How does surfactant make it easier for the baby to breathe?
4. What is the difference between the *prevention* and *rescue* procedures we have heard about?
5. What procedures must accompany the instillation of surfactant?
6. What changes in the patient's physiology should we anticipate after surfactant delivery? Describe any important side effects to watch for when administering surfactant.

Bonus.

7. Discuss the use of maternal steroid administration as an alternative to surfactant instillation in preventing or treating IRDS.

CASE 14: DIAGNOSTIC BRONCHOSCOPY (CHAPTER 16)

José A. is a 47-year-old Hispanic male who presented several days ago at his physician's office complaining of "trouble swallowing, noisy breathing and I can't breathe when I sleep." Questioning revealed a slow onset of symptoms over the past year. Mr. A has been referred to the Pulmonary Diagnostics Lab for a flexible fiberoptic bronchoscopic examination.

History and Physical Exam

Work History. The patient is a well-developed 47-year-old Hispanic male who works as a lead development technician in a chemical plant. He has held this job for 10 years. In his job, he is exposed to various chemical compounds, some of which are newly developed and whose properties are poorly, if at all, understood. Although Mr. A uses appropriate protective devices and clothing, occasional spills and circumstances expose him to these chemicals.

Vital Signs. Heart rate = 86 beats/minute; blood pressure = 126/82 mm Hg; respiratory rate = 18 breaths/minute; temperature = 37°C oral.

Cardiovascular. Within normal limits.

Respiratory. Audible stridor on both inspiration and expiration. Visibly delayed filling and emptying on right side. Reduced breath sounds in right lung. Forced expiration reveals wheezing and delayed breath sounds on right. *Impression:* Right bronchial obstruction of unknown origin.

Laboratory Values

Chest Radiograph. Apparent right mainstem mass. Evidence of air trapping on right—hyperinflated with slight mediastinal shift to left. *Impression:* Right mainstem mass.

Arterial Blood Gases. On room air: pH = 7.45; pCO_2 = 46 torr; pO_2 = 94 torr.

Hospital Orders

Diagnostic bronchoscopy. The physician asks you to set up for a bronchoscopy in the outpatient Endoscopy Lab.

1. If a bronchodilator is needed, which type of bronchodilator would you suggest: α, β_1, β_2, mixed (α/β), or an anticholinogenic agent such as atropine or Atrovent[R]. How do you support that recommendation?
2. Local anesthetics are given for several reasons. Pain reduction and gag/cough reflex control are two major rationales. Why are these important considerations and what is the usual route and method of administration?
3. In view of the enhanced possibility of vagal stimulation, what other precautions should be taken prior to introduction of the bronchoscope into the patient's airway?

CASE 15: METHACHOLINE CHALLENGE (CHAPTER 16)

Roberta S. is a 32-year-old, 56-kg, 5′5″ female who is being evaluated in the pulmonry function laboratory. She has had complaints of chronic cough, clear sputum production, and episodes of SOB for the past year. She states that she is feeling well and breathing comfortably on the day of testing.

History and Physical Exam

History. Seasonal allergic rhinitis for 14 years, treated with terfenadine (Seldane[R]) past 2 years as needed.

Vital Signs. Blood pressure 120/70 mm Hg; heart rate = 76 beats/minute; respiratory rate = 14 breaths/minute.

Respiratory. Breath sounds clear to auscultation.

Laboratory Values

Arterial Blood Gases. On room air: pH = 7.44; pCO_2 = 38 torr; pO_2 = 92 torr.

Electrolytes. HCO_3^- = 25 mEq/L.

Hospital Orders

Spirometry to be followed by bronchial provocation testing if baseline $FEV_{1.0}$ is within 20 percent of predicted value for patient's height, weight, and sex. Perform baseline arterial blood gases.

In the pulmonary function laboratory, spirometric data are obtained and the patient's flow rates are determined to be within normal range. The technician then proceeds with provocation testing according to the laboratory protocol. The following values are obtained as the methacholine test solutions are increased in concentration:

	$FEV_{1.0}$ (L)	CUMULATIVE BREATHS	PERCENT DECREASE FROM BASELINE
Predicted:	2.97	—	—
Baseline:	2.94	—	—
	2.93	5	.30
	2.90	10	1.36
	2.75	15	6.46
	2.41	20	18.03
	1.99	25	32.31

Questions

1. What instructions should be given to the patient prior to the day of testing?
2. What precautions should be taken by laboratory personnel to ensure safety during the procedure?
3. Would you perform challenge testing if the patient is symptomatic that day?
4. What pulmonary function results indicate a positive response to challenge testing?
5. What type of drug should be administered to reverse the effects of methacholine?

CASE 16: VENTRICULAR TACHYCARDIA (CHAPTER 16)

Joseph P., a 54-year-old, 80.7-kg white male, was admitted for an angioplasty. He had severe chest pains that immobilized him for approximately 30 minutes. The patient took nitroglycerine during these episodes. He had an angioplasty performed prior to this admission but his chest pains returned after 4 weeks.

History and Physical Exam

History.   Angioplasty, prostate cancer, appendectomy, pneumonia.
Social History.   Divorced, has smoked 2 packs/day for 39 years, uses alcohol.
Vital Signs.   Blood pressure = 140/90 mm Hg; heart rate = 84 beats/minute; respiratory rate = 18 breaths/minute.
Cardiovascular.   Hypertension, angina.
Respiratory.   Clear to auscultation and percussion.

Laboratory Values

Blood Chemistry. Blood urea nitrogen = 11 mg/dL; creatinine = 0.7 mg/dL.
Electrolytes. Within normal limits.
Hematology. WBC count = 6700/mm^3; Hgb = 14.6 g/dL; HCT = 44.8 percent.

Hospital Course

Day 1. The patient had a left heart catheterization using the right femoral artery approach. His left ventricular function is good.

Day 2. The patient had an angioplasty this A.M. Following the procedure, the patient developed severe chest pains with occlusion of the distal left main coronary artery. He was taken to the operating room for an emergency coronary artery bypass graft. It took two attempts to remove him from bypass. When he returned to the ICU, he was placed on controlled mechanical ventilation at 10 breaths/minute, positive end-expiratory pressure (PEEP) of 5 cm H_2O, and F_iO_2 setting of 1.0. He was in sinus tachycardia with occasional premature ventricular contractions.

Day 3. Initial vital signs: heart rate = 124–138 beats/minute; blood pressure = 140/90 mm Hg central venous pressure = 10 mm Hg, pulmonary artery pressure = 22/14 mm Hg; pulmonary capillary wedge pressure = 13 mm Hg. The F_iO_2 was decreased to 0.7, with arterial blood gases of pH = 7.50, pCO_2 = 30 torr, and pO_2 = 157 torr. The patient developed ventricular tachychardia, with a heart rate of 170 beats/minute and a blood pressure of 60/40 mm Hg.

Questions

1. What is the first step in the continuing treatment of this patient? Explain your answer.
2. Using American Heart Association (AHA) guidelines, what antiarrhythmic agent is given initially to a patient in pulsed ventricular tachycardia? What drug dose and frequency of drug administration are recommended?
3. What two other antiarrhythmic drugs are used in the treatment of pulsed ventricular tachycardia?
4. Is sodium bicarbonate indicated in this situation? Explain your answer.

ANSWERS TO CASE STUDY QUESTIONS

Case 1

1. Peak expiratory flow rate or $FEV_{1.0}$. No, misjudging the severity of attacks is recognized as an important contributing factor to many deaths from asthma.
2. The recommended dose of two puffs of albuterol is based on chronic stable asthma. The fact that this patient required three puffs suggests the asthma attack may have been at least moderate in severity. Without peak flows to evaluate the effectiveness of the bronchodilator, it is difficult to determine whether this patient was treated with

a maximal dose of bronchodilator therapy or not. There is no mention of inhaled steroid administration either in the ER or in discharge plans. There is controversy as to whether the traditional dose of ipratropium bromide in combination with β_2 agonists produces an additive effect or not.

3. The patient was intubated during the resuscitation effort at the fire station and an intravenous (IV) line was placed at that time as well. In situations where venous access is delayed, epinephrine, lidocaine, and atropine may be instilled endotracheally via a catheter passed beyond the tip of the endotracheal tube. The dose for directly instilled drugs is 2.0–2.5 times the IV dose. Chest compressions should be withheld while several quick ventilations are given. This patient's chart did not indicate that instillation of epinephrine occurred, however.

Case 2

1. The recommended dose for albuterol is 0.2–0.5 mL of 0.5% solution. However, the recommended dose may not be the optimal dose for every patient. It has been recommended that the optimal dose be determined for each patient and given QID. The dosing strategy for albuterol therapy is given in Tashkin (1991) (see reference list for Chapter 12).

2. No. Even though this patient had trouble clearing secretions, Atrovent[R] is not reported to have the side effects associated with Atropine. Had albuterol been given in an optimal dose, Atrovent[R] would not provide additional bronchodilation. However, optimal dosage of Atrovent[R] may be more beneficial than a β_2 agonist in COPD and may be ordered before starting treatment. The pre–post bronchodilator change in $FEV_{1.0}$ reflects slight reversibility in airway obstruction.

3. Yes. The recommended course of action in the treatment of COPD is 1) ipratropium MDI with spacer; 3–6 puffs QID, 2) β_2-agonist MDI with spacer q3–6h; 3) long-acting theophylline (300–900 mg/day (serum level, 8–12 μg/mL); and 4) corticosteroids—prednisone, 40 mg/day for 14 days and then reduced to minimum possible (0–10 mg SID or on alternate days use inhaled). Although steroid use is controversial in the managment of COPD, it is recommended after other agents have been tried with suboptimal results. There is no mention in this patient's chart of long-acting theophylline use. At this point, a trial of theophylline therapy may be beneficial as well.

Case 3

1. Theophylline's therapeutic blood levels range between 10 and 20 μg/mL, which is very close to the blood level associated with toxicity (>20 μg/mL). This patient's theophylline level was 13 μ-g/mL, which is acceptable. Maximal theophylline levels are not necessary in treating acute severe asthma in the emergency situation and do not achieve greater bronchodilation than repeated doses of inhaled β_2 agonists. The side effects of theophylline are more adverse than those of inhaled β_2 agonists.

2. Yes. Frequent administration of aerosolized β_2 agonists delivered at higher doses are indicated in cases of acute severe asthma in patients without cardiovascular disease

under the age of 50. The potent constrictor influences require higher doses of bronchodilators because bronchodilator potency is reduced and becomes suboptimal sooner. Although repeated doses may produce anxiety, tremulousness, palpitations, and headache, serious side effects of inhaled β_2 agonist are rare. Heart rate increases minimally and blood pressure decreases slightly. β_2 agonists can be aerosolized with significantly fewer side effects than those associated with systemic administration of β_2 agonists. The alternative course of action for a patient with such severe airway obstruction is intubation and mechanical ventilation.

3. According to Fanta (*Respiratory Care*, 37:551, 1992), PEFR or $FEV_{1.0}$ correlate inversely with arterial pCO_2. Arterial CO_2 levels generally are not elevated until the $FEV_{1.0}$ is less than or equal to 40 percent of the predicted value. The patient's arterial pCO_2 was elevated, which coincides with her $FEV_{1.0}$ of 35 percent of the predicted value.

Case 4

1. According to Kacmarek and Hess (*Respiratory Care*, 36:952–976, 1991), the patient should be instructed to: 1) warm MDI to body temperature and shake canister vigorously, 2) hold canister upright and actuate MDI into spacer, 3) place spacer mouthpiece in mouth and close lips around mouthpiece, 4) inspire slowly from spacer and continue to inspire to total lung capacity, and 5) hold breath for 4–10 seconds. A second inspiration from the spacer may be necessary depending on the recommendations of the spacer manufacturer. The patient should then wait 1–2 minutes before repeating the entire procedure for the next actuation or puff. If the patient is unable to take in a breath to total lung capacity and hold it, a SVN is indicated.

2. Proper technique in the use of the spacer and MDI should be stressed, and the patient allowed to practice under supervision. Proper care and cleaning instructions should be discussed and written instructions sent home with the patient. The patient should be shown how to determine whether the MDI is half full or empty.

3. All feasible aspects of pulmonary rehabilitation could be explored. At the very least, she should be encouraged to stop smoking and informed of the smoking cessation programs available to her. She needs to be informed of the warning signs and symptoms of a pulmonary infection (i.e., increase in sputum production, change in sputum color or odor, greater difficulty breathing despite MDI tretments, or more frequent use of her MDI).

Case 5

1. The use of a bronchodilator prior to delivery of Mucomyst[R] (*N*-acetylcysteine) helps to reduce the possibility of induced bronchospasm. It also promotes better aerosol distribution by dilating peripheral airways, allowing the mucolytic to reach the distal areas of the lung. The second MDI treatment reverses any bronchoconstriction resulting from the mucolytic and enhances secretion mobilization and removal during PD&C.

2. The order calls for the use of a cocktail made by diluting 3.0 mL of 20% Mucomyst[R] with 3.0 mL of NS and then adding 3 drops (3 gtts) of Bronkosol[R] 1 : 100. The

dilution of 3.0 mL of a 20% Mucomyst^R solution by 3.0 mL of NS yields 6.0 mL of a 10% Mucomyst^R solution. By using a 10% solution initially, the diluent (NS) is not needed, effectively reducing the nebulized volume by half. This should reduce the nebulization time by about half. This strategy will also reduce Na$^+$ intake.

3. Sodium bicarbonate has mucolytic properties because it reduces amino acid chain stability. NaHCO$_3$ (at concentrations of 2–4.5%) has relatively few side effects and generally does not cause bronchospasm. Mucomyst^R, in contrast, is a very potent mucolytic that breaks the mucopolysaccharide molecule bonds. Mucomyst has a "rotten egg" odor, whereas NaHCO$_3$ is odorless.

4. All of the treatments listed have the potential to expand the volume of or move secretions. Occasionally the mucus may expand enough to cause airway obstruction or, in weak patients, result in inability to clear secretions without mechanical assistance. Bronchospasm is also a potential problem even with the administration of prophylactic doses of bronchodilators.

5. Toby has lost weight, indicating poor nutritional status; his dry, nonelastic skin coupled with his hemoconcentration indicates dehydration. Increased fluid intake by both oral (PO) and IV routes is indicated. Increasing the fluid load will allow for better hydration of secretions, thus reducing their viscosity. With the inception of fluid therapy, a trial course of saturated solution of potassium iodide (SSKI) may be effective in lowering mucus viscosity, again aiding in secretion mobilization. The weight loss and associated reduced food intake can lead to muscle wasting and inefficiency, thus increasing the work of breathing. Food supplements and dietary counseling may be warranted.

6. Of the solutions discussed in this chapter, the only suitable and appropriate one for use in a heated high-humidity device is sterile water. Each of the other solutions will either be degraded (be destroyed or altered) by the heat or will leave deposits on the humidification device. These devices produce molecular water (vapor) and thus will not transfer the NaCL from either hypertonic or hypotonic saline.

Case 6

1. Because ribavirin is a drug with adverse effects in terms of equipment, environmental contamination, and potential teratogenicity, its use should be reserved for patients with confirmed RSV diagnosis with severe symptoms or underlying disorders such as immunodeficiency, cardiac anomalies, and bronchopulmonary dysplasia.

2. To deliver drug to the lower airways, a very small particle size is required. Ribavarin can be delivered in the appropriate particle size and quantity only by a special aerosol generator, the SPAG-II unit. Because the infant in this case is not intubated, the use of an oxygen hood or enclosure is indicated for drug administration.

3. Ribavirin is nebulized continuously for 12–18 hours/day during the course of treatment. The fine aerosol particles deposit and adhere to tubing, masks, and hoods. A severely compromised infant with life-threatening RSV infection may require intubation and mechanical ventilation. Although the drug has not been approved for in-line

delivery through ventilator circuits, the seriousness of the situation may warrant giving the drug during positive pressure ventilation. Unless appropriate measures are taken, the drug will precipitate and cause machine malfunction. Sticking of the exhalation valve is of particular concern because of the risk of high ventilation pressures with resulting barotrauma. The use of double filters proximal to the exhalation valve is recommended, as is the use of a proximal airway monitor. It is important to change the filters on a scheduled basis. Every 2 hours, the filter closest to the exhalation valve should be discarded and the other filter moved into the proximal position. A new filter is then inserted in line at the vacated position.

4. Although the long-term effects in humans are not clear, ribavirin is a known teratogen in small mammals. There is currently an awareness and concern among health care workers about the potential hazards presented by exposure to the drug. Pregnant or lactating women or those desiring to become pregnant within the near future should be excluded from the area of ribavirin delivery. Personnel should be equipped with protective barriers such as gowns, gloves, goggles, shoe covers, and properly fitted masks (nonpowered, HEPA filter). The SPAG generator should be turned off 5–10 minutes before opening the tent enclosure to allow the drug particles to be evacuated. If possible, the patient should be placed in an isolation room with filtered exhaust capability. Use of a double tent system with vacuum exhaust or a portable negative pressure system with HEPA filters is also acceptable. When a mechanical ventilator is being used, expired gases should be filtered.

Case 7

1. Although the patient does not have signs or symptoms of *Pneumocystis carinii* pneumonia (PCP) at this time, he is at high risk for incurring the infection with his deteriorating immune status. Clinical research studies have determined the importance of initiating prophylactic PCP therapy when the CD4+ lymphocyte count is less than 200/mm^3. Oral trimethoprim-sulfamethoxazole is considered to be the most effective prophylactic agent. Pentamidine aerosol is next in effectiveness and can be used for those individuals who cannot tolerate trimethoprim-sulfamethoxazole. This patient has a low CD4+ count and is allergic to sulfonamide drugs; therefore, he should begin aerosolized pentamidine treatments. For prophylaxis, 300 mg of pentamidine should be mixed with 6 ml of sterile water (a precipitate forms with saline solution) and given by special nebulizer over 30–40 minutes. Treatments should be given at 4-week intervals.

2. *Pneumocystis* infection occurs in the interstitial plasma cells of the lung. To deliver pentamidine to the alveoli, a nebulizer must be able to produce very small aerosol particles and must have the capability of delivering 6 ml of solution within a reasonable time period (20–40 minutes). In one study, the AeroTech nebulizer was shown to aerosolize significantly more drug per unit of time.

3. Concerns about health care workers delivering pentamidine therapy are twofold: 1) possible inhalation of the drug, and 2) inadvertent exposure to exhaled organisms from

patients with undiagnosed mycobacterial infections. Personnel have reported symptoms such as burning eyes, headache, stuffy nose, and bronchospasm when inadequately protected. Wearing a standard surgical mask does not protect the caregiver because the small aerosol particles of drug can penetrate the mask during inspiration. Because the probability of tuberculosis is high, all HIV-positive patients should be screened prior to pentamidine treatment; chemotherapy should be initiated when indicated. A bronchodilator may be given to the patient before pentamidine administration to minimize coughing. Caregivers may wear protective gear that meets NIOSH standards or, preferably, place the patient in a negative pressure isolation chamber with HEPA and charcoal exhaust filters. The unit should be allowed to run at least 5 minutes after therapy is terminated to clear residual aerosol particles. A patient who is coughing should not return to a common waiting area. Cleaning of surfaces and disposal of contaminated equipment should be done by personnel who are wearing appropriate barrier apparel and in an approved manner.

4. Although the parenteral administration of pentamidine may result in serious adverse effects such as hypoglycemia, hypotension, and nephrotoxicity, reactions from the aerosolized drug usually are limited to cough, bronchospasm, metallic taste, and fatigue. The occurrence of bronchospasm and cough may be decreased by the administration of a β_2-adrenergic bronchodilator prior to pentamidine nebulization.

Case 8

1. Intravenous delivery of amphotericin may not be effective for treatment of cavitary diseases such as aspergilloma. Because there is reduced blood flow to the cavitary areas, sufficient drug concentration may not be available to eradicate the organism. Should the patient be unable to continue parental administration of the drug because of adverse effects such as renal dysfunction, anemia, thrombocytopenia, convulsions, or anaphylaxis, aerosol delivery may be a viable alternative. The drug is poorly soluble in body tissues and will be confined primarily to the respiratory system.

2. Bronchospasm may result from aerosol delivery of amphotericin B, especially in asthmatics. It is recommended that a rapid-acting β_2-adrenergic bronchodilator be given immediately before or concomitantly with delivery of nebulized amphotericin.

3. The delivery of a microbial agent to target areas of the lung by aerosol is dependent on the ability of the patient to cooperate and to use optimal techniques during administration of the drug. It is the responsibility of the health care worker to assess the patient for ability to perform the procedure, to instruct the patient properly, and to monitor and coach the patient during the treatment. The drug also may not reach the desired sites areas if airway obstruction is present; pretreatment with a bronchodilator may be useful for facilitating drug distribution. Another problem is that the exact aerosol dose for maximal effectiveness has not been determined precisely. Finally, even minimal systemic absorption of amphotericin B may result in the occurrence of the adverse effects of fever, headache, gastrointestinal distress, malaise, joint pain, or renal insufficiency.

4. To protect himself or herself from exhaled drug aerosol, the health care worker should follow appropriate guidelines by wearing protective apparel or by placing the patient in a negative pressure exhaust-filtered isolation booth, chamber, or room. The use of exhaust-filtered systems also may reduce the development of drug sensitivity in practitioners and decrease the occurrence of nosocomial infection with resistant organisms.

Case 9

1. Systemic steroids are given in an acute or emergency situation. Steroids are used in an acute attack to decrease airway inflammation and potentiate the effects of β_2 agonists. An aerosolized steroid is started when oral steroids are initiated. Then the oral dose is tapered and the aerosolized dose is increased. The goal is to achieve the best lung function with the lowest systemic steroid dose.

2. Aerosolized β_2 agonists are the mainstay of bronchodilator therapy for severe exacerbations of asthma. A MDI or a wet (SVN) aerosol probably would be equally effective. If the patient is having problems with coordinating a MDI, a wet aerosol would be the better choice. Albuterol (Ventolin^R), which the patient is taking at home, would be a good choice. Because the patient is showing severe V/Q disturbances, she initially may need hourly administration with careful cardiac monitoring.

3. No, the patient should not be started on cromolyn sodium. It is a mast cell stabilizer that helps to *prevent* asthma attacks. Because this patient is currently in an asthma attack, cromolyn is not indicated. It may be considered in the development of a long-term maintenance care plan for this patient.

4. Bedside pulmonary function tests can be used to monitor the patient's response to bronchodilator therapy. Daily serial measurements of $FEV_{1.0}$ (spirometry) or PEFR (peak flow meter) before and after bronchodilator therapy are recommended to guide therapy and assess the patient's response to therapy. Because the patient is receiving oxygen, daily oximetry is recommended. Also be aware the β_2 agonists may cause the S_aO_2 to decline because they dilate pulmonary vessels and improve blood flow to less ventilated lungs units.

Case 10

1. The appearance of stridor following extubation is the result of upper airway obstruction. The patient could have glottic or subglottic edema from too large a tube, excessive cuff pressures, or traumatic injury.

2. Racemic epinephrine is the drug of choice in postextubation laryngeal edema. It is rapidly acting and can be given frequently if the patient's stridor recurs. It is an α- and β-adrenergic drug, but its primary effect by aerosol is due to its α-adrenergic activity. It constricts mucosal blood vessels and reduces tissue edema, which improves air conductance and reduces stridor.

3. Yes. Systemic steroids may reverse or prevent glottic or subglottic edema. One should be given prior to extubation.

Case 11

1. This baby was very close to respiratory failure and required aggressive therapy to avoid intubation and mechanical ventilation. Not all babies with bronchiolitis respond to bronchodilator therapy, but, in this case, the baby stabilized and improved. It is unclear if the baby improved because of continuous aerosolized albuterol or if improvement was due to the steroid therapy started at the same time.

2. Percent strength = 1:200 solution = 0.5% = 0.005. Total solution amount is 2 mL; active ingredient = x

   $0.005 = x \text{ g}/2 \text{ mL}$

   $x \text{ g} = 0.005 \times 2$

   $x = 0.01 \text{ g}$

   $0.01 \text{ g} \times 1,000 \text{ mg/g} = 10 \text{ mg}$

   $10 \text{ mg}/60 \text{ min} = x \text{ mg/min}$

   $\qquad\qquad = 0.167 \text{ mg/min}$

3. Fried's rule = (age in months/150) $\times$ adult dose:

   (5 months/150) $\times$ 2.5 mg = 0.083 mg

4. In addition to steroids and bronchodilators, another medication used to treat bronchiolitis is ribavirin. Initially, bronchodilators and steroids are given. If the baby responds, other therapy is unnecessary. If there is no improvement, ribavirin may be used. Ribavirin is reserved for high-risk infants who have either chronic cardiopulmonary disease or severe refractory bronchiolitis.

5. No. The lower airway obstruction in bronchiolitis is caused primarily by bronchiolar wall edema and increased mucus production. The drug of choice in this situation is a steroid. However, a component of the airway obstruction may be bronchospasm. In those patients with bronchospasm, bronchodilators improve airway conductance and reduce air trapping.

Case 12

1. AMS is caused by rapid changes in altitude. As the chopper rose, it gained more altitude, exacerbating the already delicate hydrostatic balance. The additional strain on the cardiopulmonary system caused the visible worsening of the patient's condition.

2. Glucocorticosteroids are potent anti-inflammatory agents and reduce cerebrovascular pressure. The reduction of cerebrovascular pressure, in turn, will help to alleviate the pulmonary edema, which is noncardiac in nature.

3. Ethyl alcohol is an antifoaming, surface tension–reducing agent that reduces the net volume of secretions in the frothy, bubble-producing edema fluid. The use of IPPB as

a delivery vehicle is warranted because the increased intrapulmonary pressures and the concomitant rise in intrathoracic pressures result in further reductions in edema fluid volume and decreased venous return, again reducing preload. The extended expiratory time increases mean intrathoracic pressure, further reducing preload. The oxygen increases F_iO_2, thus decreasing the hypoxia of altitude.

4. Yes. Decreasing wedge pressure will decrease transalveolar capillary membrane pressure gradients, thus slowing capillary "leak." Rotating tourniquets, upright seated position, and increased intrathoracic pressure (IPPB with expiratory retard) all reduce preload. Preload also may be reduced by administration of morphine (2–4 mg IV) or nitroglycerin (topical or sublingual) or by use of diuretics.

A mnemonic (memory aid) that will help you to remember the treatment strategy for pulmonary edema is *MOISTURE*:

*M*orphine
*O*xygen
*I*PPB
*S*teroids
*T*ourniquets
*U*rine output
*R*educe wedge pressure
*E*levate head

Case 13

1. There are three sources of surfactant: humans, cows (bovine), and artificial materials. Human surfactant is rarely used because of cost, as well as aesthetic/moral reasons, and because of fears of HIV or hepatitis contamination. Although bovine surfactant is less costly, has no aesthetic/moral overtones, and does not carry the risk of HIV/hepatitis B infection, fear of possible adverse immune reaction to alien protein has effectively ruled out its use in most cases. Therefore the most common source of surfactant is artificial production methods. The two forms of artificial surfactant currently available are Exosurf Neonatal[R] and Survanta[R].

2. Yes, surfactant is a detergent just like laundry soap. A detergent is a substance that lowers surface tension. Surface tension is a force of attraction that attracts or binds one structure or substance to another. By decreasing the attractive forces, it becomes easier to separate one thing from the other. Because the molecules on the alveolar surface are strongly attracted to each other, it is difficult to open closed alveoli. Surfactant decreases this attractiveness, allowing the alveoli to open more readily.

3. Surfactant provides a mechanism by which the cohesion (attractive forces) between substances in the alveolar wall can be reduced. These attractive forces are called surface tension. By reducing surface tension, surfactant allows expansion of the alveoli with much less work, and thus lower pressures. After the initial opening of the alveoli, the cohesive forces are much weaker and the residual volume is able to "splint" open the alveoli for succeeding breaths. This establishes a resting volume.

4. Prevention (prophylactic) protocols are designed to prevent IRDS development in high-risk infants (birth weight below 1250 g). The rescue protocol is used to treat infants with existing IRDS who did not meet the prevention protocol. These babies may be full term or over 1250 g at birth.

5. Immediately after surfactant is instilled into the endotracheal tube, the patient should be vigorously bag-oxygenated in order to distribute the surfactant to the peripheral airspaces. This technique also may recruit some previously closed alveoli. Rotation of the infant from side to side also is indicated to ensure that all peripheral areas are exposed to instilled surfactant. Repeat doses are given as indicated below, depending on the drug used. Hyperoxygenation is required to reduce the incidence and effects of bradycardia and oxygen denaturation.

	SURVANTA[R]	EXOSURF[R]
Prevention		
Initial dose	100 mg/kg	5 ml/kg
Time	Within 15 min of birth	ASAP after birth in two 2.5 mL/kg doses
Repeat dose	100 mg/kg	5 mL/kg
Time	q6h up to 4 times	q12h × 3
Rescue		
Initial dose	100 mg/kg	5 mL/kg
Time	Within 8 hr of IRDS onset	ASAP after IRDS onset
Repeat dose	100 mg/kg	5 mL/kg × 1
Time	q6h up to 4 times	12 h after initial dose

6. Among other changes, we should see improved pulmonary compliance, reduction of work of breathing, reduced ventilating pressures, improved pO_2, and decreased pCO_2. Additionally, heart rate should improve and the child's color, muscle tone, and reactions should be improved. The two most common side effects are bradycardia and oxygen desaturation, which may require resuscitation. These occur in about 10 percent of patients.

7. *Bonus.* Many studies have shown that administration of corticosteroids to mothers 24–72 hours before delivery stimulates normalization of the lecithin–sphingomyelin ratio and results in surfactant production by alveolar cells. These studies indicated a lower than expected number of IRDS cases and less severe IRDS in those patients whose mothers were steroid recipients than in other patients.

Case 14

1. An anticholinogenic agent, because these agents have lower potential for cardiac effects. They also are both vasoconstrictors and bronchodilators; thus, they reduce blood flow while enhancing airflow at lower resistances. Atropine-like substances also reduce bronchial secretion production, providing a drier field.

2. The usual topical anesthetics are lidocaine (1%, 2%, or 4%), cocaine (4%), or cetacaine (benzocaine and tetracaine). These are delivered initially by either a gas-powered nebulizer or, preferably, by a hand bulb–powered atomizer, then subsequently by direct instillation through the bronchoscope. Pain control and control of gag or cough reflexes reduce patient discomfort and anxiety, reduce involuntary movement, and reduce the risk of vomiting and aspiration. A hand bulb atomizer is used to produce particles of large size that will rain out in the oropharynx and upper airways. Patient anxiety can be relieved or reduced by administration of sedatives such as codeine, morphine, diazepam, or midazolam (the last two drugs also cause short-term amnesia, which may be helpful to the patient).

3. Because of increased risk of cardiac complications secondary to vagus nerve stimulation and hypoxia, an IV access route should be established before bronchoscopy and resuscitation drugs and equipment should be readily available.

Case 15

1. The patient should eliminate all β-adrenergic agents, methylxanthines, antihistamines, and other drugs that can influence airway function at least 48 hours before testing, if possible. Cromolyn sodium (Intal^R) should be withheld for 24 hours. If corticosteroids are required for maintenance therapy, the dosage should be stable before the patient undergoes the procedure. Patients also should be cautioned to avoid exercise, smoking, coffee, cola, and chocolate during the 6 hours prior to testing. Nursing mothers, persons who are receiving β blockers, or individuals with known parasympathomimetic hypersensitivity should be excluded from pharmacologic challenge testing.

2. If the test solutions are prepared in the pulmonary function laboratory, they should not be mixed by a technician who has asthma. A scavenging device should be used to prevent inadvertant inhalation of the agent by personnel or contamination of the environment. Emergency resuscitative equipment should be in the testing laboratory; personnel should be trained in CPR and use of the equipment. A physician should be present or immediately available in the event of a serious adverse reaction to the test solution. A rapid-onset β-adrenergic bronchodilator such as albuterol (Proventil^R) should be prepared and ready for administration.

3. Pharmacologic challenge agents such as methacholine are used to identify hyperreactive airways disease in patients who experience symptoms of airway obstruction but who may have normal or equivocal spirometry and bronchodilator studies. For the safety of the patient and for accuracy of the test results, methacholine challenge should not be performed during a period of symptom exacerbation.

4. Although other parameters (FVC, FEF 25–75%, FEF_{max}, PEF, Raw) have been examined, the $FEV_{1.0}$ customarily is used as the index of response. A 20 percent reduction in $FEV_{1.0}$ from baseline value is indicative of a positive response. The test is terminated when a positive response occurs or when the maximum dose of methacholine has been delivered.

5. An inhaled dose of a β-adrenergic agent should be given to reverse the methacholine when a 20 percent or greater reduction in $FEV_{1.0}$ occurs. A bronchodilator also may be given when less than a 20 percent decrease occurs if the patient complains of difficulty breathing after completion of the test.

Case 16

1. Assessing the ABCs of resuscitation is always the first step in any emergency situation. Because the patient already has a stable airway, ventilation, oxygen, and monitors, this step has been performed. Therefore, the first step would be to prepare for immediate unsynchronized countershock. According to AHA guidelines, the patient who is hypotensive, unconscious, pulseless, or in pulmonary edema should receive unsynchronized shock to avoid the delay associated with synchronization. The patient should receive electrical shock using 100 J, then 200 J, then 300 J, then 360 J. If the patient's arrhythmia converts after any shock, additional shock is not given. Also, a brief trial of medications may be given. The physician must exercise his or her judgment in determining if the patient should receive immediate electrical therapy, drug therapy, or a combination.

2. The first antiarrhythmic drug recommended for use in pulsed ventricular tachycardia is lidocaine. According to AHA guidelines, procainamide may be used, but it takes longer to work and may decrease blood pressure. The dose for lidocaine is 1–1.5 mg/kg by IV push, with a maximum total dose of 3 mg/kg. Lidocaine is given every 5–10 minutes until resolution of the tachycardia or the patient has received the maximum dosage.

3. The other two antiarrhythmic drugs used to treat patients with pulsed ventricular tachycardia are procainamide and bretylium.

4. No, sodium bicarbonate is not indicated. Bicarbonate use is limited to patients with pre-existing metabolic acidosis or hyperkalemia. This patient does not have these problems.

APPENDIX C

PROBLEM SOLVING/DRUG CALCULATIONS

INTRODUCTION

The most common drug administration problem-solving skills needed by the respiratory care practitioner are those that require the conversion of a volume (solution) to a weight, or vice versa. In other words, the practitioner must be able to determine how many *milligrams* (mg) of a drug are contained in a specific solution with a known concentration, such as "how many milligrams of racemic epinephrine are contained in 0.50 mL of Vaponefrin^R?" Another application of this concept is calculating how many milliliters (ml, or cubic centimeters [cc]) of a drug will be needed to fill a physician's order that is stated in milligrams, such as "how much Ventolin^R should be given if the physician has ordered 1.5 mg of albuterol per treatment?"

To solve these problems, the practitioner must know two things: 1) what is the **concentration** of the drug solution being used, and 2) how is this concentration calculated?

DRUG CONCENTRATIONS

The concentration is the **percent solution** of the *active ingredient* in the drug. This is found on the label or in the product information.

CONCENTRATION CALCULATIONS

In drug solutions, a 1% solution means that **1 gram** of the solute (*drug*) is dissolved in **100 cubic centimeters** of the solvent (usually water). It is commonly assumed that 1 mL = 1 cc.

This information can be used to set up a simple mathematical relationship, or algebraic formula. Because most of the drugs administered by respiratory care practitioners are given in small dosages, milligrams rather than grams, the first conversion should be from **grams** to **milligrams**:

$$1 \text{ gram} = 1,000 \text{ milligrams} = 1,000 \text{ mg}$$
$$0.50 \text{ gram} = 500 \text{ milligrams} \quad = 500 \text{ mg}$$
$$0.10 \text{ gram} = 100 \text{ milligrams} \quad = 100 \text{ mg}$$

SETTING UP THE PROBLEM

Suppose the problem is: "How many **milligrams** of salt are contained in 3.0 mL of normal saline?" To solve this problem, set up a series of easily solved steps:

Step 1: What is the **concentration** of normal saline?
Answer: 0.9% NaCl (salt)
Step 2: How many milligrams of salt are contained in **1 mL** of normal saline?
Answer: 0.9% means that there are 0.9 **grams** of salt **per 100 mL** of solution. This can be stated mathematically as:

$$\frac{0.9 \text{ grams}}{100 \text{ mL}} = \frac{900 \text{ mg}}{100 \text{ mL}} = \frac{9 \text{ mg}}{1 \text{ mL}}$$

Step 3: If 1 mL contains 9 mg of salt, how much is contained in 3 mL?
Answer:

$$x = \frac{9 \text{ mg}}{1 \text{ mL}} (3 \text{ mL}) = 9 \text{ mg } (3) = 27 \text{ mg}$$

Thus, the answer is 3 ml of normal saline contains 27 mg of NaCl.

SAMPLE PROBLEMS

1. How many milligrams of isoproterenol are contained in 0.25 mL of Isuprel[R] 1:100?

Step 1: What is the **concentration** of Isuprel[R] 1:100?
Answer: 1:100 means 1/100, which is equal to 1%
Step 2: How many milligrams of isoproterenol are contained in **1 mL** of Isuprel[R] 1:100?
Answer: 1.0% means that there is 1.0 **gram** of isoproterenol **per 100 mL** of solution. This can be stated mathematically as:

$$\frac{1.0 \text{ grams}}{100 \text{ mL}} = \frac{1,000 \text{ mg}}{100 \text{ mL}} = \frac{10 \text{ mg}}{1 \text{ mL}}$$

Step 3: If 1 mL contains 10 mg of isoproterenol, how much is contained in 0.25 mL?
Answer:

$$x = \frac{10 \text{ mg}}{1 \text{ mL}} (0.25 \text{ mL}) = 10 \text{ mg } (0.25) = 2.5 \text{ mg}$$

Thus, the answer is 0.25 mL of Isuprel[R] 1:100 contains 2.5 mg of isoproterenol.

2. How many cc of Alupent^R must be given if the physician has ordered 10 mg of metaproterenol per treatment?

Step 1: What is the **concentration** of Alupent^R?

Answer: Both Alupent^R and Metaprel^R are supplied in 5% solution.

Step 2: How many milligrams of metaproterenol are contained in **1 mL** of Alupent^R?

Answer: 5.0% means that there are 5.0 **grams** of metaproterenol **per 100 mL** of solution. This can be stated mathematically as:

$$\frac{5.0 \text{ grams}}{100 \text{ mL}} = \frac{5000 \text{ mg}}{100 \text{ mL}} = \frac{50 \text{ mg}}{1 \text{ mL}}$$

Step 3: If 1 mL contains 50 mg of metaproterenol, how much is needed to provide 10 mg?

Answer:

$$\frac{x \text{ mL}}{10 \text{ mg}} = \frac{1.0 \text{ mL}}{50 \text{ mg}}$$

$$x \text{ mL} = \frac{10 \text{ mg}}{50 \text{ mg}} = 10/50 = 1/5 = 0.20 \text{ mL}$$

Thus, the answer is 0.20 mL of Alupent^R contains 10.0 mg of metaproterenol.

APPENDIX **D**

LIST OF DRUGS BY GENERIC AND TRADE NAMES

acetaminophen (Tylenol^R)

acetylcholine

acetylcysteine (Mucomyst^R, Mucosil^R)

activated charcoal

acyclovir (Zovirax^R)

Adsorbocarpine^R (**pilocarpine**)

Advil^R (**ibuprofen**)

Aerobid^R (**flunisolide**)

Aftate^R (**tolnaftate**)

albuterol (Proventil^R, Ventolin^R, [C] Salbutamol)

Aldactone^R (**spironolactone**)

Aldomet^R (α methyldopa)

α-methyldopa (Aldomet^R)

alprazolam (Xanax^R)

aluminum hydroxide (Amphojel^R)

Alupent^R (**metaproterenol**)

amantadine (Symmetrel^R)

amikacin

amiloride (Midamor^R)

amiodarone

amitriptyline (Elavil^R)

amoxicillin

amoxicillin + clavulanic acid (Augmentin^R)

Amphojel^R (**aluminum hydroxide**)

amphotericin B (Fungizone^R)

ampicillin (Unasyn^R)

Ancobon^R (**flucytosine**)

Anectine^R (**succinylcholine**)

Antivert^R (**meclizine**)

Apresoline^R (**hydralazine**)

Aramine^R (**metaraminol**)

Artane^R (**trihexyphenidyl**)

atenolol (Tenormin^R)

atracurium (Tracrium^R)

Atromid^R (**clofibrate**)

atropine (Atropisol^R)

Atropisol^R (**atropine**)

Augmentin^R (**amoxicillin + clavulanic acid**)

Azactam^R (**aztreonam**)

azlocillin

Azmacort^R (**triamcinolone**)

aztreonam (Azactam^R)

Azulfidine^R (**sulfasalazine**)

Bactrim^R (**trimethoprim-sulfamethoxazole**)

Baking Soda^R (**sodium bicarbonate**)

beclomethasone (Beclovent^R, Vanceril^R)

Beclovent^R (**beclomethasone**)

Bentyl^R (**dicyclomine**)

benzylpenicillin (penicillin G)

betamethasone

bethanechol (Urecholine^R)

bisacodyl

bishydroxycoumarin (Dicumarol^R, Warfarin^R)

bismuth salts

bismuth subsalicylate (Pepto-Bismol^R)

Blenotaine^R (**bleomycin**)

bleomycin (Blenotaine^R)

Blocadren^R (**timolol**)

Brethine^R (**terbutaline**)

bretylium

Bricanyl^R (**terbutaline**)

bromocriptine mesylate (Parlodel^R)

Bronkometer^R (**isoetharine**)

Bronkosol^R (**isoetharine**)

budesonide

bupropion (Welbutrin[R])
BuSpar[R] (buspirone)
buspirone (BuSpar[R])
busulfan (Myleran[R])

Calan[R] (verapamil)
calcium carbonate (Tums[R], Tempo[R])
Capoten[R] (captopril)
captopril (Capoten[R])
Carafate[R] (sucralfate)
carbamazepine (Tegretol[R])
carbenicillin (Geopen[R])
carboxymethylcellulose
Cardilate[R] (erythrityl tetranitrate)
Cardizem[R] (diltiazem)
carisoprodol (Soma[R])
castor oil
Catapres[R] (clonidine)
Ceclor[R] (cefaclor)
cefaclor (Ceclor[R])
cefotaxime (Claforan[R])
cephalexin (Keflex[R])
chlordiazepoxide (Librium[R])
chlorothiazide (Diuril[R])
chlorpromazine (Thorazine[R])
chlortetracycline
chlorthalidone (hygroton[R])
cholestyramine (Questran[R])
Choloxin[R] (dextrothyroxine)
ciclopirox (Loprox[R])
cimetidine (Tagamet[R])
Cipro[R] (ciprofloxacin)
ciprofloxacin (Cipro[R])
cisplatin (Platinol[R])
Claforan[R] (cefotaxime)
clavulanic acid
Cleocin[R] (clindamycin)
clindamycin (Cleocin[R])
clofibrate (Atromid[R])
clonidine (Catapres[R])
clotrimazole (Lotrimin[R])
cloxacillin
codeine
Colestid[R] (colestipol)

colestipol (Colestid[R])
colistin (Coly-Mycin S[R])
Corgard[R] (nadolol)
cortisone
Cosmegen[R] (dactinomycin)
cromolon sodium (Intal[R], Nasalcrom[R])
Curare[R] (d-tubocurarine)
cyclobenzaprine (Flexeril[R])
cyclophosphamide (Cytoxan[R])
cyclopropane
Cytotec[R] (misoprostol)
Cytoxan[R] (cyclophosphamide)

d-tubocurarine (Curare[R])
dactinomycin (Cosmegen[R])
Dantrium[R] (dantrolene)
dantrolene (Dantrium[R])
Decadron[R] (dexamethasone)
demeclocycline
Demerol[R] (meperidine)
Depakene[R] (valproic acid)
deprenyl (Selegiline[R])
Desenex[R] (undecylenic acid)
Desyrel[R] (trazodone)
dexamethasone (Decadron[R] Respihaler[R])
dextrothyroxine (Choloxin[R])
diazepam (Valium[R])
diazoxide and sodium nitroprusside
Dibenzyline[R] (phenoxybenzamine)
dicloxacillin
Dicumarol[R] (bishydroxycoumarin)
dicyclomine (Bentyl[R])
dietary fiber
diethyl ether
digitalis
digitoxin (Purodigin[R])
digoxin (Lanoxin[R])
Dilantin[R] (phenytoin)
Dilaudid[R] (hydromorphone)
diltiazem (Cardizem[R])
dimenhydrinate (Dramamine[R])
dinitrate
diphenoxylate + atropine (Lomotil[R])
Diprivan[R] (propofol)

Diuril[R] (chlorothiazide)
docusate
dopamine (Intropin[R])
doxepin (Sinequan[R])
doxycycline
Dramamine[R] (dimenhydrinate)
Dyrenium[R] (triamterene)

E-Mycin[R] (erythromycin)
Edecrin[R] (ethacrynic acid)
edrophonium (Tensilon[R])
Elavil[R] (amitriptyline)
enalapril (Vasotec[R])
enflurane (Ethrane[R])
ephedrine
epinephrine Asthmahaler[R], Bronitin Mist[R], Bronkaid
    Mist[R], Medihaler-Epi[R], Primatene Mist[R]
erythrityl tetranitrate (Cardilate[R])
erythromycin (E-Mycin[R])
Eserine[R] (physostigmine)
Esidrix[R] (hydrochlorothiazide)
ethacrynic acid (Edecrin[R])
ethosuximide (Zarontin[R])
Ethrane[R] (enflurane)

famotidine (Pepcid[R])
fentanyl
Flagyl[R] (metronidazole)
Flexeril[R] (cyclobenzaprine)
flucytosine (Ancobon[R])
Fluothane[R] (halothane)
fluoxetine (Prozac[R])
Foranel[R] (isoflurane)
Fulvicin[R] (griseofulvin)
Fungizone[R] (amphotericin B)
furosemide (Lasix[R])

Gantrisin[R] (sulfsoxazole)
Garamycin[R] (gentamicin)
gemfibrozil (Lopid[R])
gentamicin (Garamycin[R])
Geopen[R] (carbenicillin)
glipizide (Glucotrol[R])
Glucotrol[R] (glipizide)
glyburide (Micronase[R])

griseofulvin (Fulvicin[R])
guanethidine (Ismelin[R])

Halcion[R] (triazolam)
halothane (Fluothane[R])
heparin
Herplex[R] (idoxuridine)
hydralazine (Apresoline[R])
hydrochlorothiazide (Esidrix[R], Hydropres[R])
hydrocortisone
hydromorphone (Dilaudid[R])
Hydropres[R] (hydrochlorothiazide)
Hygroton[R] (chlorthalidone)

ibuprofen (Advil[R], Motrin[R])
idoxuridine (Herplex[R])
imipenem
imipramine (Tofranil[R])
Imodium[R] (loperamide)
Inderal[R] (propranolol)
Intal[R] (cromolon sodium)
Intropin[R] (dopamine)
Ismelin[R] (guanethidine)
isocarboxazid (Marplan[R])
isoetharine (Bronkometer[R], Bronkosol[R])
isoflurane (Foranel[R])
isoproterenol (Isuprel[R], Vapo-N-Iso[R])
Isordil[R] (isosorbide)
isosorbide (Isordil[R])
Isuprel[R] (isoproterenol)

kanamycin (Kantrex[R], Klebcil[R])
Kantrex[R] (kanamycin)
kaolin
Kaopectate[R] (pectin)
Keflex[R] (caphalexin)
ketamine (Phencycline[R])
ketoconazole (Nizoral[R])
Klebcil (kanamycin)

Lanoxin[R] (digoxin)
Lasix[R] (furosemide)
levodopa
levodopa plus carbidopa (Sinemet[R])
Levophed[R] (norepinephrine)
Librium[R] (chlordiazepoxide)

lidocaine (Xylocaine[R])
lisinopril (Prinivil[R])
Lomotil[R] (diphenoxylate atropine)
Loniten[R] (minoxidil)
loperamide (Imodium[R])
Loped[R] (gemfibrozil)
Lopressor[R] (metoprolol)
Loprox[R] (ciclopirox)
Lorelco[R] (probucol)
Lotrimina[R] (clotrimazole)
lovastatin (Mevacor[R])
Luminal[R] (phenobarbital)

magnesium citrate
magnesium hydroxide (Milk of Magnesia[R])
magnesium sulfate
Marplan[R] (isocaroxazid)
mechlorethamine (Mustargen[R])
meclizine (Antivert[R])
meperidine (Demerol[R])
mercaptopurine (Purinethol[R])
Mestinon[R] (pyridostigmine)
metaproterenol (Alupent[R], Metaprel[R])
Metaprel[R] (metaproterenol)
metaraminol (Aramine[R])
methacholine (Provocholine[R])
methicillin
methocarbamol (Robaxin[R])
methotrexate (Methotrexate[R])
Methotrexate[R] (methotrexate)
methoxyflurane (Penthrane[R])
methylcellulose
methylphenidate (Ritalin[R])
metolazone (Zeroxolyn[R])
metoprolol (Lopressor[R])
metronidazole (Flagyl[R])
Mevacor[R] (lovastatin)
mezlocillin
Micatin[R] (miconazole)
miconazole (Micatin[R], Monistat[R])
Micronase[R] (glyburide)
Midamor[R] (amiloride)
Milk of Magnesia[R] (magnesium hydroxide)
mineral oil

Minipress[R] (prazosin)
minoxidil (Loniten[R])
misoprostol (Cytotec[R])
Monistat[R] (miconazole)
morphine
Motrin[R] (ibuprofen)
Mucomyst[R] (acetylcysteine)
Mucosil[R] (acetylcysteine)
Mustargen[R] (mechlorethamine)
Mycostatin[R] (nystatin)
Mydriacyl[R] (tropicamide)
Myleran[R] (busulfan)

nadolol (Corgard[R])
nafcillin
naloxone (Narcan[R])
Narcan[R] (naloxone)
Nardil[R] (phenelzine)
Nasalcrom[R] (cromolyn sodium)
nedocromil sodium (Tilade [C])
Nembutal[R] (pentobarbital)
neostigmine (Prostigmin[R])
netilmicin
niacin (Nicolar[R])
Nicolar[R] (niacin)
nifedipine (Procardia[R])
nitroglycerin (Nitrol[R], Nitrostat[R])
Nitrol[R] (nitroglycerin)
Nitrostat[R] (nitroglycerin)
nitrous oxide
Nizoral[R] (ketoconazole)
Norcuron[R] (vecuronium)
norepinephrine (Levophed[R])
norfloxacin (Noroxin[R])
Noroxin[R] (norfloxacin)
nystatin (Mycostatin[R])

olive oil
omeprazole (Prilosec[R])
Oncovin[R] (vincristine)
Orinase[R] (tolbutamide)
oxacillin

Paregoric[R] (tincture of opium)
Parlodel[R] (bromocriptine mesylate)

Parnate[R] (tranylcypromine)
pectin (Kaopectate[R])
penicillin G (benzylpenicillin)
penicillin V (phenoxymethylpenicillin)
pentamidine (Pentam[R], Pentacarinat [C], Phenmopent [C])
Penthrane[R] (methoxyflurane)
pentobarbital (Nembutal[R])
Pentothal[R] (thiopental)
Pepcid[R] (famotidine)
Pepto-Bismol[R] (bismuth subsalicylate)
pergolide (Permax[R])
Permax[R] (pergolide)
phenacetin
Phencycline[R] (ketamine)
phenelzine (Nardil[R])
phenobarbital (Luminal[R])
phenolphthalein
phenoxybenzamine (Dibenzyline[R])
phenoxymethylpenicillin (penicillin V)
phentolamine (Regitine[R])
phenylephrine
phenylpropanolamine
phenytoin (Dilantin[R])
physostigmine (Eserine[R])
pilocarpine (Adsorbocarpine[R])
piperacillin
Platinol[R] (cisplatin)
polycarbophil
potassium salts
prazosin (Minipress[R])
prednisone
Prilosec[R] (omeprazole)
Prinivil[R] (lisinopril)
Priscolin[R] (tolazoline)
Pro-Banthīne (propantheline)
probucol (Lorelco[R])
Procardia[R] (nifedipine)
propantheline (Pro-Banthīne[R])
propofol (Diprivan[R])
propranolol (Inderal[R])
Prostagmin[R] (neostigmine)
Proventil[R] (albuterol)

Provocholine[R] (methacholine)
Prozac[R] (fluoxetine)
psyllium
Purinethol[R] (mercaptopurine)
Purodigin[R] (digitoxin)
pyridostigmine (Mestinon[R])

Questran[R] (cholestyramine)
Quinaglute[R] (quinidine)
quinidine (Quinaglute[R])

ranitidine (Zantac[R])
Regitine[R] (phentolamine)
reserpine (Serpasil[R])
Retrovir[R] (zidovudine)
ribavirin (Virazole[R])
Ritalin[R] (methylphenidate)
Robaxin[R] (methocarbamol)

scopolamine
Seldane[R] (terfenadine)
Selegiline[R] (deprenyl)
senna
Septra[R] (trimethoprim-sulfamethoxazole)
Serpasil[R] (reserpine)
Silvadene[R] (silver sulfadiazine)
silver sulfadiazine (Silvadene[R])
simethicone
Sinemet[R] (levodopa plus carbidopa)
Sinequan[R] (doxepin)
sodium bicarbonate (Baking Soda[R])
sodium phosphate
sodium sulfate
Soma[R] (carisoprodol)
spironolactone (Aldactone[R])
succinylcholine (Anectine[R])
succinylsulfathiazole (Sulfasuxidine[R])
sucralfate (Carafate[R])
Sulamyd[R] (sulfacetemide)
sulbactam
sulfacetemide (Sulamyd[R])
sulfamethoxazole-trimethoprim (Bactrim[R])
sulfasalazine (Azulfidine[R])
Sulfasuxidine[R] (succinylsulfathiazole)

sulfisoxazole (Gantrisin^R)
Symmetrel^R (amantadine)

Tagamet^R (cimetidine)
Tegretol^R (carbamazepine)
Tempo^R (calcium carbonate)
Tenormin^R (atenolol)
Tensilon^R (edrophonium)
terbutaline (Brethine^R, Bricanyl^R, Brethaire^R)
terfenadine (Seldane^R)
tetranitrate
thiopental (Pentothal^R)
Thorazine^R (chlorpromazine)
ticarcillin (Timentin^R)
Timentin^R (ticarcillin)
timolol (Blocadren^R)
tincture of opium (Paregoric^R)
tobramycin
Tofranil^R (imipramine)
tolazamide (Tolinase^R)
tolazoline (Priscoline^R)
tolbutamide (Orinase^R)
Tolinase^R (tolazamide)
tolnaftate (Aftate^R)
Tracrium^R (atracurium)
tranylcypromine (Parnate^R)
trazodone (Desyrel^R)
triamcinolone (Azmacort)
triamterene (Dyrenium^R)
triazolam (Halcion^R)
trihexyphenidyl (Artane^R)
trimethoprim sulfamethoxazole (Bactrim^R, Septra^R)

tropicamide (Mydriacyl^R)
Tums^R (calcium carbonate)
Tylenol^R (acetaminophen)

Unasyn^R (ampicillin)
undecylenic acid (Desenex^R)
Urecholine^R (bethanechol)

Valium^R (diazepam)
valproic acid (Depakene^R)
Vanceril^R (beclomethasone)
Vancocin^R (vancomycin)
vancomycin (Vancocin^R)
Vasotec^R (enalapril)
vecuronium (Norcuron^R)
Velban^R (vinblastine)
verapamil (Calan^R)
Vidarabine (Vira-A^R)
vinblastine (Velban^R)
vincristine (Oncovin^R)
Vira-A^R (vidarabine)
Virazole^R (ribavirin)

Warfarin^R (bishydroxycoumarin)
Wellbutrin^R (bupropion)

Xanax^R (alprazolam)
Xylocaine^R (lidocaine)

Zantac^R (ranitidine)
Zarontin^R (ethosuximide)
Zaroxolyn^R (metolazone)
zidovudine (Retrovir^R)
Zovirax^R (acyclovir)

GLOSSARY

acetylcholinesterase   An enzyme that hydrolyzes acetylcholine within the central nervous system and at peripheral neuroeffector sites.

actin   One of the contractile protein components in muscle cells.

acuity   The relative severity of an illness or injury; relating to the need for hospitalization (e.g. "the higher the *acuity* of the patient, the more resources will be needed to care for the patient").

adrenergic   Nerve fibers that release epinephrine when stimulated; sympathomimetic.

agonist   A drug capable of combining with receptors to initiate a drug action.

akinesia   Absence or loss of the power of voluntary motion.

aldosterone   A steroid hormone produced by the adrenal cortex; its major action is to facilitate potassium exchange for sodium in the distal convoluted tubule, causing sodium reabsorption and potassium and hydrogen loss.

alkylation   An irreversible chemical bonding to nucleic acids (DNA)

allergenic   Having the properties of an antigen, a substance that can potentially initiate an allergic antigen–antibody reaction.

allergenicity   The ability of an allergen to produce an allergic reaction.

alopecia   Loss of hair.

α-adrenergic   Sympathetic stimulation of *alpha* receptors, usually leading to vasoconstriction of smooth muscle.

analogue   A compound or drug that resembles another in structure.

anaphylactic shock   A severe, often fatal form of shock characterized by smooth muscle contraction and capillary dilation initiated by a strong antigen–antibody reaction.

anorexia   Diminished appetite; aversion to food.

antagonist   A drug that combines with a receptor and causes no drug action.

anticholinergic   A drug that is antagonistic to or blocks the action of parasympathetic nerves or other cholinergic sites; parasympatholytic.

anticholinesterase   A drug that inhibits or inactivates acetylcholinesterase.

antidiuretic hormone   A hormone that reduces the output of urine or prevents diuresis.

antimuscarinic   A drug that blocks muscarinic receptor sites.

antispasmodic   A drug that prevents spasms of either smooth or skeletal muscle.

anuria   Absence of urine formation.

APC   An abbreviation for aspirin, phenacetin, and caffeine.

aplastic   Pertaining to defective regeneration, as in aplastic anemia.

arrhythmia   Loss of rhythm; denoting especially an irregularity or an atypical heart beat.

ataxia   Inability to coordinate the muscles in voluntary movement.

atherosclerosis   Disease characterized by irregularly distributed lipid deposits in the lining of large and medium-sized arteries; associated with fibrosis and calcification.

atomizer A device that generates an aerosol; an apparatus that changes a jet of liquid into a spray. An atomizer differs from a nebulizer in that it has no baffles and therefore the quality of the aerosol produced is less uniform and particle sizes have more variation.

atony Lack of muscle tone.

autodigestion Destruction of cells as a result of pepsin and HCl in the stomach or small intestine.

autoimmune The condition in which one's own tissues are subject to deleterious effects of the immune system.

autolytic Pertaining to or causing autolysis or self-destruction of cells.

autorhythmicity Automatic rhythm set by the sinoatrial node in the heart.

β-endorphin A protein substance released in brain tissue that combines with morphine receptors, causing analgesia.

bilipid Two layers of lipid material.

biotransformation Conversion of molecules from one form to another; refers especially to drugs.

bland aerosol An aerosol used primarily for hydrating the airway or for thinning mucus secretions, without a mucolytic effect. Bland aerosols include sterile distilled water and various saline concentrations (most often 0.45% NaCl and 0.9% NaCl).

bradykinesia Extreme slowness in movement.

bronchoconstriction Narrowing of the internal diameter (lumen) of the airways, especially the bronchi; may be caused by mucosal edema, pulmonary secretions, or bronchospasm.

bronchorrhea Excessive or abnormal secretion of mucus from bronchial submucosal glands.

bronchospasm Bronchoconstriction (narrowing) of bronchi and bronchioles as a result of spasm of peribronchial smooth muscle.

cAMP cyclic $3'5'$-adenosine monophosphate; intracellullar substance that promotes smooth muscle relaxation; adenosine triphosphate is converted to cAMP when sympathetic β_2 receptors are stimulated (e.g., in bronchial smooth muscle cells).

carbonic anhydrase An enzyme that converts water and CO_2 to carbonic acid.

carcinogen Any cancer-producing substance.

cathartic An agent causing active movement of the bowels.

cation An ion carrying a positive charge.

cavitating Disease process that leads to the formation of hollow spaces (cavities); pulmonary tuberculosis is typically a cavitating disease.

cGMP Cyclic $3'5'$-guanosine monophosphate; Intracellular substance that promotes smooth muscle contraction; adenosine triphosphate is converted to cGMP when parasympathetic muscarinic receptors are stimulated (e.g., in bronchial smooth muscle cells).

ceiling effect The point at which further increase in dosage of a drug causes no increase in effect.

cerebral palsy   Bilateral, symmetrical nonprogressive paralysis from development defects in brain or trauma at birth.

chelation   Combining of a metal ion with other compounds.

chemoreceptor   A receptor that is activated by other chemicals.

cholestatic   A decrease or stop in the flow of bile.

cholinergic   Acetylcholine-like.

chronotropic   Affecting the rate or rhythm of the heart beat.

colic   Spasmodic contractions of smooth muscle.

competitive antagonist   A drug that competes with other drugs (other antagonists) for a common receptor site.

creatine   A compound that occurs in the urine, generally as creatinine, and in muscle, generally as phosphocreatine.

cretinism   A condition combining dwarfism with mental retardation; associated with low levels of thyroxine.

dementia   A general mental deterioration resulting from organic or psychological factors.

digitalization   Administration of digitalis by a dosage schedule until sufficient amounts are present in the body to produce the desired therapeutic effects.

diluent   A liquid used to dilute a drug without changing its composition; usually sterile distilled water or 0.9% NaCl (normal saline).

diverticulosis   Presence of a number of diverticula or outpouchings of the large intestine.

drug action   The physiological modification or alteration that occurs in a cell or an organ as a result of a drug combining with its receptor site.

dual innervation   Innervation by both sympathetic and parasympathetic nervous system; occurs in most organs of the body.

dynorphin   A polypeptide in brain tissue with analgesic properties.

dysphoria   A feeling of unpleasantness or discomfort.

ectopic   In cardiography, denotes a heart beat that has its origin in a focus other than the sinoatrial node.

ED_{50}   Effective dose in 50 percent of population.

edema   An accumulation of an excessive amount of watery fluid in cells, tissues, or serous cavities.

ELISA test   Enzyme-linked immunosorbent assay; specific laboratory analysis to determine the presence of respiratory syncytial virus.

embolus   A plug, composed of a detached clot or vegetation, mass of bacteria, or other foreign body, occluding a blood vessel.

emollient   A substance that helps prevent water loss.

endorphin   One of a family of opioid-like polypeptides originally isolated from the brain but now found in many parts of the body; in the brain, it binds to the same receptors as other opioids.

endoscope   An instrument for the examination of the interior of a canal or hollow organ cavity.

epistaxis   Nosebleed; hemorrhage from the nose.

euphoria A feeling of well-being commonly exaggerated and not necessarily well founded.

exocrine Pertaining to a gland that secretes outwardly through excretory ducts.

expectorant A drug that improves the clearance of pulmonary secretions.

expectorate/expectoration The process of clearing pulmonary secretions from the airway by coughing and spitting out saliva and mucus. Secretions that are swallowed are not expectorated.

extrapyramidal Movements or activities outside the central nervous system.

facultative In the kidney, the ability to control H_2O reabsorption using antidiurectic hormone.

FAS Fetal alcohol syndrome.

fasciculations Involuntary contractions, or twitchings, of groups of muscle fibers.

feedback control The situation in which, at a proper level, a hormone feeds back information that shuts off its own release.

fibrin An elastic filamentous protein derived from fibrinogen by the action of thrombin, leading to the formation of a blood clot.

fight or flight A condition of the body when it is under dominant control of the sympathetic nervous system.

fluid mosaic Refers to the cell membrane, which is constantly changing in regard to the pattern of proteins in relation to the bilipid layers.

fulminant Rapidly occurring; coming in lightning-like flashes.

fungicidal A drug that destroys fungi.

fungistatic Having an inhibiting action on the growth of fungi.

ganglion A collection of nerve cell bodies and synapses outside of the central nervous system.

gastrin A hormone released by the intestine causing a release of HCl and pepsin.

generic name The official contracted chemical name of a drug.

gluconeogenesis Formation of glucose from sources other than carbohydrates.

glucosuria Increased levels of glucose in urine.

glycogenolysis The hydrolysis (breakdown) of glycogen to glucose.

growth-onset diabetes The type of diabetes mellitus that is insulin dependent.

gynecomastia Excessive development of the male mammary glands.

half-normal saline Saline solution that is one half the osmotic pressure of body fluids; a solution that is 0.45% NaCl.

hangover Excess central nervous system depression following use of central nervous system depressants.

hematocrit The percentage of red blood cells in a given volume of blood.

hemostatic Arresting the flow of blood within the vessels; arresting hemorrhage.

hygroscopic Possessing the ability to absorb moisture; inhaled particles that are hygroscopic will attract water in the airway and will increase in size as they absorb this water.

hypercalcemia An abnormally high concentration of calcium in the circulating blood.

hyperlipidemia Elevated levels of fat or lipids in the blood.

hypertonic saline Saline solution that has a greater osmotic pressure than body fluids (e.g., 5.0% or 10% NaCl); hypertonic saline is hygroscopic.

hypervitaminosis A condition resulting from the ingestion of an excessive amount of vitamin preparations.

hypocalcemia Abnormally low levels of calcium in the circulating blood.

hypolipidemia Low levels of fat or lipids in the blood.

hypothalamus An important part of the diencephalon anatomically located under the thalamus.

hypoxemia Insufficient oxygenation of the blood.

idiopathic Of unknown cause.

idiosyncrasy An unusual or unpredictable effect of a drug.

infarct Infarction; an area of necrosis resulting from a sudden insufficiency of arterial or venous blood supply.

inotropic Influencing the contractility of cardiac muscle.

inspissated Thickened; term is used to describe pulmonary secretions that are thickened by dehydration or evaporation.

instillation/instilled Introduction of a liquid into a cavity or surface; term is used to describe administration of drugs drop by drop or as a bolus into a catheter or endotracheal tube (in contrast to aerosol or injection).

interstitial The space between or surrounding cells.

IV intravenous or intravenously.

ketosis A condition characterized by the enhanced production of ketone bodies, as in diabetes mellitus.

key–lock A description of a specific drug fitting or combining with a specific receptor.

laxative A remedy that moves the bowels slightly without pain or violent action.

LD$_{50}$ Lethal dose in 50 percent of population.

L/S ratio Lecithin–sphingomyelin ratio; the ratio of lecithin to sphingomyelin in the amniotic fluid, used to assess fetal lung maturity (when there is less lecithin than sphingomyelin, the likelihood of respiratory distress is much greater).

macro Large or long.

macrolide A class of antibiotics characterized by molecules made up of large-ring lactones.

malignant hyperthermia An undetermined rapid rise in body temperature, usually associated with general anesthetic use.

medulla An area in the center of a gland.

meningitis Inflammation of the membranes of the brain or spinal cord.

minor tranquilizers A class including drugs such as diazepines or various antianxiety drugs.

miosis Contraction of the pupil.

monotherapy The use of one medication rather than multiple drugs.

mucolysis The process of dissolving mucus.

mucolytic A drug that has the action of dissolving mucus.

muscarinic The parasympathetic receptor site found in organ sites affected by acetylcholine.

mutagenic Having the power to cause mutations.

mydriasis Dilation of the pupil.

myosin A contractile protein in muscle.

myositis Inflammation of a muscle.

negative feedback Same as feedback control, reversing the direction of the original action.

nephrogenic Having to do with the kidney nephron.

nephrotoxic Toxic to the kidney.

neuroeffector junction The location where a nerve interacts with another organ.

neurotransmitter Any chemical released by a presynaptic cell that crosses the synapse to stimulate or inhibit the postsynaptic cell or organ.

nicotinic The receptor in cholinergic nerves, either at the ganglion or at the neuromuscular junction of the striated muscle.

normal saline A saline solution that has the same osmotic pressure as body fluids; a solution that is 0.9% NaCl.

nosocomial Pertaining to or originating in a hospital.

oliguria Scanty urine formation.

opioid Any synthetic narcotic that resembles morphine and codeine in action or is derived from opium.

orthostatic hypotension Lightheadness or syncope when moving from a prone or sitting position to a standing position.

osmotic pressure Pressure that develops when two solutions of different concentrations are separated by a semipermeable membrane; two solutions with the same pressure are isotonic.

osteoporosis Reduction in the quantity of bone or atrophy of skeletal tissue.

ototoxicity Toxic effect in ear.

palpate To examine by feeling and pressing with the palms of the hands or the fingers.

parasympatholytic Anticholinergic; refers to a drug that blocks the transmission of impulses through parasympathetic nerve fibers.

parasympathomimetic Imitates the parasympathetic nervous system.

parenteral By some other means than through the gastrointestinal tract or lungs; referring particularly to the introduction of substances into an organism by intravenous, subcutaneous, or intramuscular injection.

paresthesia A tingling sensation or partial feeling in the skin or mucous membrane.

paroxysmal Of sudden onset.

peptidoglycan A compound containing amino acids (or peptides) linked to sugars, and forming the cell wall of bacteria.

peritonitis Inflammation of the peritoneum.

petechiae Minute hemorrhage spots in the skin.

pH The amount of acidity or alkalinity.

phosphodiesterase Enzyme present in bronchial smooth muscle cells that promotes the conversion of cAMP to AMP; intracellular levels of cAMP promote bronchodilation.

pK$_a$ The pH at which half of a compound is in the undissociated (un-ionized) state and half in the dissociated or ionized state.

placebo An inert compound identical in appearance with material being tested in experimental research, wherein the patient, and possibly the physician, may not know which is which.

PO By mouth.

polydipsia Frequent drinking because of extreme thirst.

polypeptide A peptide formed by the union of an indefinite (usually large) number of amino acids.

polyphagia Excessive eating.

postjunctional The area after the innervation of a nerve to its organ site or after a synapse.

postsynaptic The nerve membrane after the synapse.

postural hypotension Same as orthostatic hypotension.

Potency In therapeutics, the pharmacological activity of a compound.

preganglion The nerve fiber before the synapse in a ganglion.

proprioception The awareness of the position of the body with respect to the external environment.

proteolytic A drug or substance that has the effect of dissolving protein.

pruritis Itching.

releasing hormones Hormones that are released by the hypothalamus and travel through a portal system to the anterior lobe of the pituitary, causing release of other hormones.

REM Rapid eye movement, a stage of sleep.

renin A hormone released by the juxtaglomerular apparatus, operating in the kidney to provide constant blood pressure to ensure glomerular filtration.

rescue protocol A sequence of responses for a specific disease or condition; in newborn resuscitation, it refers to the use of surfactant replacement therapy for an infant who develops infant respiratory distress syndrome (in contrast to a premature or low-birth-weight infant, who meets the prophylactic protocol criteria).

reuptake The process that terminates the effect of norepinephrine at the nerve ending wherever norepinephrine is released.

schizophrenia The most common type of psychosis, characterized by a disorder in the thinking processes, such as delusions and hallucination, and extensive withdrawal of the individual's interest from other people and the outside world.

senility Old age; the sum of the physical and mental changes occurring in advanced life.

serotonin 5-Hydroxytryptamine

site of action The location in the body where a drug creates its drug action.

spastic A type of uncoordinated muscle contraction.

status asthmaticus   Persistent and intractable asthmatic attack; refers to the asthmatic patient who develops severe respiratory distress and does not respond to typical medical and pharmacological interventions. May be a life-threatening event.

stereotypic   A predictable or expected action.

suprarenal   On top of or above the kidney.

supraventricular   Above the ventricles; especially applied to rhythms originating from centers proximal to the ventricles, in the atrium or atrioventricular node.

sympathomimetic   Sympathetic-like, adrenergic; term referring to nerve fibers that release epinephrine when stimulated.

synaptic cleft   A gap or space between a presynaptic nerve fiber and a postsynaptic membrane.

syncope   A fainting; a sudden fall of blood pressure resulting in cerebral anoxia and subsequent loss of consciousness.

tardive dyskinesia   A late-appearing defect in voluntary movement.

tenacious   Adhesive; sticky.

teratogen   An agent that causes abnormal fetal development.

teratogenic   Leading to the development of abnormal structures in an embryo, resulting in a severely deformed fetus.

tetanic   Sustained contractions.

therapeutic index   The ratio of LD_{50} to ED_{50}. The higher the number the higher the relative safety of a drug.

thrombin   An enzyme that converts fibrinogen into fibrin.

thrombocytopenia   An abnormally small number of platelets in the circulating blood.

thrombophlebitis   Venous inflammation with thrombus formation.

thromboplastin   A substance that is necessary for the conversion of prothrombin to thrombin.

thrombus   A stationary clot.

thyroid storm   A condition of exaggerated sympathetic activity causing elevated blood pressure and possible death. Associated with high levels of thyroxin.

tight junction   The proximal borders of cell membranes that allow only very small particles or molecules to pass.

tolerance   A condition in which the dose of a drug must be increased to obtain the desired effect.

trade name   The name assigned to a drug by the manufacturer. The name is a registered trade name and can only be used by the original company that registers that name.

transdermal   A method of administering a drug by application to the skin; drug is slowly absorbed.

trigeminal neuralgia   A rare idiopathic disorder of the trigeminal nerve (Vth cranial nerve) causing extreme pain.

tropic   A hormone that stimulates another endocrine gland to release its hormone.

ulcerogenic   A substance that causes ulcers.

urticaria   Hives; an eruption of itching and localized edema, usually of systemic origin. May be due to a state of hypersensitivity to foods or drugs, foci of infection, physical agents, or psychic stimuli.

vasospasm   Angiospasm; contraction or hypertonia of the muscular coats of the blood vessels.

vertigo   A sensation of irregular or whirling motion, either of oneself (subjective) or of external objects (objective).

xanthine   Slow and long-acting bronchodilators that inhibit phosphodiesterase; Refers to the methylated xanthines (caffeine, theophylline, and theobromine).

xerostomia   Dryness of the mouth, resulting from diminished or arrested salivary secretion.

zombie   A person who is in a state of excessive sedation or central nervous system depression.

INDEX

Note: Page numbers followed by t indicate tables; page numbers followed by f indicate illustrations.

Absorbant drugs, 114, 115t
Absorption, drug, 8–9
ACE inhibitors, 99t, 100, 100f
Acetaminophen, 70–71
Acetazolamide, 97t
Acetohexamide, 135t
Acetylcholine, 35, 35t
Acetylcholinesterase, 33
Acetylsalicylic acid, 70–71
  as anticoagulant, 104t
Activated charcoal, 114
Acute mountain sickness, 283–284. *See also* Surface active
    agents
Acyclovir, 154–155
Administration, drug
  routes of, 7, 8t
  time of, 14
Adrenergic, definition of, 24
Adrenergic drugs
  adrenergic antagonists, 99, 99t
  aerosols, 224–226
  alpha-adrenergic drugs, 26–27, 26t
  alpha-blocking drugs, 29–30, 29t
  beta-adrenergic drugs, 27–29, 28t
  beta-blocking drugs, 30–31, 30t
  definitions of, 26
  neuronal activators and blockers, 31–32, 31t
  sites of action of, 25–26
Adrenergic receptors, location and action of, 25, 25t
Adrenocorticoids, 162t
Adrucil, 161t
Adsorbocarpine, 35t, 36
Advil, 72t
AeroBid, 229–230
Aerosolized medications, 167–172
  advantages of, 167–168
  alpha-adrenergic drugs, 224–226
  anti-asthmatic drugs, 230–234
  in antimicrobial therapy, 208–217
  bland, 197–198
  case study, 269–270
  corticosteroids, 226–230
  disadvantages of, 167–168
  factors in delivery, 168–169
  metered dose inhalers, 169–171, 170f, 171f
  powder aerosols, 171
Aerosporin, 214
Aftate, 153
Age, and drug effects, 14
Agonists, definition of, 11
Albuterol, 28t, 29, 184t, 185
  as aerosol, 171

  dosage for children, 255t
Alcohol
  in alveolar pulmonary edema, 244–245
  central nervous system effects, 51–52
Aldactone, 97t
Aldomet, 100
  as hypertensive, 99t, 100
  mechanism of action, 31t, 32
Aldosterone, 127t
  and blood pressure, 94, 95
Alkylating drugs, in chemotherapy, 160–161, 161t
Allergic response
  defined, 6
  and histamine release, 229, 230f
Alpha-adrenergic drugs, 26–27, 26t. *See also* Adrenergic
    drugs
Alpha-blocking drugs, 29–30, 29t. *See also* Adrenergic
    drugs
Alprazolam, 52t, 59t
Aluminum hydroxide, 111
Alupent, 28t, 29, 184t, 186
  dosage for children, 255t
Amantadine
  as antiviral agent, 154
  in parkinsonism, 62
Amikacin, 151
Amiloride, 97t
Aminoglycosides, 151
Aminophylline, 191, 191t
Amiodarone, 91t
Amitriptyline, 55t
Amoxapine, 55t, 57t
Amoxicillin, 146, 149t
  as aerosol, 212
Amoxil, 212
Amphojel, 111
Amphotericin B, 154
  as aerosol, 215
Ampicillin, 146, 149t
Amyl nitrite, 92t
Anaerobic infections, antibiotics in, 150
Analgesics. *See* Narcotic analgesics; Nonnarcotic analgesics
Ancobon, 154
Anectine, 78, 78t
Anesthetics, general, 62–66
  classification of, 64t
  inhalation, 63–65
  intravenous, 65
  preanesthetic medications, 66, 66t
  properties of, 63, 64t
  stages of anesthesia, 63t
Angina pectoris, 91

Angiotensin-converting enzyme, and blood pressure, 94
Antacids, 111, 111t
Antagonists, definition of, 11
Antianxiety drugs, 49, 58, 59t
Antiarrhythmic drugs, 90–91, 91t
Anti-asthmatic drugs, 230–235
Antibiotics
    aerosol administration of, 211–215
    in anaerobic infections, 150
    basic principles, 142–143
    beta-lactams, 144–150, 149t
    broad-spectrum, 151–152
    case study, 277
    categories of, 144
    causes of failure in, 143–144
    in gram-negative organisms, 151
    in gram-positive infections, 150
    sulfonamides, 152–153
Anticholinergic drugs, 37–38, 38t
    bronchodilators, 181f, 188–190
Anticholinesterase drugs, 36–37, 36t
Anticoagulant drugs, 100–102,103t,104t
Antidepressants, 54–56, 54t
    monoamine oxidase inhibitors, 55–56, 55t
    new generation, 56, 57t
    tricyclic, 55–56, 55t
Antidiarrheal drugs, 114–116, 115t
Antidiuretic hormone, 95
Antiepileptic drugs, 60–61
Antifungal drugs, 153–154
    aerosol administration of, 215–216
Antigen-antibody reactions, 135–138
    antihistamines, 137–138, 137t
    histamine effects, 135–136, 136t
    histamine receptors, 136
Antihistamines, 137–138, 137t. See Also Histamine
    as antiasthmatic, 230
Antihypertensive drugs, 97–100, 97t, 99t
    central-acting, 100
Anti-inflammatory drugs. See also Corticosteroids
    aerosol, 226–230
Antimetabolite drugs, in chemotherapy, 161, 161t
Antimicrobial therapy, 140–155
    aerosol, 208–217
        case study, 277–279
        deposition of, 210f
        disadvantages of, 209–211
        drug categories of, 211
        indications for, 209
        limitations of, 209–211
        pulmonary infectious processes and, 211
    agents and definitions, 141
    antibacterial therapy failure, 143–144
    antibiotics, 143–153, 211–215. See also Antibiotics
    antifungal drugs, 153–154, 215–216
    antiprotozoal drugs, 217–218
    antiviral drugs, 154–155, 216–217
    in diarrhea, 115–116, 115t

Antimuscarinic drugs
    as antidiarrheal agent, 114, 115t
    in ulcer therapy, 111–112
Antiprotozoal drugs, 217–218
Antipsychotics, 53–54, 54t
Antivert, 137t, 138
Antiviral drugs, 154–155
    aerosols, 216–217
Apresoline, 99t, 100
Aramine, 26t, 27
Armour Thyroid, 128t
Arrhythmias, 88–91
    antiarrhythmic drugs, 90–91, 91t
    causes of, 89–90
    characteristics of, 89t
    reasons for converting, 89
Artane, 62
Asendin, 55t, 57t
Asparaylnase, 162t
Aspergillosis, 278–279. See also Antimicrobial therapy, aerosol
Aspirin, 70–71
    as anticoagulant, 104t
Asthma, 230–235. See also Anti-asthmatic drugs
    case studies
        acute, 280–281
        acute severe, 272–273
    management in children, 254–255, 255t
Asthmahaler, 225–226
Atenolol
    clinical usage, 30t, 31
    in hypertension, 99, 99t
Atherosclerosis, 104
Atracurium, 78, 78t
Atripison. See Atropine
Atromid, 105
Atropine
    as antidiarrheal agent, 114
    as bronchodilator, 189
    in cardiac life support, 256t
    therapeutic usage, 37, 38t
    in ulcer therapy, 112
Atrovent, 189–190
Augmentin, 146, 149t
Autodigestion, 109
Autoimmune disease, 128
Autonomic nervous system, 18–40
    adrenergic drugs and, 25–32
        alpha-adrenergic drugs, 26–27, 26t
        alpha-blocking drugs, 29–30, 39t
        beta-adrenergic drugs, 27–29, 28t
        beta-blocking drugs, 30–31, 30t
        definitions of, 26
        neuronal activators and blockers, 31–32, 31t
        site of action of, 25–26
    adrenergic receptors and, 25, 25t
    cholinergic drugs and, 34–38
        anticholinergic drugs, 37–38, 37f

anticholinesterase drugs, 36–37, 36t
choline esters, 35–36, 35t
definitions of, 35
mechanism of action, 34
function and anatomy of, 19–20
general physiological functions and, 22, 23t
neurotransmitters and, 20–21, 23t
origin and distribution of, 22f
parasympathetic division effect, 23t, 32
parasympathetic nerve endings, 33–34, 33f
receptors, 23t
sites of action, 23t
sympathetic division effect, 23–24, 23t
sympathetic nerve ending, 24–25
synapses and ganglia of, 21f
Azactam, 148, 149t
Azlocillin, 149t
Azmacort, 230
Aztreonam, 148, 149t
Azulfidine, 153

Bactrim
as antidiarrheal agent, 116
in urinary infection, 153
Baking soda. *See* Sodium bicarbonate
Barbituates, 49–51, 50t
Beclomethasone
as aerosol, 229
deposition by metered dose inhalers, 170
dosage for children, 255t
Beclovent, 229
Belladonna alkaloids, 112
Benadryl, 137t
Bentyl
clinical use of, 38, 38t
in ulcer therapy, 112
Benzodiazepines, 50–51, 52t
Beta-adrenergic drugs, 27–29, 28t. *See also* Adrenergic
drugs
Beta-blocking drugs, 30–31, 30t. *See also* Adrenergic drugs
in angina therapy, 92–93
Beta-endorphins, 66
Beta-lactam antibiotics, 144–150, 145f, 149t. *See also*
Antibiotics
beta-lactamase inhibitors, 146–147
carbapenem, 148
cephalosporins, 147–148, 147f, 147t
monobactam, 148
penicillins, 145–146
Beta-lactamase inhibitors, 146–147, 149t
Betamethasone, 126t
Bethanechol, 35t, 36
BiCNU, 161t
Biotransformation, 12
Bisacodyl, 117
Bishydroxycoumarin, 102–103, 103t

Bismuth salts, 114
Bismuth subsalicylate compounds, 112–113
Bitolterol mesylate, 184t, 188
Bland aerosols, 197–198
hypertonic saline, 198
hypotonic saline, 198
normal saline, 197–198
sterile distilled water, 198
therapeutic indications for, 197–198
Blenotaine, 162t
Bleomycin, 162t
Blocadren, 30t, 31
Blood flow, and drug distribution, 12
Blood pressure, factors controlling, 94
Bowel function, 113–117. *See also* Constipation; Diarrhea
Brain stem, anatomy of, 45
Brethine, 184t, 187–188
Bretylium
in cardiac arrhythmia, 91t
in cardiac life support, 256t
Bricanyl, 184t, 187–188
Broad-spectrum antibiotics, 151–152
Bromocriptine mesylate, 62
Bronchial cells
parasympathetic stimulation in, 180f
sympathetic stimulation in, 180f
Bronchial challenge testing, 257–258
Bronchiolitis, 282–283. *See also* Bronchodilator therapy
Bronchoconstriction, 179, 223–224, 224f. *See also*
Bronchodilator therapy
Bronchodilator therapy, 178–192
anticholinergic bronchodilators, 188–190
bronchoconstriction, 179
bronchospasm and, 180–181
case study, 282–283
methods of, 179–182
mucosal edema and, 179
neurochemical mediators in, 182
sympathomimetic bronchodilators, 183–190, 184t
xanthines and, 190–192
Bronchorrheic agents, 203
Bronchoscopy, 257–258
case study, 286–287
Bronitin mist, 225–226
Bronkaid, 185, 225–226
Bronkometer, 28t, 29
Bronkosol, 184t, 185–186, 225
Budesonide, 230
Bu-lak, 117t
Bulk-forming agents, 117
Buprenex, 69t
Buprenorphine, 69t
Bupropion, 55t, 57t
Buspar, 52t, 58, 59t
Buspirone, 52t, 58, 59t
Busulfan, 161t
Butazolidin, 72t
Butorphanol, 69t

Calan
  in angina therapy, 93
  in arrhythmia therapy, 91t
  in hypertension therapy, 99t, 100
Calcium, hormones controlling, 130t
Calcium carbonate, 111
Calcium channel blockers, 93
Calcium chloride, 131t
Calcium gluconate, 131t
Calcium lactate, 131t
Cancer. *See also* Chemotherapy
  basic principles of, 159
  treatment approach, 159–160
Capoten, 99t, 100
Captopril, 99t, 100
Carafate, 112
Carbamazepine, 57, 60Carbapenem, 148, 149t
Carbenicillin, 149t
  aerosol, 212–213
Carbidopa, 61–62
Carbonic anhydrase inhibitors, 97t, 98
Carboxycellulose, 117, 117t
Carcinogens, 7
Cardiac life support, 255–257
  primary advanced, 256t
  secondary advanced, 257t
Cardilate, 92t
Cardiovascular pharmacology
  antianginal drugs, 91–93
  arrhythmias, 88–91
  coagulation process, 100–104
  glycosides and congestive heart failure, 86–88, 88t
  heart disease, 85–86
  high blood lipids, 104–105
  hypertension, 93–100
Cardizem
  in angina therapy, 93
  in hypertension therapy, 100
Carisoprodol, 79, 79t
Carmustine, 161t
Castor oil, 117
Catapres, 31t, 32, 100
  in hypertension therapy, 99t, 100
  in opium addiction, 60t
Ceclor, 147t, 149t
Cefaclor, 147t, 149t
Cefotaxime, 147t, 149t
Cefoxitin, 147t, 149t
Celusil, 111t
Central nervous system, 43–74
  additive drug effects in, 48f
  alcohol and, 51–52
  anatomy of, 44–45, 45f
  anesthetics and, 62–66
  antianxiety drugs defined, 48–49
  barbiturates and, 49–51, 50t
  common drug characteristics for, 46–48
  drug antagonism in, 48f

drug effects in, 46
drug potency and efficacy in, 47f
epilepsy treatment, 58–61
excitability and depression levels in, 47f
general anesthetics and, 62–66
mental disorder treatment, 52–58
narcotic analgesics and, 66–69
nonnarcotic analgesics and, 69–72
parkinsonism treatment, 61–62
sedative hypnotics and, 48–49
Cepacol, 226
Cephalexin, 147t, 149t
Cephalosporins, 147–148, 147f, 147t, 149t
Cephalothin, 147t, 149t
Cerebellum, anatomy of, 45
Cerebrum, anatomy of, 44
Cetyl alcohol, 244–245
Chemotherapy, 158–162, 161t, 162t
  agent categories, 160–161
Children
  asthma management in, 254–255, 255t
  dosage guidelines for, 253–254
Chloral hydrate, 50t
Chloramphenicol, 151–152
Chlordiazepoxide, 51, 52t
Chlorothiazide, 97t
Chlorpheniramine, 137t
Chlorpromazine, 53, 54t, 55t
Chlorpropamide, 135t
Chlortetracycline, 152
Chlorthalidone, 97t
Chlortrimaton, 137t
Cholestyramine, 105
Choline esters, 35–36, 35t
Cholinergic drugs, 34–38
  anticholinergic drugs, 37–38, 38t
  anticholinesterase drugs, 36–37, 36t
  choline esters, 35–36, 35t
  definition of, 32
  definitions of, 35
  mechanism of action, 34
Cholinergic receptors
  classification of, 33
  location and action of, 34t
Choloxin, 105
Chronic obstructive pulmonary disease. *See also* Mucolytics;
      Wetting agents
  case study, 271–272
  home care for, 273–275
Ciclopirox, 153
Cimetidine, 110
Cipro, 151
Ciprofloxacin, 151
Cisplatin, 161t
Citrate, 117
Claforan, 147t, 149t
Clavulanic acid, 146, 149t
Cleocin, 150

Clindamycin, 150
Clofibrate, 105
Clonidine, 31t, 32, 100
 in hypertension therapy, 99t, 100
 in opium addiction, 60t
Clotrimazole, 153
Clotting mechanism, 102f
Cloxacillin, 149t
Coagulation process, 100–104
Codeine, 69t
 as antidiarrheal agent, 115
 comparison with other narcotics, 70t
Colestid, 105
Colestipol, 105
Colfosceril palmitate, 244–245
Colic, and morphine, 68
Colistin, 213
Coly-Mycin S, 213
Compliance, patient, and drug effects, 13
Comprehensive Drug Abuse Prevention and Control Act,
 15, 15t
Conduction system of heart, 83–85, 84f
Congestive heart failure, 85–86
 cardiac glycosides and, 86–88
Constipation, 116–117
 causes, 116
 laxatives/cathartics in, 116–117, 117t
Contact cathartics, 117, 117t
Corgard, 30t, 31
 in hypertension therapy, 99
Coronary artery disease, 86
Corticosteroids, 124–127
 aerosol, 226–229
  advantages of, 227
  contraindications for, 228
  disadvantages of, 227
  indications for, 227–228
  side effects of, 228–229
 function of, 125t
 glucocorticoids, 125–126, 126t, 127t
 mineralocorticoids, 126–127, 127t
Cortisone, 126t
Cosmegen, 162t
Coumarins, 102–103, 103t
Cromolyn sodium
 as aerosol, 171
 in asthma therapy, 231–232, 231f
 dosage for children, 255t
Curare, 77, 78t
Curarin, 77, 78t
Cyclobenzaprine, 79, 79t
Cyclophosphamide, 161t
Cyclopropane, 64
Cystic fibrosis
 aerosal administered antibiotics and, 211–212
 case study, 275–277
Cytarabine, 161t
Cytomel, 128t

Cytosar, 161t
Cytotec, 112
Cytoxan, 161t

Dactinomycin, 162t
Dalmane, 52t
Danthron, 117
Dantrium, 78–79, 78t
Dantrolene, 78–79, 78t
Darvon, 69t
Decadron Respihaler, 229
Demeclocycline, 152
Demerol, 69t
Depakene, 60
Deprenyl, 62
Desenex, 153
Desoxycorticosterone, 127t
Desoxyn, 59t
Desyrel, 55t, 57t
Detergents, and surface active agents, 241
Dexamethasone
 as aerosol, 229
 anti-inflammatory dosage, 126t
Dexedrine, 59t
Dextroamphetamine, 59t
Diabetes mellitus, 132–135
 insulin preparations in, 134t
 oral hypoglycemic agents, 135t
 overall treatment of, 132
 symptoms of, 133t
 type I, 132–134
 type II, 134–135
Diabinese, 135t
Diamox, 97t
Diarrhea, 113–116
 antidiarrheal drugs, 114–116, 115t
 causes, 113–114, 114t
 treatment of, 113–114, 114t
Diazepam
 as anesthetic agent, 65
 in anxiety therapy, 59t
 duration of action, 52t
 in epilepsy therapy, 61
Diazoxide, 99t, 100
Dibenzyline, 29, 29t
Diclofenac, 72t
Dicloxacillin, 149t
Dicumarol, 102
Dicyclomine
 clinical use of, 38, 38t
 in ulcer therapy, 112
Diencephalon, anatomy of, 45
Diethyl ether, 64–65
Digestion, 109
Digitalis, 87–88, 88t
 in cardiac life support, 257t
Digitoxin, 88t

Digoxin, 88t
Dihydrocodeine, 69t
Dihydrotachysterol, 131t
Dilantin
    in arrhythmia therapy, 91t
    in epilepsy therapy, 60
Dilaudid, 69t
Diltiazem
    in angina therapy, 93
    in hypertension therapy, 100
Dimenhydrinate, 137t, 138
Diphenhydramine, 137t
Diphenoxylate-atropine, 115
Diprivan, 65
Dipyridamole, 104t
Disopyramide, 91t
Distribution, drug, 11–12
Diuretics, 97–99, 97t
Diuril, 97t
Diverticulosis, 117
Dobutamine, 257t
Docusate, 117
Dolophine, 69t
Dopamine, 28, 28t
    in cardiac life support, 257t
Dorbane, 117t
Doriden, 50t
Dornavac, 198
Dose-response curve, 4–5, 4f
Doxepin, 55t, 57t
Doxycycline, 152
    as antidiarrheal agent, 116
Dramamine, 137t
Droperidol, 65
Drug dependence, 7
Drug information, sources of, 3–4
Drug nomenclature, 6
D-Tubocurarine, 77, 78t
Dual innervation, 22, 23t
Dulcolax, 117
Dymelor, 135t
Dynorphines, 66
Dyrenium, 97t
Dysphoria, and morphine, 67

Edecrin, 97t
Edema
    mucosal, 223–224, 224f, 225t
    pulmonary, 245–246
        case study, 283–284
Edrophonium, 36, 36t
Elavil, 55t
Eldepry, 62
Emesis, and morphine, 67
E-Mycin, 150
Enalaprilat, 99t, 100

Endocrine system, 120–139
    antigen-antibody reactions, 135–138
    corticosteroids and, 124–127
    diabetes mellitus, 132–135
    hormone release, 123–124
    hypothalamus, 122–123, 122f
    pancreas, 131–132
    parathyroid gland, 129–131
    pituitary gland, 122–123, 122f, 123f
    thyroid gland, 127–129
Enflurane, 65
Enzyme induction, 12
Ephedrine, 26t, 27, 28, 28t
Epilepsy, 58–61
Epinephrine
    as alpha-adrenergic drug, 26t, 27, 226
    as beta-adrenergic drug, 28, 28t
    as bronchodilator, 187
    in cardiac life support, 256t
    racemic, 226
Ergocalciferol, 131t
Erythrityl tetranitrate, 92t
Erythromycin, 150
Eserine, 36t, 37
Estrogen, 162t
Ethacrynic acid, 97t
Ethanol
    central nervous system effects, 51–52
    in pulmonary edema, 245–246
Ethosuximide, 61
Ethrane, 65
Ethyl alcohol, 246–247
Ethylchlorvynol, 50t
Ethylenediaminetetraacetic acid, 104t
Euphoria, and morphine, 67
Euthroid, 128t
Excretion, drug, 12–13
Ex-Lax, 117t
Exosurf neonatal, 244–245
Expectorants, 203
Extrapyramidal movements, and antipsychotics, 53

Famotidine, 110
Feldene, 72t
Fenoprofen, 72t
Fentanyl, 65
Fiber, dietary, 117
Fight or flight response, 23–24
Flagyl, 150
Fleet enema, 117
Fletcher's Castoria, 117t
Flexeril, 79, 79t
Florone, 127t
Flucytosine, 154
Fludrocortisone acetate, 127t
Fluid mosaic model, 9–10, 10f

Flunisolide, 229–230
Fluoroquinolones, 151
Fluorouracil, 161t
Fluothane, 65
Fluoxetine, 55t, 57t
Fluphenazine, 55t
Flurazepam, 52t
Forane, 65
Fulminant alveolar pulmonary edema, 245–246, 246f
Fulvicin, 153
Fungizone, 154
    as aerosol, 215–216
Furosemide
    in cardiac life support, 257t
    in hypertension therapy, 97t

Ganglia, of autonomic nervous system, 20, 21f
Gantrisin, 152
Garamycin, 213–214
Gastrin, and digestion, 109
Gastrointestinal tract, 108–118
    constipation, 116–117
    diarrhea, 113–116
    digestion, 109
    overall bowel function, 113
    ulcer disease, 109–113
Gemfibrozil, 105
Genetic variations, and drug effects, 14
Gentamicin, 151
    aerosol, 213–214
Geopen, 149t
    aerosol, 212–213
Glipizide, 135t
Glucocorticoids, 125–126
    adverse effects, 127t
    dosage, 126t
    function of, 125t
Gluconeogenesis, 132
Glucotrol, 135t
Glutethimide, 50t
Glyburide, 135t
Glycogenolysis, 131
Glycosides, cardiac, 86–88, 88t
    digitalis, 87–88
    mechanism of action, 86–87
Gonadocorticoids, 125t
Gram-negative organisms, antibiotics in, 151
Gram-positive infections, antibiotics in, 150
Griseofulvin, 153
Guanethidine, 31t, 32
    in hypertension therapy, 99, 99t

Halcion, 52t, 59t
Haldol, 60t

Haleys MO, 117t
Haloperidol, 60t
Halothane, 65
Hangover effect, barbiturates and, 50
Heart, conduction system of, 83–85, 84f
Heart disease, 85–86
Heparin, 101–101, 103t
Heroin, 69t
Herplex, 155
Histamine. *See also* Antihistamines
    and allergic response, 230–231, 230f
    blockers, 110
    overall effects of, 135–136, 136t
    receptors, 136
Hormone release control, 123–124, 124f
Human immunodeficiency virus, 278. *See also* Antibiotics
Hydralazine, 99t, 100
Hydrochloric acid, 109
Hydrochlorothiazide, 97t
Hydrocodone, 69t
Hydrocortisone, 126t
Hydromorphone, 69t
Hydropres, 97t
Hydroxide, 117
Hydroxyurea, 162t
Hygroton, 97t
Hypercalcemia, 129
Hyperlipidemia, 104–105
Hypertension, 93–100
    antihypertensive drugs, 99–100, 99t
    diuretics in, 97–99
    factors determining, 94
    levels of, 93t
    nephron physiology and, 95–96
    therapeutic approach to, 94–95
Hyperthyroidism, 129, 130t
Hypnotics, definition of, 49
Hypocalcemia, 129
Hypoglycemic agents, 134, 135t
Hypolipidemic agents, 104–105
Hypoparathyroidism, 130–131, 131t
Hypothalamus, 122–123, 122f
Hypothyroidism, 128–129, 128t
Hypoxemia, and instilled medications, 173
Hytakerol, 131t

Ibuprofen, 72t
Idiosyncrasy, and drug action, 6
Idoxuridine, 155
Imipenem, 149t
Imipramine
    in depression therapy, 55t
    in nocturnal enuresis, 60t
Imodium, 115
Inderal, 30, 30t
    in angina therapy, 93

in anxiety therapy, 60t
in arrhythmia therapy, 91t
in cardiac life support, 257t
in hypertension therapy, 99, 99t
Indocin, 72t
Indomethacin, 72t
Infant respiratory distress syndrome, 243–245
  case study, 285–286
Infants, dosage guidelines for, 253–254
Inhalation route of drug administration, 8t
Instilled medications, 171–173
Insulin, 133–134, 134t
Intal
  as aerosol, 171
  in asthma therapy, 232, 234f
Interaction, drug, 14–15
Interstitial pulmonary edema, 245–246, 245f
Intraarterial route of drug administration, 8t
Intramuscular route of drug administration, 8t
Intravenous route of drug administration, 8t
Iodine, 162t
Ion exchange resins, 114
Ionization, drug, 9
Ipratropium bromide, 189–190
Ismelin, 31t, 32
  in hypertension therapy, 99, 99t
Isocarboxazid, 55t
Isoetharine
  as bronchodilator, 184t, 185–186
  clinical uses, 28t, 29
Isoflurane, 65
Isoproterenol
  and bronchodilator, 184t, 186
  in cardiac life support, 257t
  clinical uses, 28, 28t
Isordil, 92t
Isosorbide dinitrate, 92t
Isuprel, 28, 28t, 184t, 186

Kanamycin, 214
Kantrex, 214
Kaolin, 114
Kaopectate, 114
Keflex, 147t, 149t
Keflin, 147t, 149t
Ketamine, 65
Ketoconazole, 154
Klebcil, 214

Lanoxin, 88t
Larotid, 212
Lasix, 97t
Laxatives, 116–117, 117t
Levodopa, 61–62

Levo-Dromoran, 69t
Levophed, 26, 26t
Levorphanol, 69t
Levothroid, 128t
Levothyroxine sodium, 128t
Librium, 51, 52t
Lidocaine
  in arrhythmia therapy, 91t
  in bronchoscopy, 258
  in cardiac life support, 256t
Liothyronine sodium, 128
Liotrix, 128
Lipid solubility, and drug absorption, 9
Lisinopril, 99t, 100
Lithium, 56–57
Lomotil, 115
Loniten, 99t, 100
Loop diuretics, 97t, 98
Loped, 105
Loperamide, 115
Lopressor, 30t, 31
  in hypertension therapy, 99, 99t
Loprox, 153
Lorelco, 105
Lotrimin, 153
Lovastatin, 105
Lugol solution, 130t
Luminal
  in anxiety therapy, 59t
  in epilepsy therapy, 61
  as hypnotic, 50t

Maalox, 111t
Magnesium hydroxide, 111
Magnesium sulfate, 117
Mannitol, 97t
Marplan, 55t
Maxair, 186
Mechanism of action, drugs, 11
Mechlorethamine, 161t
Meclizine, 137t, 138
Meclofenamate, 72t
Meclomen, 72t
Median effective dose, 5
Median lethal dose, 5
Medihaler-Epi, 225–226
Medihaler-Iso, 186
Mefoxin, 147t, 149t
Mellaril, 55t
Membranes, drug passage across, 9–10, 10f
Mental disorders, 52–58
  antianxiety drugs in, 58
  antipsychotics in, 53–54
  depression, 54–56, 55t, 57t
  mood stabilizers in, 56–57
  psychopharmacological drugs in, 54t

psychostimulant drugs in, 57–58
Meperidine, 69t
    comparison with other narcotics, 70t
Meprobamate
    in anxiety, 59t
    as hypnotic, 50t
Mercaptopurine, 161t
Mestinon, 36t, 37
Metabolism, drug, 12
Metamucil, 117t
Metaprel, 184t, 186–187
Metaproterenol, 28t, 29, 184t, 186–187
    dosage for children, 225t
Metaraminol, 26t, 27
Metered dose inhalers, 169–171, 170f, 171f
Methacholine, 35, 35t
    challenge, 259
        case study, 287–288
Methadone, 69t
Methamphetamine, 59t
Methicillin, 149
Methimazole, 130t
Methocarbamol, 79, 79t
Methotrexate, 161t
Methoxyflurane, 65
Methyl-Ccnu, 161t
Methylcellulose, 117
Methyldopa
    as hypertensive, 99t, 100
    mechanism of action, 31t, 32
Methylphenidate, 59t
Methylsalicylate, 70–71
Metolazone, 97t
Metoprolol, 30t, 31
    in hypertension therapy, 99, 99t
Metronidazole, 150
Mevacor, 105
Mezlocillin, 149t
Micatin, 153
Miconazole, 153
Micronase, 135t
Micronefrin, 184t, 187, 226
Microsomal enzyme system, 12
Midamor, 97t
Milk of Magnesia, 111, 111t, 117t
Miltown, 50t, 59t
Mineralocorticoids, 126–127, 127t
Mineral oil, 117
Minipress, 29t, 30
    in hypertension therapy, 99, 99t
Minoxidil, 99t, 100
Misoprostol, 112
Mistometer, 185
Monistat, 153
Monoamine oxidase inhibitors, 55–56, 55t
Monobactam, 148, 149t
Mood stabilizers, 56–57
Morphine, 69t

in cardiac life support, 256t
    comparison with other narcotics, 70t
    physiological effects of, 67–68
Motrin, 72t
Moxalactam, 147t, 149t
Moxan, 147t, 149t
Mucolytics, 199–203
    contradictions and, 201–202
    dosage and concentrations of, 202
    indications for, 201
    mucus molecule and, 199–201, 199f
Mucomyst, 199, 201–203
Mucosal edema. See Edema, mucosal
Mucosil, 199, 201–203
Mucoviscidosis, case study, 275–277
Muscarine receptors, 33
Muscle relaxants. See Skeletal muscle relaxants
Mustargen, 161t
Mycostatin, 153
    aerosol, 216
Mydrasil, 38, 38t
Mylanta, 111t
Myleran, 161t

N-Acetylcysteine, 199, 200f, 201–202
Nadolol, 30t, 31
    in hypertension therapy, 99
Nafcillin, 149t
Nalbuphine, 69t
Nalfon, 72t
Naloxone, 68, 69t
Naltrexone, 69t
Naprosyn, 72t
Naproxen, 72t
Narcan, 68, 69t
Narcotic analgesics, 66–69, 69t
    classification of, 68
    comparison of, 68, 70t
    narcotic antagonists, 68
    physiological effects of morphine, 67–68
Narcotic antagonists, 68
Narcotic derivatives, 115, 115t
Nardil, 55t
Nasalcrom, 232
National Formulary, 4
Nebulizers, and aerosol drug delivery, 168–169
Nedocromil sodium, 233
Nembutal, 50t
Neostigmine, 36t, 37
Neo-Synephrine, 225
Nephron, and hypertension, 95–96
Netilmicin, 151
Neuronal blocking drugs, 31–32, 31t
Niacin, 105
Nicolar, 105
Nicotinic receptors, 33

Nifedipine
in angina therapy, 93
in hypertension therapy, 99t, 100
Nitrates, 91–92, 92t
Nitrites, 91–92, 92t
Nitroglycerin, 92t, 257t
Nitrous oxide, 64
Nizoral, 154
Noctec, 50t
Nocturnal enuresis, 60t
Nonbarbiturate sedative hypnotics, 50, 50t
Nonnarcotic analgesics, 69–72
nonsalicylate nonnarcotic drugs, 71–72
nonsteroidal anti-inflammatory drugs, 72, 72t
salicylates, 70–71
Nonsalicylate nonnarcotic drugs, 71–72
Nonsteroidal anti-inflammatory drugs, 72, 72t
Norcuron, 78, 78t
Norepinephrine, 26, 26t, 253t
Norfloxacin, 151
Noroxin, 151
Norpace, 91t
Novocain, 258
Nubain, 69t
Numorphan, 69t
Nystatin, 153
aerosol, 216

Oliguria, and morphine, 68
Olive oil, 117
Omeprazole, 112
Onconvin, 162t
Opiate addiction, 60t
Oral route of drug administration 7, 8t
Orinase, 135t
Osmitrol, 97t
Osmotic diuretics, 97, 97t
Oxacillin, 149t
Oxycodone, 69t
Oxymorphone, 69t

Pancreas, 131–132. *See also* Diabetes mellitus
Pancreatic dornase, 200
Panic attack, 60t
Parasympathetic division of autonomic nervous system, 32
overall effects of, 23t
Parasympathetic nerve ending, 33–34, 33f
Parathyroid gland, 129–131
hormones controlling blood calcium, 130t
hypoparathyroidism, 130–131, 131t
structure and function of, 129–130
Parathyroid hormone, 130t
Paregoric, 115
Parenteral route of drug administration, 7, 8t

Parkinsonism, 61–62
Parlodel, 62
Parnate, 55t
Pathological state, and drug effects, 14
Pectin, 114
Penicillins, 145–146, 149t
Pentacarinat, 218
Pentaerythritol, 92t
Pentam, 218
Pentamidine isethionate, 218
Pentazocine, 69t
Penthrane, 65
Pentobarbital, 50t
Pentothal, 50t
Pepcid, 110
Pepsin, 109
Pepto-Bismol, 114
Percocet, 69t
Percodan, 69t
Percorten, 127t
Pergolide, 62
Peritonitis, 109
Peritrate, 92t
Permax, 62
Perphenazine, 55t
Persantine, 104t
Pharmacology, definition of, 3
Phenacetin, 70–71
Phencycline, 65
Phenelzine, 55t
Phenergan, 137t
Phenobarbital
in anxiety therapy, 59t
in epilepsy therapy, 61
as hypnotic, 50t
Phenolphthalein, 117
Phenothiazines, 55t
Phenoxybenzamine, 29, 29t
Phenprocoumon, 102
Phentolamine, 29, 29t
Phenylbutazone, 72t
Phenylephrine, 26t, 27, 223
Phenylpropanolamine, 26t, 27
Phenytoin
in arrhythmia therapy, 91t
in epilepsy therapy, 60
Phosphorous, 162t
Physicians' Desk Reference, 4
Physostigmine, 36t, 37
Pilocarpine, 35t, 36
Piperacillin, 149t
Pirbuterol, 184t, 188
Piroxicam, 72t
Pituitary gland, 122–123, 122f, 123f
Placebo effect, 6, 14
Placidyl, 50t
Plasma protein binding, and drug distribution, 11
Platinol, 161t

Pneumopent, 218
Polycarbophil, 117
Polymox, 212
Polymyxin B, 214–215
Postextubation stridor, 281–282
Potassium iodide, 130t
Potassium salts, 117
Potassium-sparing diuretics, 97t, 98
Potency, drug, 5
Powder aerosols, 171
Prazosin, 29t, 30
    in hypertension therapy, 99, 99t
Prednisone, 126t
Prescription drugs, abuse of, 15–16
Prilosec, 112
Primatene mist, 185, 225–226
Primaxin, 149t
Prinivil, 99t, 100
Priscoline, 29, 29t
Pro-Banthine, 38, 38t
    in ulcer therapy, 112
Probucol, 105
Procainamide
    in arrhythmia therapy, 91t
    in coronary crisis, 256t
Procaine, 258
Procardia, 100
    in angina therapy, 93
    in hypertension therapy, 99t, 100
Prolixin, 55t
Proloid, 128t
Promethazine, 137t
Pronestyl, 91t
Propantheline, 38, 38t
    in ulcer therapy, 112
Propofol, 65
Propoxyphene, 69t
Propranolol, 30, 30t
    in angina therapy, 93
    in anxiety therapy, 60t
    in arrhythmia therapy, 91t
    in cardiac life support, 257t
    in hypertension therapy, 99, 99t
Propylthiouracil, 130t
Prostigmin, 36t, 37
Proton pump inhibitors, 112
Proventil, 28t, 29, 184t, 185
Provocholine, 35, 35t
    in bronchial challenge testing, 259
Prozac, 55t, 57t
Psychostimulant drugs, 57–58, 59f
Psyllium, 117
Pulmonary diseases, and aerosol anti-infectives, 211
Pulmonary edema, 245–246
    case study, 283–284
Purinethol, 161t
Puritis, and morphine, 68
Purodigin, 87–88, 88t

Pyribenzamine, 137t
Pyridostigmine, 36t, 37

Questran, 105
Quinaglute, 91t
Quinidine, 91t

Racemic epinephrine, 184t, 187, 224–225, 226
Racepinephrine, 184t, 187, 224–225, 226
Radioactive iodine, 130t
Ranitidine, 110
Receptors, drug action and, 10–11, 12f
Rectal route of drug administration, 8t
Redistribution, barbiturates and, 49–50
Regitine, 29, 29t
Renin, and blood pressure, 92
Reserpine, 31t, 32
Retrovin, 155
Ribavirin, 155, 216–217
Ritalin, 59t
Robaxin, 79, 79t
Rotohaler, 171, 173f

Salbutamol, 184t, 185
Sal Hepatica, 117t
Salicylamide, 70–71
Salicylates, 70–71
    adverse effects, 71
    therapeutic effects, 70–71
Saline
    cathartics, 117, 117t
    hypertonic, 198
    hypotonic, 198
    normal, 197–198
Saturated solution of potassium iodide, 203
Scopolamine
    as antidiarrheal, 114
    in motion sickness, 37, 38t
    in ulcer therapy, 112
Sedatives, definition of, 48
Seldane, 137, 137t
Selegiline, 62
Semustine, 161t
Senna, 117
Septra, 153
Serpasil, 31t, 32
Sex of individual, and drug effects, 14
Silvadene, 153
Silver sulfadiazine, 153
Sinemet, 61–62
Sinequan, 55t, 57t
Site of action, and drug effects, 11

Skeletal muscle relaxants, 77–80
  central nervous system, 79–80
  peripheral-acting, 77–79, 77t
    depolarizing, 78
    direct-acting, 78–79
    nondepolarizing, 77–78
Small-volume nebulizer, 168–169
Sodium bicarbonate
  in cardiac resuscitation, 256t
  as mucolytic, 199, 200f, 201–202
  in ulcer therapy, 111
Sodium iodide, 130t
Sodium nitroprusside
  in cardiac life support, 257t
  in hypertension therapy, 99t, 100
Sodium phosphate, 117
Soma, 79, 79t
Somatic nervous system, 20f
Spinhaler, 171, 172f, 234f
Spironolactone, 97t
Sputum induction, 198
Stadol, 69t
Sterile distilled water, 198
Subcutaneous route of drug administration, 8t
Sublingual route of drug administration, 8t
Succinylcholine, 78, 78t
Succinylsulfathiazole, 152
Sucralfate, 112
Sulamyd, 153
Sulbactam, 146, 149t
Sulfamethoxazole-trimethoprim, 116
Sulfaninylacetamide, 153
Sulfasalazine, 153
Sulfasuxidine, 152
Sulfisoxazole, 152
Sulfonamides, 152–153
Surface active agents, 240–246
  case study, 283–284
  fulminant alveolar pulmonary edema and, 245–246
  infant respiratory distress syndrome and, 243–245
  surface tension and, 241
  surfactant, 242
Surface tension, and surface active agents, 241
Surfactant, 242. *See also* Surface active agents
  and infant respiratory distress syndrome, 243–245
  lack of, 243f
  normal, 242f
Survanta, 244
Symmetrel
  as antiviral agent, 154
  in parkinsonism, 62
Sympathetic effect, and autonomic nervous system, 23t
Sympathetic nerve ending, 24, 24f
Sympathomimetic bronchodilators, 181, 183–190
  calculating drug dosages, 183
  therapeutic indications, 183–184
Synalgos, 69t
Synapses, of autonomic nervous system, 20, 21f

Syncytial virus infection, 277–278
Synthroid, 128t

Tachycardia, ventricular, 288–289
Tachyphylaxis, 6
Tagamet, 110
Talwin, 69t
Tapazole, 130t
Tardive dyskinesia, and chlorpromazine, 53–54
Tegretol, 57, 60
Tempo, 111
Tenormin
  clinical usage, 30t, 31
  in hypertension, 99, 99t
Tensilon, 36, 36t
Teratogens, 7
Terbutaline, 28t, 29, 184t, 187–188
Terfenadine, 137, 137t
Tetracyclines, 152
Theophylline, 191t, 192
Therapeutic dose, 5
Therapeutic effect, 6
Therapeutic index, 5
Thiazide and thiazide-like diuretics, 97t, 98
Thiopental, 50t
Thioridazine, 55t
Thorazine, 53, 54t, 55t
Thyrar, 128t
Thyrocalcitonin, 130t
Thyrogolubin, 128
Thyroid gland, 127–129
  hyperthyroidism, 129
  hypothyroidism, 128–129
Thyroid hormones, 128t
Thyroid storm, 129
Thyroxine, 105
Ticarcillin, 146, 149t
Tilade, 233
Timentin, 146
Timolol, 30t, 31
Tincture of opium, 115
Tissue affinity, and drug distribution, 11–12
Tobramycin, 151
Tofranil
  in depression therapy, 55t
  in nocturnal enuresis, 60t
Tolazamide, 135t
Tolazoline, 29, 29t
Tolbutamide, 135t
Tolerance, 6
Tolinase, 135t
Tolnaftate, 153
Tornalate, 184t, 188
Tourette syndrome, 60t
Toxic effect, 7
Tracrium, 78, 78t

Transdermal route of drug administration, 8t
Transderm-Nitro, 92t
Transport mechanisms, and drug absorption, 8
Tranylcypromine, 55t
Trazodone, 55t, 57t
Trexan, 69t
Triamcinolone
    aerosol, 230
    anti-inflammatory dose, 126t
Triamterene, 97t
Triazolam, 52t, 59t
Tricyclic antidepressants, 54–56, 55t
Trihexyphenidyl, 62
Trilafon, 55t
Trimenton, 149t
Trimethoprim-sulfamethoxazole
    as antidiarrheal agent, 116
    in urinary infections, 153
Trimox, 212
Tripelennamine, 137t
Tropicamide, 38, 38t
Tums, 111
Turbo-Inhaler, 234f
Tylenol, 70–71
Tylox, 69t
Tyloxapol, 244–245

Ulcer disease, 109–113
    decreasing attack factors, 110–112
    increasing defense factors, 112–113
    treatment objectives, 110
Unasyn, 146, 149t
Undecylenic acid, 153
United States Pharmacopeia, 3
Urecholine, 35t, 36
Urticaria, and morphine, 68

Valium
    in anxiety therapy, 59t
    duration of action, 52t
    in epilepsy therapy, 61
Valproic acid, 60
Vanceril
    as aerosol, 229
    deposition by metered dose inhalers, 170
    dosage for children, 255t
Vancocin, 150

Vancomycin, 150
Vaponefrin, 184t, 187, 226
Vapo-N-Iso, 186
Vasodilator drugs, 99t, 100
Vasotec, 99t, 100
Vecuronium, 78, 78t
Velban, 162t
Ventolin, 171, 184t, 185
Verapamil
    in angina therapy, 93
    in arrhythmia therapy, 91t
    in cardiac life support, 256t
    in hypertension, 100
    in hypertension therapy, 99t, 100
Vidarabine, 155
Vinblastine, 162t
Vincristine, 162t
Vira A, 155
Virazole, 155, 216–217
Visceral pain, 67
Vitamin D, 131t
Voltaren, 72t

Warfarin sodium, 102
Water, sterile distilled, and humidification, 198
Wellbutrin, 55t, 57t

Xanax, 52t, 59t
Xanthines, 182f, 190–193
    aminophylline, 191t
    description of, 192
    mechanism of bronchodilation, 190
    side effects of, 190–191
    theophylline, 191t
    therapeutic use of, 190–191
Xylocaine
    in arrhythmia therapy, 91t
    in bronchoscopy, 258
    in cardiac life support, 256t

Zantac, 110
Zarontin, 61
Zaroxolyn, 97t
Zidovudine, 155
Zovirax, 154–155

albuterol	isoproterenol
metaproterenol	pirbuterol
isoetharine	bitolterol

Isuprel[R], Vapo-N-Iso[R], Medihaler-Iso[R]
Sympathomimetic bronchodilator
β agonist
Adrenergic

Ventolin[R], Proventil[R], (C) Salbutamol
Sympathomimetic bronchodilator
β agonist
Adrenergic

Maxair[R] MDI
Sympathomimetic bronchodilator
β agonist
Adrenergic
VERY LONG ACTING

Alupent[R], Metaprel[R]
Sympathomimetic bronchodilator
β agonist
Adrenergic

Tornalate[R] MDI
Sympathomimetic bronchodilator
β agonist
Adrenergic
VERY LONG ACTING

Bronkosol[R], Bronkometer[R]
Sympathomimetic bronchodilator
β agonist
Adrenergic

racemic epinephrine	ipratropium bromide
terbutaline	beclomethasone
atropine sulfate	dexamethasone

Atrovent[R]
Parasympatholytic bronchodilator
Anticholinergic

Vaponefrin[R], **Micronefrin**[R], **Racepinephrine**[R]
Sympathomimetic bronchodilator
β agonist and α effects
Adrenergic
Weak bronchodilator, strong vasoconstrictor

Vanceril[R], **Beclovent**[R] **MDI**
Anti-inflammatory (antiasthmatic)
NO BRONCHODILATING EFFECTS

Brethine[R], **Bricanyl**[R]
Sympathomimetic bronchodilator
β agonist
Adrenergic

Decadron Respihaler[R] **MDI**
Anti-inflammatory (antiasthmatic)
NO BRONCHODILATING EFFECTS

atropine sulfate
Parasympatholytic bronchodilator
Anticholinergic

flunisolide	nedocromil sodium
triamcinolone	ethyl alcohol
cromolyn sodium	beractant

(C) Tilade
Mast cell stabilizer, prevents allergic asthmatic
  response
PROPHYLACTIC ONLY, NO
  BRONCHODILATING EFFECTS

AeroBid^R MDI
Anti-inflammatory (antiasthmatic)
NO BRONCHODILATING EFFECTS

ethyl alcohol (30–50%)
Surface active agent, use only for acute alveolar
  pulmonary edema

Azmacort^R MDI
Anti-inflammatory (antiasthmatic)
NO BRONCHODILATING EFFECTS

Survanta^R
Phospholipid surfactant replacement
NONAEROSOL; use by ENDOTRACHEAL
  INSTILLATION ONLY

Intal^R
Mast cell stabilizer, prevents allergic asthmatic
  response
PROPHYLACTIC ONLY, NO
  BRONCHODILATING EFFECTS

colfosceril, tyloxapol	lidocaine
N-acetylcysteine	ribavirin
methacholine	pentamidine

Xylocaine[R]
Local anesthetic and antitussive
Use by aerosol; instill during or before
bronchoscopy

Exosurf Neonatal[R]
Phospholipid surfactant replacement
NONAEROSOL; use by ENDOTRACHEAL
INSTILLATION ONLY

Virazole[R]
Antiviral
Aerosol given by SPAG nebulizer
Specifically for respiratory syncytial virus
(RSV)

Mucomyst[R], Mucosil[R]
Mucolytic
May cause bronchospasm; use with
bronchodilator recommended

Pentam[R], (C) Pentacarinat, (C) Pneumopent
Antiprotozoal
Aerosol given for *Pneumocystis carinii*
pneumonia

Provocholine[R]
Parasympathomimetic
STIMULATES BRONCHOSPASM
No therapeutic uses; diagnostic only